Lung Transplantation

Editors

JASLEEN KUKREJA
AIDA VENADO

THORACIC SURGERY CLINICS

www.thoracic.theclinics.com

Consulting Editor
VIRGINIA R. LITLE

May 2022 • Volume 32 • Number 2

ELSEVIER

1600 John F. Kennedy Boulevard • Suite 1800 • Philadelphia, Pennsylvania, 19103-2899

http://www.thoracic.theclinics.com

THORACIC SURGERY CLINICS Volume 32, Number 2
May 2022 ISSN 1547-4127, ISBN-13: 978-0-323-89768-6

Editor: John Vassallo (j.vassallo@elsevier.com)
Developmental Editor: Jessica Nicole B. Cañaberal

Thoracic Surgery Clinics (ISSN 1547-4127) is published quarterly by Elsevier Inc., 360 Park Avenue South, New York, NY 10010-1710. Months of publication are February, May, August, and November. Business and editorial offices: 1600 John F. Kennedy Boulevard, Suite 1800, Philadelphia, PA 19103-2899. Periodicals postage paid at New York, NY, and additional mailing offices. Subscription prices are $405.00 per year (US individuals), $875.00 per year (US institutions), $100.00 per year (US students), $473.00 per year (Canadian individuals), $893.00 per year (Canadian institutions), $100.00 per year (Canadian students), $225.00 per year (international students), $494.00 per year (international individuals), and $893.00 per year (international institu-tions). Foreign air speed delivery is included in all Clinics' subscription prices. All prices are subject to change without notice. **POSTMASTER:** Send address changes to Thoracic Surgery Clinics, Elsevier Health Sciences Division, Subscription Customer Service, 3251 Riverport Lane, Maryland Heights, MO 63043. **Customer Service (orders, claims, online, change of address): Telephone: 1-800-654-2452 (U.S. and Canada); 314-447-8871 (outside U.S. and Canada). Fax: 314-447-8029. E-mail: jour-nalscustomerservice-usa@elsevier.com (for print support); journalsonlinesupport-usa@elsevier.com (for online support).**

Reprints. For copies of 100 or more, of articles in this publication, please contact Commercial Rights Department, Elsevier Inc., 360 Park Avenue South, New York, NY 10010-1710. Tel: 212-633-3874; Fax: 212-633-3820; E-mail: reprints@elsevier.com.

Thoracic Surgery Clinics is covered in *MEDLINE/PubMed (Index Medicus), EMBASE/Excerpta Medica, Science Citation Index Expanded (SciSearch®), Journal Citation Reports/Science Edition,* and *Current Contents®/Clinical Medicine.*

Contributors

CONSULTING EDITOR

VIRGINIA R. LITLE, MD
Section Chief of Thoracic Surgery,
Cardiovascular Surgery, Medical Director of
Thoracic Surgery, Intermountain Healthcare,
Murray, Utah, USA

EDITORS

JASLEEN KUKREJA, MD, MPH
Program and Surgical Director of Lung
Transplantation, Professor of Surgery, Division
of Cardiothoracic Surgery, University of
California, San Francisco, San Francisco,
California, USA

AIDA VENADO, MD, MAS
Transplant Pulmonologist, Assistant Professor
of Medicine, Division of Pulmonary, Critical
Care, Allergy, and Sleep Medicine, University
of California, San Francisco, San Francisco,
California, USA

AUTHORS

AADIL ALI, PhD
Toronto Lung Transplant Program, Division of
Thoracic Surgery, Department of Surgery,
University Health Network, University of
Toronto, Toronto General Hospital, Toronto,
Ontario, Canada

SELIM M. ARCASOY, MD, MPH
Columbia University Irving Medical Center,
Lung Transplant Program, New York, New
York, USA

ASHWINI ARJUNA, MD
Norton Thoracic Institute, St. Joseph's
Hospital and Medical Center, Assistant Clinical
Professor of Medicine, Creighton University
School of Medicine–Phoenix, Phoenix,
Arizona, USA

AMIT BERY, MD
Division of Pulmonary and Critical Care
Medicine, Department of Medicine,
Washington University School of Medicine, St
Louis, Missouri, USA

ANKIT BHARAT, MD
Professor of Surgery, Division of Thoracic
Surgery, Northwestern University
Feinberg School of Medicine, Chicago,
USA

ROSS M. BREMNER, MD, PhD
Norton Thoracic Institute, St. Joseph's Medical
Center, Creighton University School of
Medicine–Phoenix, Phoenix, Arizona,
USA

MAREK BRZEZINSKI, MD, PhD
Department of Anesthesia and Perioperative
Care, University of California, San Francisco,
San Francisco VA Medical Center,
Anesthesiology Service, San Francisco,
California, USA

MARIE M. BUDEV, DO, MPH, FCCP
Professor, Lerner College of Medicine,
Respiratory Institute, Cleveland Clinic,
Cleveland, Ohio, USA

LAURENS J. CEULEMANS, MD, PhD
Department of Thoracic Surgery, University
Hospitals Leuven, UZ Gasthuisberg,
Department of Chronic Diseases and
Metabolism, KU Leuven University, Leuven,
Belgium

MARCELO CYPEL, MD, MSc, FACS, FRCSC
Toronto Lung Transplant Program, Division of
Thoracic Surgery, Department of Surgery,
University Health Network, University of
Toronto, Toronto General Hospital, Toronto,
Ontario, Canada

EDUARDO FONTENA, MD
Lung Transplant Program, Hospital COPA D'Or,
Rede D'Or Sao Luiz, Rio de Janeiro, Brazil

MATTHEW GALEN HARTWIG, MD, MHS
Associate Professor of Surgery with Tenure,
Division of Cardiovascular and Thoracic
Surgery, Department of Surgery, Duke
University School of Medicine, Duke University
Medical Center, Durham, North Carolina, USA

HILARY J. GOLDBERG, MD, MPH
Brigham and Women's Hospital, Harvard
Medical School, Boston, Massachusetts, USA

HARPREET SINGH GREWAL, MD
Columbia University Irving Medical Center,
Lung Transplant Program, New York,
Massachusetts, USA

JOHN R. GREENLAND, MD, PHD
Associate Professor of Medicine, Division of
Pulmonary, Critical Care, Allergy, and Sleep
Medicine, University of California, San
Francisco, Staff Physician, San Francisco VA
Health Care System, San Francisco, USA

RAMSEY R. HACHEM, MD
Division of Pulmonary and Critical Care
Medicine, Washington University in St. Louis,
St Louis, Missouri, USA

KONRAD HOETZENECKER, MD
Professor of Surgery, Department of Thoracic
Surgery, Medical University of Vienna, Vienna,
Austria

DANIEL KREISEL, MD, PhD
Departments of Surgery, and Pathology and
Immunology, Washington University School of
Medicine, St Louis, Missouri, USA

JASLEEN KUKREJA, MD, MPH
Program and Surgical Director of Lung
Transplantation, Professor of Surgery, Division
of Cardiothoracic Surgery, University of
California, San Francisco, San Francisco,
California

ERIKA D. LEASE, MD, FCCP
Associate Professor, Department of Medicine,
Division of Pulmonary, Critical Care, and Sleep
Medicine, University of Washington, Seattle,
Washington, USA

DEBORAH J. LEVINE, MD
Division of Pulmonary and Critical Care
Medicine, University of Texas Health San
Antonio, San Antonio, Texas, USA

BRONWYN LEVVEY, RN
Lung Transplant Service, The Alfred Hospital
and Monash University, Melbourne, Victoria,
Australia

GABRIEL LOOR, MD
Department of Surgery and Baylor Lung
Institute, Baylor College of Medicine, Division
of Cardiothoracic Transplantation and
Circulatory Support, Texas Heart Institute,
Houston, Texas, USA

TIAGO N. MACHUCA, MD PhD
Chief, Division of Thoracic Surgery, Surgical
Director, UF Lung Transplant Program,
Director of Adult ECMO, University of Florida,
Division of Thoracic Surgery, Gainesville,
Florida, USA

LUCIANA MASCIA, MD
Dipartimento di Scienze Biomediche e
Neuromotorie, Associate Professor of
Anesthesia and Intensive Care, Director of the
Residency Program in Anaesthesia, Intensive
Care and Pain, University of Bologna, Bologna,
Italy

ALADDEIN MATTAR, MD
Department of Surgery, Baylor Lung Institute,
Baylor College of Medicine, Houston, Texas,
USA

ANNA TERESA MAZZEO, MD
Associate Professor of Anesthesia and
Intensive Care, Department of Adult and
Pediatric Pathology, University of Messina,
Messina, Italy

ERIBERTO MICHEL, MD
Division of Cardiac Surgery, Department of Surgery, Massachusetts General Hospital, Boston, Massachusetts, USA

DOMAGOJ MLADINOV, MD, PhD
Department of Anesthesiology and Perioperative Medicine, The University of Alabama at Birmingham, Birmingham, Alabama, USA

ARNE NEYRINCK, MD, PhD
Department of Anesthesiology, University Hospitals Leuven, UZ Gasthuisberg, Department of Cardiovascular Sciences, KU Leuven University, Leuven, Belgium

JOSEPH M. PILEWSKI, MD
Division of Pulmonary, Allergy, and Critical Care Medicine, Department of Medicine, University of Pittsburgh, Pittsburgh, Pennsylvania, USA

JUAN C. SALGADO, MD
Associate Professor of Medicine, Division of Pulmonary, Allergy and Critical Care Medicine, Department of Medicine, Perelman School of Medicine, University of Pennsylvania, Philadelphia, Pennsylvania, USA

MARCOS N. SAMANO, MD PhD
Division of Thoracic Surgery, University of Sao Paulo, Lung Transplant Program, Hospital Israelita Albert Einstein, Sao Paulo, Brazil

DAVID M. SAYAH, MD, PhD
Division of Pulmonary, Critical Care, Allergy and Sleep Medicine, Department of Medicine, David Geffen School of Medicine, University of California, Los Angeles, Los Angeles, California, USA

LARA SCHAHEEN, MD
Norton Thoracic Institute, St. Joseph's Medical Center, Creighton University School of Medicine–Phoenix, Phoenix, Arizona, USA

ABBAS SHAHMOHAMMADI, MD
Lung Transplant and ECMO Program, Division of Pulmonary, Critical Care and Sleep Medicine, Department of Medicine, University of Florida, Gainesville, Florida, USA

GREGORY I. SNELL, MBBS, MD
Lung Transplant Service, The Alfred Hospital and Monash University, Melbourne, Victoria, Australia

STEPHAN A. SODER, MD
Division of Thoracic Surgery and Lung Transplant Program, Irmandade da Santa Casa de Misericordia de Porto Alegre, Porto Alegre, RS, Brazil

WIEBKE SOMMER, MD
Department of Cardiac Surgery, University of Heidelberg, Heidelberg, Germany

TANY THANIYAVARN, MD
Brigham and Women's Hospital, Harvard Medical School, Boston, Massachusetts, USA

TOMMASO TONETTI, MD
University of Bologna, Department of Medical and Surgical Sciences, Anesthesia and Intensive Care Medicine, Sant'Orsola Research Hospital - Bologna, Bologna, Italy

BINH N. TRINH, MD, PhD
Division of Cardiothoracic Surgery, University of California, San Francisco, San Francisco, California, USA

DIRK VAN RAEMDONCK, MD, PhD
Department of Thoracic Surgery, University Hospitals Leuven, UZ Gasthuisberg, Department of Chronic Diseases and Metabolism, KU Leuven University, Leuven, Belgium

AIDA VENADO, MD, MAS
Transplant Pulmonologist, Assistant Professor of Medicine, Division of Pulmonary, Critical Care, Allergy, and Sleep Medicine, University of California, San Francisco, San Francisco, California, USA

RAJAT WALIA, MD
Norton Thoracic Institute, St. Joseph's Hospital and Medical Center, Professor of Medicine, Creighton University School of Medicine–Phoenix, Phoenix, Arizona, USA

Contents

The medical care of patients awaiting lung transplantation is complex and requires the treatment of active medical conditions, including lung disease, while at the same time maintaining candidacy for transplantation. Some medications that would otherwise be considered routine may create undesirable challenges or complications in the perioperative setting. Therefore, a comprehensive assessment of the risks and benefits of these medications must take into account both their potential utility in managing a patient's current disease state, as well as the risks of compromising postlung transplant outcomes. In this review, we summarize the available data regarding several medications that are commonly used to treat patients with a variety of lung diseases, but that may impact a patient's course on the waiting list or in the posttransplant period.

Lung allocation in the US changed nearly 15 years ago from time accrued on the waiting list to disease severity and likelihood of posttransplant survival, represented by the lung allocation score (LAS). Notably, the risk of death within a year plays a stronger role on the score calculation than posttransplant survival. While this change was associated with the intended decrease in waitlist mortality (most recently reported at 14.6%), it was predictable that transplant teams would have to care for increasingly older and complex candidates and recipients. This urgency-based allocation also led centers to routinely consider transplanting patients with higher acuity, often hospitalized and, not infrequently, in the intensive care unit (ICU). According to the Scientific Registry for Transplant Recipients, from 2009 to 2019, the proportion of lung recipients hospitalized and those admitted to the ICU at the time of transplant increased from 18.9% to 26.8% and from 9.2% to 16.5%, respectively..

In this review, we discuss the outcomes of patients with severe acute respiratory distress syndrome (ARDS). We discuss evidence that suggests that a significant proportion of patients with ARDS develop end-stage lung disease and die of pulmonary complications. In carefully selected patients with permanent lung damage, lung transplant can be a life-saving treatment.

function. Cardiovascular, gastrointestinal, renal, and hematologic derangements are common and require close management to limit their negative sequelae.

Lung transplantation is a life-saving intervention and the most effective therapy for select patients with irreversible lung disease. Despite the effectiveness of lung transplantation, it is a major operation with several opportunities for complications. For example, recipient and donor factors, technical issues, early postoperative events, and immunology can all contribute to potential complications. This article highlights some of the key surgery-related complications that can undermine a successful lung transplantation. The authors offer their expert opinion and experience to help practitioners avoid such complications and recognize and treat them early should they occur.

Infection remains a common cause of death throughout the lifespan of a lung transplant recipient. The increased susceptibility of lung transplant recipients is multifactorial including exposure of the graft to the external environment, impaired mucociliary clearance, and high levels of immunosuppression. Long-term outcomes in lung transplant recipients remain poor compared with other solid organ transplants largely due to deaths from infections and chronic allograft dysfunction. Antibacterial, antifungal, and antiviral prophylaxis may be used after lung transplantation to target a number of different opportunistic infections for varying durations of time. The first-month posttransplant is most commonly characterized by nosocomial infections and donor-derived infections. Following the first month to the first 6 months after transplant—a period of intense immunosuppression—is associated with opportunistic infections. While immunosuppression is reduced after the first year posttransplant, infection remains a risk with community-acquired and rarer infectious agents. Clinicians should be vigilant for infection at all time points after transplant. The use of patient-tailored prophylaxis and treatments help ensure graft and patient survival.

Rejection is a major complication following lung transplantation. Acute cellular rejection (ACR), and antibody-mediated rejection (AMR) are risk factors for the subsequent development of chronic lung allograft dysfunction and worse outcomes after transplantation. Although ACR has well-defined histopathologic diagnostic criteria and grading, the diagnosis of AMR requires a multidisciplinary diagnostic approach. This article reviews the identification, clinical and pathologic features of, and therapeutic options for ACR and AMR.

Chronic lung allograft dysfunction (CLAD) is a syndrome of progressive lung function decline, subcategorized into obstructive, restrictive, and mixed phenotypes. The trajectory of CLAD is variable depending on the phenotype, with restrictive and mixed phenotypes having more rapid progression and lower survival. The mechanisms driving CLAD development remain unclear, though allograft injury during primary graft dysfunction, acute cellular rejection, antibody-mediated rejection, and infections trigger immune responses with long-lasting effects that can lead to CLAD months or years later. Currently, retransplantation is the only effective treatment.

Long-term exposure to immunosuppressive therapy may exacerbate pre-existing medical comorbidities or result in the development of new chronic medical conditions after lung transplantation. This article focuses on common nonallograft complications with the highest impact on short- and long-term outcomes after transplantation. These include diabetes mellitus, hypertension, dyslipidemia, kidney disease (acute and chronic), and malignancy. We discuss evidence-based strategies for the prevention, diagnosis, and management of these nonallograft complications in this article.

Lung retransplantation remains the standard treatment of irreversible lung allograft failure. The most common indications for lung retransplantation are acute graft failure, chronic lung allograft dysfunction, and postoperative airway complications. Careful patient selection with regards to indications, anatomy, extrapulmonary organ dysfunction (specifically renal dysfunction), and immunologic consideration are of utmost importance. The conduct of the lung retransplantation operation is arduous with special considerations given to operative approach, type of surgery (single vs bilateral), use of extracorporeal circulatory support, and hematological management. Outcomes have improved significantly for most patients, nearing short and midterm outcomes of primary lung recipients in select cases.

THORACIC SURGERY CLINICS

SERIES OF RELATED INTEREST

Advances in Surgery
http://www.advancessurgery.com/

Surgical Clinics
http://www.surgical.theclinics.com/

Surgical Oncology Clinics
https://www.surgonc.theclinics.com/

THE CLINICS ARE AVAILABLE ONLINE!
Access your subscription at:
www.theclinics.com

Foreword

Lung Transplantation: Moving Forward yet Still Impeded by Infection and Rejection

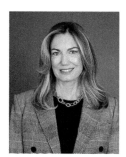

Virginia R. Litle, MD
Consulting Editor

We are excited to bring you the "Lung Transplantation: Advances Through Collaboration" issue for the *Thoracic Surgery Clinics*. Invited guest editors, UCSF Thoracic Surgeon Jasleen Kukreja, MD, MPH, and Transplant Pulmonologist Aida Venado, MD, MAS, have brought together a panoply of current topics about lung transplantation. Through invited experts in the field, our editors provide a state-of-the-union summary for surgical management of advanced lung disease, including chronic problems like pulmonary fibrosis and COPD, and acute indications, like acute respiratory distress syndrome, including, selectively, as a complication of COVID-19. Approximately 2500 US and 4000 global patients receive lung transplants annually, yet that's not enough. Per Sayah and Pilewski, only 70% of patients are transplanted after 1 year of being listed. Approaches to increasing the donor pool include identifying more donors after circulatory death (DCD) and ex vivo lung perfusion to allow use of extended criteria donor lungs and to improve geographic disparities for smaller programs. The former has associated ethical, legal, and professional challenges; however, the transplant community is making efforts to address this and increase the DCD pool. The envelope continues to be pushed with an ~400% increase in transplantation of those over 65 years with improved outcomes attributed to better organ preservation and

perioperative intensive care unit management. Transplant challenges ripe for clinical trials include novel immunosuppression protocols to make headway into the allograft acute cellular rejection rate of ~50% in first year and cause of 30-day posttransplant mortality of ~3%. Infectious complications also remain a challenging postoperative morbidity and mortality with 35% of deaths at 1 year attributed to infections. Lots of progress in improving organ pool but some persistent posttransplant challenges remain.

Thank you to all the contributors and to guest editors Drs Kukreja and Venado. Enjoy and appreciate the content and please share with your trainees to foster enthusiasm and interest in this intellectually and clinically complex microcosm of thoracic surgery. We hope you will enjoy this issue!

Sincerely,

Virginia R. Litle, MD
Section Chief of Thoracic Surgery
Cardiovascular Surgery
Medical Director of Thoracic Surgery,
Intermountain Healthcare
5169 So. Cottonwood St., Ste 640
84107 Murray, UT, USA

E-mail address:
virginia.litle@imail.org

Twitter: @vlitlemd (V.R. Litle)

Thorac Surg Clin 32 (2022) xiii
https://doi.org/10.1016/j.thorsurg.2022.02.002
1547-4127/22/© 2022 Published by Elsevier Inc.

thoracic.theclinics.com

Preface

Lung Transplantation: Advances Through Collaboration

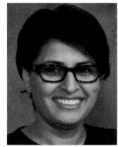 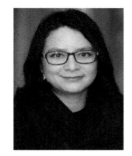

Jasleen Kukreja, MD, MPH   Aida Venado, MD, MAS

Editors

It "takes a village" to care for a lung transplant recipient. With advances in surgical technique for implantation, donor organ preservation and recovery, immunosuppression, and medical management over the past six decades, there has been a remarkable improvement in outcomes following lung transplantation. Today, the overall median survival following lung transplantation is 6.7 years. In fact, at some centers, the median survival has approached 10 years with a handful of lung recipients surviving close to 30 years posttransplant. This feat has been possible due to a multidisciplinary collaboration among surgeons, pulmonologists, anesthesiologists, nurses, pharmacists, immunologists, respiratory therapists, physical therapists, nutritionists, and social workers. Despite this success, preserving lung allograft function over time and achieving long-term survival remain a challenge. Early events, such as primary graft dysfunction and acute cellular rejection, can lead to chronic lung allograft dysfunction (CLAD), which in turn limits organ and recipient viability in the long run. As of 2022, half of the recipients develop CLAD within 5 years after transplant. Furthermore, complications of chronic immunosuppression, such as infections, chronic kidney disease, cardiovascular morbidity, and malignancy, can truncate life expectancy following lung transplantation. In addition, unexpected challenges, such as the current SARS-CoV-2 pandemic, can pose a threat to recipients and healthcare systems alike. Therefore, innovation and collaboration remain the key to achieving long-term success in the future. With that spirit in mind, we, a transplant surgeon and a pulmonologist, got together to edit this issue of "Lung Transplantation" for *Thoracic Surgery Clinics*.

To provide a balanced perspective of lung transplant care worldwide, when possible, we invited experts from different parts of the world to collaborate in writing each article. Similarly, we were intentional about selecting topics—both medical and surgical—to attract the broader audience and deliver a "one-stop-shop" experience for the reader (i.e., a single resource to get a comprehensive look at state-of-the-art in lung transplantation).

Thorac Surg Clin 32 (2022) xv–xvi
https://doi.org/10.1016/j.thorsurg.2022.01.006
1547-4127/22/© 2022 Published by Elsevier Inc.

We learned much from our colleagues' contributions to this issue of "Lung Transplantation" and believe that it will similarly help others advance toward our common goal of improving the outcomes for lung recipients worldwide.

Jasleen Kukreja, MD, MPH
Division of Cardiothoracic Surgery
500 Parnassus Avenue, MU 405W
San Francisco, CA 94143, USA

Aida Venado, MD, MAS
Division of Pulmonary, Critical Care
Allergy, and Sleep Medicine
University of California, San Francisco
505 Parnassus Avenue, M1093A
San Francisco, CA 94143, USA

E-mail addresses:
Jasleen.Kukreja@ucsf.edu (J. Kukreja)
Aida.Venado@ucsf.edu (A. Venado)

Outpatient Pharmacologic Management of Lung Transplant Candidates on the Waiting List

David M. Sayah, MD, PhD[a],*, Joseph M. Pilewski, MD[b]

KEYWORDS

- Lung transplantation • Glucocorticoids • Corticosteroids • Antifibrotics • Nintedanib • Pirfenidone
- mTOR inhibitors • Sirolimus

KEY POINTS

- Many medications that are routine therapies for lung diseases can potentially impact the peritransplant course of lung transplant recipients.
- Successful medical management of lung transplant candidates on the waiting list must take into account the effects of pretransplant medications on intra- and postoperative outcomes such as wound healing, bleeding, and infection.
- Medication classes that are of note with respect to their posttransplant impact include glucocorticoids, antifibrotics, mechanistic target of rapamycin (mTOR) inhibitors, cystic fibrosis transmembrane conductance regulator (CFTR) modulators, targeted therapies for pulmonary arterial hypertension (PAH), and anticoagulants.

INTRODUCTION

Lung transplantation is an increasingly used therapy for end-stage lung disease, with more than 2500 transplants completed in the United States annually, and more than 4000 worldwide.[1,2] In 2019 in the United States alone, more than 3000 individuals were added to the lung transplant waiting list, the vast majority of these being outpatients.[2] While median waiting time until transplant for these patients is approximately 2 to 3 months, there is substantial variation in waiting time between individuals.[2] Many factors contribute to this variation, including the underlying pulmonary disease diagnosis, severity of illness as determined by the lung allocation score (LAS), blood type, height, and geographic disparities in organ availability. As a result, only 60% of candidates

are transplanted by 6 months after listing, and only 70% by 1 year.[2] Therefore, ongoing outpatient medical care of these patients with end-stage lung disease on the lung transplant waiting list is an essential component of successful transplantation.

Goals of pretransplant medical care are first and foremost preserving the well-being and, in many cases, survival of patients while they await lung transplantation. Patients with end-stage lung disease are susceptible to debilitation and other medical complications. Anticipating and preventing complications that may temporarily or permanently disqualify patients from transplant candidacy is fundamental to pretransplant care.

However, some therapies that would otherwise be considered routine may create undesirable challenges or complications in the perioperative

[a] Division of Pulmonary, Critical Care, Allergy and Sleep Medicine, Department of Medicine, David Geffen School of Medicine, University of California, 10833 Le Conte Avenue, Box 951690, Los Angeles, CA 90095-1690, USA; [b] Division of Pulmonary, Allergy, and Critical Care Medicine, Department of Medicine, University of Pittsburgh, NW 628 MUH, 3459 Fifth Avenue, Pittsburgh, PA 15213, USA
* Corresponding author.
E-mail address: dsayah@mednet.ucla.edu

Thorac Surg Clin 32 (2022) 111–119
https://doi.org/10.1016/j.thorsurg.2022.01.002

setting. Therefore, in contrast to patients with similar lung diseases who are not awaiting lung transplantation, medical decision making must take into account not only the optimal therapies for the disease and specific patient but also the impact of these therapies on the immediate postoperative period after lung transplantation.

Adding further complexity, the timing of when a particular patient will receive an appropriate donor offer and undergo lung transplantation is unpredictable. This unpredictability must be taken into account to avoid jeopardizing either a patient's posttransplant outcome, or their candidacy for a given offer if, for example, they are temporarily ineligible for transplantation because of a medication or other therapy has created a perioperative risk that is unacceptable to the transplant program. Therefore, a comprehensive assessment of the risks and benefits of these medications must consider both their potential utility in managing a patient's current disease state and the risks of compromising postlung transplant outcomes.

In this review, we will aim to summarize the available data and consensus opinions regarding the optimal medical management of lung transplant candidates on the transplant waiting list. As this topic is potentially vast, our focus will be on specific medications and scenarios that frequently arise in the prelung transplant population.

Glucocorticoids

Glucocorticoids are used ubiquitously in the treatment of a multitude of lung diseases for which lung transplantation may ultimately be indicated, including chronic obstructive pulmonary disease (COPD), sarcoidosis, connective tissue disease-associated interstitial lung disease (CTD-ILD), allergic bronchopulmonary aspergillosis (ABPA) among others. These medications have a multitude of anti-inflammatory and immunosuppressive effects which makes them useful in the treatment of a wide variety of pulmonary diseases.[3] They unfortunately also cause a wide range of adverse effects, in particular with long-term use, many of which (such as impaired wound healing) could be detrimental in the postlung transplant setting.[4,5]

While glucocorticoids are now a mainstay of maintenance immunosuppressive therapy after lung transplantation,[1] there have been significant concerns about long-term systemic glucocorticoid therapy before lung transplantation. Early preclinical studies suggested an increased risk of bronchial anastomosis dehiscence associated with glucocorticoid exposure.[6,7] Indeed, early expert opinion in lung transplantation suggested that chronic glucocorticoid treatment was a contraindication.[8]

Subsequent clinical experience in human lung transplantation, likely along with refinements in surgical technique, led to retrospective, observational studies demonstrating that chronic, "low dose" glucocorticoid therapy before transplantation (variably defined as doses ranging up to 20 mg/d of prednisone,[9] prednisolone up to 0.3 mg/kg/d,[10] or prednisone up to 0.42 mg/kg/m²,[11] among others) did not negatively impact posttransplant outcomes.

Conversely, McAnally and colleagues reported increased early posttransplant mortality in patients chronically taking more than 0.42 mg/kg/m² of prednisone daily, an effect driven by an increase in early posttransplant infections and anastomotic complications.[11] In their patient population, with an average BMI of 22.5 kg/m², this threshold corresponded to an average prednisone dose of just under 10 mg/d. Using the same definition of high versus low-dose pretransplant glucocorticoids, Sugimoto and colleagues reported their experience with a small group of patients who received living lobar lung transplants after allogeneic hematopoietic stem cell transplants.[12] They also found decreased survival in the high-dose group.

An analysis of the International Society for Heart and Lung Transplantation (ISHLT) registry found that recipient pretransplant glucocorticoid use is associated with an increased risk of 1-year posttransplant mortality.[13] Interestingly, this effect seemed limited to recipients with COPD and not those with idiopathic interstitial pneumonia (IIP). However, a study using the Scientific Registry of Transplant Recipients (SRTR) did not identify pretransplant glucocorticoids as a risk factor for airway dehiscence,[14] so the potential mechanism by which pretransplant glucocorticoids may adversely impact posttransplant survival is uncertain.

Given the ambiguities surrounding the question of pretransplant glucocorticoid therapy, it is perhaps not surprising that the field has not reached a consensus on what the maximum dose of these medications, if any, should be for lung transplant candidates. Indeed, while early international guidelines specifically advised minimizing the glucocorticoid dose before lung transplant,[15] subsequent iterations do not address this topic.[16–18]

ANTIFIBROTICS

Pirfenidone and nintedanib, both antifibrotic medications, were approved for use by the US Food and Drug Administration (FDA) in 2014, following studies demonstrating efficacy in reducing the rate of decline of lung function in patients with idiopathic pulmonary fibrosis (IPF).[19,20] Nintedanib has subsequently shown similar effects in the treatment of scleroderma-associated interstitial lung disease (ILD), as well as a diverse group of progressive, chronic fibrosing ILDs.[21,22] Use of antifibrotic therapy to treat IPF has rapidly been adopted, with a recent US registry study finding more than 70% of patients were receiving one of these therapies at registry enrollment.[23]

As both pirfenidone and nintedanib impair fibroblast function and proliferation, there are theoretic concerns that these agents could impair wound healing and therefore lead to postoperative complications after lung transplantation.[24] Furthermore, nintedanib inhibits vascular endothelial growth factor, which could increase the risk of perioperative bleeding.[25]

Despite the hypothetical, mechanistic concerns regarding the safety of continuing antifibrotic therapies in patients actively awaiting lung transplantation, multiple observational studies have found no evidence that these medications increase the risk of postoperative complications. In one of the earliest studies, Leuschner and colleagues found no difference in blood product utilization, wound-healing or anastomotic complications, or post-transplant mortality among 30 patients with IPF receiving antifibrotic (23 pirfenidone, 7 nintedanib) therapy before transplantation, as compared with 32 control patients who did not receive antifibrotics.[26] These findings were despite the fact that the patients receiving antifibrotic therapy were significantly older. The largest study to date examined the outcomes of 40 patients receiving antifibrotic therapy up until the time of transplant (29 pirfenidone, 11 nintedanib) out of a group of 226 patients with pulmonary fibrosis who underwent lung transplantation.[27] While there was a nonsignificant trend toward an increased rate of airway dehiscence in the antifibrotic group versus the comparator group (7.5% vs 2.2%), the absolute number of events was small and the difference was not statistically significant. 30-day survival was not significantly different, while 1-year survival favored the antifibrotic group over the controls (93% vs 88%). Several smaller studies, examining either pirfenidone, nintedanib, or both, have found no meaningful differences in wound healing or other surgical complications.[28–31]

Given the consistent absence of association between antifibrotic therapy and postoperative complications after lung transplantation, the consensus in the field is that patients can safely continue these medications up until the time of transplantation.[18]

Veit and colleagues examined outcomes after single lung transplantation in 17 patients with IPF who had previously received pirfenidone, as compared with 26 patients who had not received antifibrotics.[32] Consistent with other studies, there were no differences in blood loss, wound healing, or anastomotic complications. Interestingly, however, the severity of primary graft dysfunction, duration of mechanical ventilation, and duration of ICU stay were all reduced in the pirfenidone group, suggesting a potential beneficial effect of pirfenidone in this group of patients. Lastly, a recent retrospective analysis suggested that the use of either nintedanib or pirfenidone at the time of transplant was associated with improved resolution of primary graft dysfunction and fewer anastomotic complications without an increase in complications. [33] Whether additional, larger studies show similar findings, and whether effects are similar with nintedanib compared with pirfenidone, remains to be determined.

MECHANISTIC TARGET OF RAPAMYCIN INHIBITORS

Sirolimus, and its derivative everolimus, are potent immunosuppressive that acts via the inhibition of the mechanistic target of rapamycin (mTOR).[34,35] In addition to their immunosuppressive effects, these medications disrupt the proliferation of a number of cell types, including fibroblasts, and have antineoplastic effects that are useful in the treatment of some malignancies.[36]

Because of their combined immunosuppressive and potentially antifibrotic effects, mTOR inhibitors were thought to be promising agents for immunosuppression after lung transplantation. However, early reports describing experience with sirolimus-containing immunosuppression regimens in the immediate postlung transplant period found a high rate of catastrophic, often fatal, bronchial anastomosis dehiscence.[37,38] This led the FDA to specifically warn against the use of sirolimus for *de novo* immunosuppression after lung transplantation.[39]

While mTOR inhibitors are not often used in the treatment of end-stage lung disease, a notable exception is lymphangioleiomyomatosis (LAM), a rare, progressive cystic lung disease that can lead to respiratory failure and is an established indication for lung transplantation. Treatment with sirolimus stabilizes lung function, improves symptoms, and improves the quality of life in patients with LAM.[40]

The potential hazard of airway dehiscence caused by sirolimus in the early postlung transplant period has led to questions about whether it is safe for patients with LAM to continue sirolimus therapy while awaiting lung transplantation, or whether sirolimus should be stopped before listing for transplant.[41] Studies of patients undergoing lung transplant while taking mTOR inhibitors are limited. In one study of 3 patients with LAM who continued sirolimus therapy up until the time of transplantation, there were no cases of bronchial dehiscence.[42] Another study described 7 patients with LAM treated with sirolimus until the time of transplantation, 1 of whom developed fatal anastomotic dehiscence 12 days after transplant.[43] Finally, a report described the experience of 2 patients who were receiving everolimus for maintenance immunosuppression after lung transplantation for diseases other than LAM, and who continued everolimus up until the time of lung retransplantation.[44] Neither patient suffered airway dehiscence.

Everolimus has a shorter half-life than sirolimus (30 vs 60 hours).[39,45] Some have suggested everolimus may, therefore, be a safer option for the treatment of LAM in patients awaiting lung transplantation because the shorter half-life may reduce the risk of airway dehiscence.[18,41] Studies supporting this approach have not yet been conducted.

Ultimately, the optimal approach to mTOR inhibitor therapy in patients with LAM awaiting transplantation remains uncertain, and decisions should be based on individualized discussions of risks and benefits.[18] At our centers, we generally advise patients to stop mTOR inhibitors before active listing for transplantation as our average waiting time for a transplant is relatively short, making concerns about declining lung function off of therapy in patients with LAM less relevant. Each transplant center, and potentially each patient, however, may have a different risk/benefit calculation in this regard so center- or patient-specific approaches are advisable.

CYSTIC FIBROSIS TRANSMEMBRANE CONDUCTANCE REGULATOR MODULATORS

The development of cystic fibrosis transmembrane conductance regulator (CFTR) modulators has been a remarkable story in respiratory medicine. Defining the genetic, molecular, and cellular biology of CF mutations enabled high throughput screening to identify compounds that partially restore CFTR function. The first highly effective CFTR modulator became available in 2012 when the FDA approved Ivacaftor (Kalydeco, IVA) for individuals with the G551D CFTR mutation. IVA substantially decreased sweat chloride, increased respiratory function, promoted weight gain, reduced exacerbation frequency, and improved the quality of life for patients with an FEV_1 40% to 90% predicted.[46] As that time, IVA was approved for several other gating mutations, providing opportunity by early 2020 for ~20% of individuals with CF to be treated with a disease-modifying oral medication. Several studies have examined the effect of IVA on patients with advanced lung disease and demonstrated similar improvements to what was observed in patients with modest lung disease.[47–50]

In late 2019, the second highly effective CFTR modulator therapy, Elexacaftor/Tezacaftor/Ivacaftor (Trikafta, ETI) was approved for individuals with the F508del CFTR mutation. ETI also dramatically improves sweat chloride, FEV_1 (by ~14% absolute predicted), nutritional status, exacerbation frequency, and quality of life for individuals with an FEV_1 40% to 90% predicted.[51–53] Because F508del is the most common CFTR mutation, now ~90% of individuals with CF have access to an efficacious disease-modifying therapy. While the transformative effects of ETI have been extensively studied in individuals with mild to moderate CF lung disease, the clinical impact for individuals with severe lung disease has been less well described.

In early 2021, the effect of ETI for individuals with CF and advanced lung disease who received ETI through an early access program in France was reported.[54] Consistent with prior studies, ETI was well tolerated in individuals with an FEV_1 less than 40% predicted, and there were dramatic improvements in lung function and weight. The 15% mean increase in absolute % predicted FEV_1 was consistent with the subset of patients in the Phase 3 studies whose FEV_1 was just less than 40% predicted.[52] This study provided additional evidence for a transformative effect of ETI for individuals with severe lung disease, as ETI use reduced the need for supplemental O_2 by 50%, noninvasive ventilation (NIV) by 30%, and enteral tube feeding by 50%. Perhaps more important for lung transplant programs, before the initiation of ETI in this population, 16 patients were on the lung transplant waiting list and 37 were undergoing transplant evaluation. Although somewhat confounded by the COVID-19 pandemic, 2 patients underwent lung transplantation, 1 died, and only 5 remained on the path to transplant. Given the duration of the study, these results are extraordinary and have contributed to a marked reduction in the number of individuals with CF referred for lung transplant, and in the number of lung transplants for CF in countries where ETI is available. The effects of ETI also have implications for decisions when to list for lung transplant.

Long-term studies recently demonstrated that IVA significantly reduced the progression of CF lung disease over 5 years.[55] This, coupled with the short-term effects of both IVA,[49] and ETI[54] for individuals with CF and advanced disease, suggests that survival with advanced CF lung disease will increase significantly. Although additional studies are needed, experience thus far suggests that those on ETI are less likely to suffer rapid progression to respiratory failure and death. ETI may slow the progression of lung disease such that individuals with CF on ETI will progress more like individuals with bronchiectasis due to diseases other than CF, such as primary ciliary dyskinesia or immune deficiency. Survival with advanced CF lung disease is likely to occur slowly, suggesting that for this population, decisions on listing for transplant should be made carefully to avoid early transplant that may decrease life span.

In contrast, for the ~10% of individuals without F508del, who are not on IVA or ETI, disease progression is likely to approximate the 6.6-year median survival when FEV_1 is less than 30% predicted, with up to 10% of individuals dying or undergoing transplant each year after going below that threshold during periods of clinical stability.[56] For this subgroup of individuals with CF, decisions on transplant listing do not require practice change.

CFTR modulators have improved the nutritional status of many with CF, and fewer individuals with CF will approach transplant with an abnormally low body mass index. In fact, obesity is an emerging challenge in CF. Moreover, with the slowing of the decline in lung function, individuals with CF will come to transplant older, perhaps with additional comorbidities like coronary disease that historically have rarely been an issue in CF.

The improvements in lung function, reduction in pulmonary exacerbation frequency, increase in weight, and improved quality of life associated with IVA and ETI suggest that they should be continued until the transplant operation. This is particularly important due to reports that the discontinuation of IVA in individuals with advanced CF lung disease is associated with rapid progression, in some individuals to death.[57]

A more difficult decision is whether and when to resume highly effective CFTR modulators after transplant. Most individuals with CF have improved nutrition after transplant without the use of a CFTR modulator, and there are drug interactions with azoles and calcineurin inhibitors that make use of IVA or ETI after transplant complex and potentially risky. As the recipient lungs are genetically normal, the potential indications for resuming IVA or ETI after transplant are for improved nutrition, sinus disease refractory to medical and surgical therapy, and in rare circumstances, glycemic control. Experience thus far suggests that the initiation of ETI is associated with modest weight gain. Notably, early experience suggests that ETI is not tolerated in up to a third of lung transplant recipients, in marked contrast to use before transplant whereby the intolerance rate is less than 5%. Additional registry data are necessary to better define the use of IVA or ETI after lung transplant.

PULMONARY VASODILATORS

Pulmonary arterial hypertension (PAH, group 1) is a common primary indication for lung transplantation, and elevated pulmonary artery pressure often complicates other end-stage lung diseases (group 3 pulmonary hypertension).[1,2] FDA-approved indications for the treatment of group 3 pulmonary hypertension are currently limited to a single agent (inhaled treprostinil) so most data and recommendations are driven by PAH. While a comprehensive overview of the treatment of PAH is beyond the scope of this review, patients with PAH awaiting lung transplantation are often receiving targeted therapies for the treatment of PAH. Therefore, management of these agents while patients await lung transplantation is an essential component of pretransplant care.

Several different medical therapies are now available for the treatment of PAH. Current targeted therapies are directed at one of the 3 pathways: endothelin-1 (bosentan, macitentan, and ambrisentan), prostacyclin (epoprostenol, treprostinil, iloprost, and selexipag), and nitric oxide (sildenafil, tadalafil, and riociguat), with patients typically receiving treatment targeting more than one pathway by the time of transplant consideration.[58] There are no high-quality studies evaluating specific agents, or combinations of these agents, with respect to outcomes after lung transplantation, but no significant hypothetical concerns exist regarding continuing any of these medications up until the point of transplantation. Importantly, elevated pulmonary artery pressure at the time of lung transplantation, whether due to PAH, or secondary (group 3) pulmonary hypertension, is a significant risk factor for primary graft dysfunction after transplant.[59,60] Therefore, most centers, including ours, follow an approach of optimizing targeted medical therapy for PAH before and during listing for transplantation, then stopping these medications in the immediate posttransplant setting.

The development of right heart failure, despite optimal medical therapy, is an ominous sign and may portend rapid decompensation and death.[58,61,62] Therefore, our approach is to have a low threshold to hospitalize patients with PAH who are awaiting lung transplantation if they develop signs or symptoms of worsening right heart failure. Such patients sometimes improve with adjustments to their diuretic regimens, but frequently may require vasopressor and/or ionotrope support as a bridge to transplantation. In selected cases, atrial septostomy or veno-arterial extracorporeal membrane oxygenation may be required to bridge patients with severe PAH to successful lung transplantation,[61,63] though the specific approaches to patients in this crisis are highly patient- and center-specific and should be undertaken only by centers with significant experience in this area.

ANTICOAGULANTS

Patients on the active lung transplant list and on anticoagulants require special attention to minimize the risk of bleeding due to residual anticoagulant effects. The timing of organ offers is unpredictable, as is the time between organ offer and start of the lung transplant operation. Consequently, it is important to have a plan for reversal of anticoagulant before admission for surgery. As higher intra- and postoperative blood transfusion may increase the risk of primary graft dysfunction and the development of donor-specific human leukocyte (HLA) antibodies, minimizing intraoperative bleeding is a high priority.

For patients on warfarin, there are several approaches to reverse the anticoagulated state. In addition to discontinuing warfarin, Vitamin K may be given by slow intravenous infusion at a dose of 5 or 10 mg, with anticipation that vitamin K-dependent clotting factor levels will be restored in no less than 6 hours assuming normal hepatic function. Thus, for patients with a < 24-h window between admission and operation time, the prothrombin time and international normalized ratio (INR) should be repeated before surgery, and if the INR remains in the therapeutic range, a rapid reversal agent should be administered. Options for rapid reversal include fresh frozen plasma, or a 3- or 4-factor prothrombin complex concentrate (PCC). Of the PCCs, despite the lack of comparative trials, 4-factor is favored over 3-factor due to the lack of Factor VII in the 3-factor PCC. More importantly, a randomized trial comparing a 4-factor PCC to fresh frozen plasma demonstrated more effective hemostasis and rapid INR reduction compared with plasma, with a similar safety profile and lower risk of volume overload with 4-factor PCC compared with plasma.[64,65] Thus, 4-factor PCC is the preferred reversal agent. If a PCC is not available, plasma should be used for rapid reversal of warfarin-induced anticoagulated state.

An increasing number of lung transplant candidates are on chronic direct-acting oral anticoagulants (DOACs). Until recently, there were no effective reversal agents for the approved DOACs, so many if not all transplant programs transitioned patients from a DOAC to warfarin at the time of transplant listing to allow for rapid reversal before surgery. With the development and FDA-approval of idarucizumab, patients on dabigatran could potentially remain on this DOAC and receive idarucizumab at the time of admission for transplant. Recent data from both heart and lung transplant programs suggest that idarucizumab reversal is a reasonable approach. In one single-center retrospective review, 4 patients on dabigatran who were not anticipated to have a sufficient time off dabigatran before surgery received idarucizumab in the preoperative holding area after the donor organs were deemed acceptable for transplant.[66] The 4 patients required 4 or fewer units of packed red blood cells, had grade 0 or 1 PGD, and no in-hospital mortality. However, 3 of the 4 had lower or upper extremity deep venous thrombosis on surveillance Doppler ultrasound postoperatively. Collectively, this experience and those from heart transplant programs,[67,67] suggest that for some transplant candidates on the active list who require anticoagulation, the use of dabigatran with a plan for reversal with idarucizumab is a reasonable alternative to warfarin.

DISCUSSION

Over the last decade, several newer medical therapies have become available for advanced lung diseases that have important implications for lung transplant preparation. Outpatient care of individuals approaching the need for lung transplant requires communication and collaboration with the referring physician(s) and longitudinal care providers to ensure that medical regimens are optimized to improve survival on the waiting list while ensuring that components of the patient's medical regimen do not increase the risk for a worse outcome after transplant. Particular attention is required to corticosteroid use and dosing, antifibrotics now often used for pulmonary fibrosis, mTOR inhibitors for patients with LAM and potentially other diseases, CFTR modulators for those with CF, and anticoagulants. Based on careful risk/benefit analysis and preparation, often in collaboration with a transplant pharmacist, medical management of lung transplant candidates before and at the time of listing with the drugs reviewed in this article will not adversely impact transplant outcomes.

DISCLOSURE

D.M. Sayah: No commercial or financial conflicts of interest to disclose. No funding sources are relevant to this work. J.M. Pilewski: No commercial or financial conflicts of interest. Dr J.M. Pilewski has received research grants for multi-center studies of CFTR modulators from Vertex.

CLINICS CARE POINTS

In patients awaiting lung transplantation

- The maximal safe dose of glucocorticoids is not defined, so the chronic dose should be minimized.
- Antifibrotics (pirfenidone and nintedanib) are likely safe and can be continued.
- Data for mTOR inhibitors (sirolimus and everolimus) are limited so risks versus benefits should be weighed for individual patients. Everolimus has a shorter half-life and may be preferred.
- CFTR modulators should be continued as withdrawal may be dangerous.
- PAH therapies should be continued and adjusted to optimize right heart function
- Anticoagulants are preferably reversed with 4-factor prothrombin complex concentrate (PCC) for warfarin or idarucizumab for-direct-acting oral anticoagulants when urgent reversal is needed before transplant surgery.

REFERENCES

1. Chambers DC, Cherikh WS, Harhay MO, et al. The International Thoracic Organ Transplant Registry of the International Society for Heart and Lung Transplantation: Thirty-sixth adult lung and heart-lung transplantation Report-2019; Focus theme: Donor and recipient size match. J Heart Lung Transpl 2019;38(10):1042–55.
2. Valapour M, Lehr CJ, Skeans MA, et al. OPTN/SRTR 2019 Annual Data Report: Lung. Am J Transplant 2021;21(Suppl 2):441–520.
3. Rhen T, Cidlowski JA. Antiinflammatory action of glucocorticoids–new mechanisms for old drugs. N Engl J Med 2005;353(16):1711–23.
4. Wang AS, Armstrong EJ, Armstrong AW. Corticosteroids and wound healing: clinical considerations in the perioperative period. Am J Surg 2013;206(3): 410–7.
5. Rice JB, White AG, Scarpati LM, et al. Long-term Systemic Corticosteroid Exposure: A Systematic Literature Review. Clin Ther 2017;39(11):2216–29.
6. Lima O, Cooper JD, Peters WJ, et al. Effects of methylprednisolone and azathioprine on bronchial healing following lung autotransplantation. J Thorac Cardiovasc Surg 1981;82(2):211–5.
7. Goldberg M, Lima O, Morgan E, et al. A comparison between cyclosporin A and methylprednisolone plus azathioprine on bronchial healing following canine lung autotransplantation. J Thorac Cardiovasc Surg 1983;85(6):821–6.
8. Patterson GA, Cooper JD. Status of lung transplantation. Surg Clin North Am 1988;68(3):545–58.
9. Park SJ, Nguyen DQ, Savik K, et al. Pre-transplant corticosteroid use and outcome in lung transplantation. J Heart Lung Transpl 2001;20(3):304–9.
10. Schafers HJ, Wagner TO, Demertzis S, et al. Preoperative corticosteroids. A contraindication to lung transplantation? Chest 1992;102(5):1522–5.
11. McAnally KJ, Valentine VG, LaPlace SG, et al. Effect of pre-transplantation prednisone on survival after lung transplantation. J Heart Lung Transpl 2006; 25(1):67–74.
12. Sugimoto S, Miyoshi K, Kurosaki T, et al. Favorable survival in lung transplant recipients on preoperative low-dose, as compared to high-dose corticosteroids, after hematopoietic stem cell transplantation. Int J Hematol 2018;107(6):696–702.
13. Yusen RD, Edwards LB, Dipchand AI, et al. The Registry of the International Society for Heart and Lung Transplantation: Thirty-third Adult Lung and Heart-Lung Transplant Report-2016; Focus Theme: Primary Diagnostic Indications for Transplant. J Heart Lung Transpl 2016;35(10):1170–84.
14. Malas J, Ranganath NK, Phillips KG, et al. Early airway dehiscence: Risk factors and outcomes with the rising incidence of extracorporeal membrane oxygenation as a bridge to lung transplantation. J Card Surg 2019;34(10):933–40.
15. Maurer JR, Frost AE, Estenne M, et al. International guidelines for the selection of lung transplant candidates. The International Society for Heart and Lung Transplantation, the American Thoracic Society, the American Society of Transplant Physicians, the European Respiratory Society. Heart Lung 1998; 27(4):223–9.
16. Orens JB, Estenne M, Arcasoy S, et al. International guidelines for the selection of lung transplant candidates: 2006 update–a consensus report from the Pulmonary Scientific Council of the International Society for Heart and Lung Transplantation. J Heart Lung Transpl 2006;25(7):745–55.
17. Weill D, Benden C, Corris PA, et al. A consensus document for the selection of lung transplant

candidates: 2014–an update from the Pulmonary Transplantation Council of the International Society for Heart and Lung Transplantation. J Heart Lung Transpl 2015;34(1):1–15.

18. Leard LE, Holm AM, Valapour M, et al. Consensus document for the selection of lung transplant candidates: An update from the International Society for Heart and Lung Transplantation. J Heart Lung Transpl 2021;40(11):1349–79.

19. Richeldi L, du Bois RM, Raghu G, et al. Efficacy and safety of nintedanib in idiopathic pulmonary fibrosis. N Engl J Med 2014;370(22):2071–82.

20. King TE Jr, Bradford WZ, Castro-Bernardini S, et al. A phase 3 trial of pirfenidone in patients with idiopathic pulmonary fibrosis. N Engl J Med 2014; 370(22):2083–92.

21. Wells AU, Flaherty KR, Brown KK, et al. Nintedanib in patients with progressive fibrosing interstitial lung diseases-subgroup analyses by interstitial lung disease diagnosis in the INBUILD trial: a randomised, double-blind, placebo-controlled, parallel-group trial. Lancet Respir Med 2020;8(5):453–60.

22. Distler O, Highland KB, Gahlemann M, et al. Nintedanib for Systemic Sclerosis-Associated Interstitial Lung Disease. N Engl J Med 2019;380(26):2518–28.

23. Salisbury ML, Conoscenti CS, Culver DA, et al. Antifibrotic Drug Use in Patients with Idiopathic Pulmonary Fibrosis. Data from the IPF-PRO Registry. Ann Am Thorac Soc 2020;17(11):1413–23.

24. Lehtonen ST, Veijola A, Karvonen H, et al. Pirfenidone and nintedanib modulate properties of fibroblasts and myofibroblasts in idiopathic pulmonary fibrosis. Respir Res 2016;17:14.

25. Wollin L, Wex E, Pautsch A, et al. Mode of action of nintedanib in the treatment of idiopathic pulmonary fibrosis. Eur Respir J 2015;45(5):1434–45.

26. Leuschner G, Stocker F, Veit T, et al. Outcome of lung transplantation in idiopathic pulmonary fibrosis with previous anti-fibrotic therapy. J Heart Lung Transpl 2017;37(2):268–74.

27. Mackintosh JA, Munsif M, Ranzenbacher L, et al. Risk of anastomotic dehiscence in patients with pulmonary fibrosis transplanted while receiving anti-fibrotics: Experience of the Australian Lung Transplant Collaborative. J Heart Lung Transpl 2019;38(5):553–9.

28. Mortensen A, Cherrier L, Walia R. Effect of pirfenidone on wound healing in lung transplant patients. Multidiscip Respir Med 2018;13:16.

29. Delanote I, Wuyts WA, Yserbyt J, et al. Safety and efficacy of bridging to lung transplantation with antifibrotic drugs in idiopathic pulmonary fibrosis: a case series. BMC Pulm Med 2016;16(1):156.

30. Tanaka S, Miyoshi K, Higo H, et al. Lung transplant candidates with idiopathic pulmonary fibrosis and long-term pirfenidone therapy: Treatment feasibility influences waitlist survival. Respir Investig 2019; 57(2):165–71.

31. Lambers C, Boehm PM, Lee S, et al. Effect of antifibrotics on short-term outcome after bilateral lung transplantation: a multicentre analysis. Eur Respir J 2018;51(6).

32. Veit T, Leuschner G, Sisic A, et al. Pirfenidone exerts beneficial effects in patients with IPF undergoing single lung transplantation. Am J Transplant 2019; 19(8):2358–65.

33. Combs MP, Fitzgerald LJ, Wakeam E, et al. Pretransplant antifibrotic therapy is associated with resolution of primary graft dysfunction. Ann Amer Thorac Soc 2022;19(2):335–8.

34. Kahan BD. Sirolimus: a comprehensive review. Expert Opin Pharmacother 2001;2(11):1903–17.

35. Nashan B. Review of the proliferation inhibitor everolimus. Expert Opin Investig Drugs 2002;11(12):1845–57.

36. Hua H, Kong Q, Zhang H, et al. Targeting mTOR for cancer therapy. J Hematol Oncol 2019;12(1):71.

37. King-Biggs MB, Dunitz JM, Park SJ, et al. Airway anastomotic dehiscence associated with use of sirolimus immediately after lung transplantation. Transplantation 2003;75(9):1437–43.

38. Groetzner J, Kur F, Spelsberg F, et al. Airway anastomosis complications in de novo lung transplantation with sirolimus-based immunosuppression. J Heart Lung Transpl 2004;23(5):632–8.

39. Pfizer Inc. Rapamune (sirolimus) [package insert]. U.S. Food and Drug Administration website. 2021. Available at: https://www.accessdata.fda.gov/spl/data/411b5f71-515a-431e-ae12-5db5ea5a06fd/411b5f71-515a-431e-ae12-5db5ea5a06fd.xml. Accessed August 28, 2021.

40. McCormack FX, Inoue Y, Moss J, et al. Efficacy and safety of sirolimus in lymphangioleiomyomatosis. N Engl J Med 2011;364(17):1595–606.

41. El-Chemaly S, Goldberg HJ, Glanville AR. Should mammalian target of rapamycin inhibitors be stopped in women with lymphangioleiomyomatosis awaiting lung transplantation? Expert Rev Respir Med 2014;8(6):657–60.

42. Baldi BG, Samano MN, Campos SV, et al. Experience of Lung Transplantation in Patients with Lymphangioleiomyomatosis at a Brazilian Reference Centre. Lung 2017;195(6):699–705.

43. Zhang J, Liu D, Yue B, et al. A Retrospective Study of Lung Transplantation in Patients With Lymphangioleiomyomatosis: Challenges and Outcomes. Front Med (Lausanne) 2021;8:584826.

44. Costa AN, Baldi BG, de Oliveira Braga Teixeira RH, et al. Can patients maintain their use of everolimus until lung transplantation? Transplantation 2015; 99(6):e42–3.

45. Novartis Inc. Zortress (everolimus) [package insert]. U.S. Food and Drug Administration website. 2018. Available at: https://www.accessdata.fda.gov/drugsatfda_docs/label/2018/021560s021lbl.pdf. Accessed December 20th, 2021.

46. Ramsey BW, Davies J, McElvaney NG, et al. A CFTR potentiator in patients with cystic fibrosis and the G551D mutation. N Engl J Med 2011;365(18): 1663–72.

47. Barry PJ, Plant BJ, Nair A, et al. Effects of ivacaftor in patients with cystic fibrosis who carry the G551D mutation and have severe lung disease. Chest 2014;146(1):152–8.

48. Polenakovik HM, Sanville B. The use of ivacaftor in an adult with severe lung disease due to cystic fibrosis (DeltaF508/G551D). J Cyst Fibros 2013; 12(5):530–1.

49. Taylor-Cousar J, Niknian M, Gilmartin G, et al. Effect of ivacaftor in patients with advanced cystic fibrosis and a G551D-CFTR mutation: Safety and efficacy in an expanded access program in the United States. J Cyst Fibros 2016;15(1):116–22.

50. Salvatore D, Terlizzi V, Francalanci M, et al. Ivacaftor improves lung disease in patients with advanced CF carrying CFTR mutations that confer residual function. Respir Med 2020;171:106073.

51. Keating D, Marigowda G, Burr L, et al. VX-445-Tezacaftor-Ivacaftor in Patients with Cystic Fibrosis and One or Two Phe508del Alleles. N Engl J Med 2018;379(17):1612–20.

52. Middleton PG, Mall MA, Drevinek P, et al. Elexacaftor-Tezacaftor-Ivacaftor for Cystic Fibrosis with a Single Phe508del Allele. N Engl J Med 2019;381(19): 1809–19.

53. Heijerman HGM, McKone EF, Downey DG, et al. Efficacy and safety of the elexacaftor plus tezacaftor plus ivacaftor combination regimen in people with cystic fibrosis homozygous for the F508del mutation: a double-blind, randomised, phase 3 trial. Lancet 2019;394(10212):1940–8.

54. Burgel PR, Durieu I, Chiron R, et al. Rapid Improvement after Starting Elexacaftor-Tezacaftor-Ivacaftor in Patients with Cystic Fibrosis and Advanced Pulmonary Disease. Am J Respir Crit Care Med 2021; 204(1):64–73.

55. Volkova N, Moy K, Evans J, et al. Disease progression in patients with cystic fibrosis treated with ivacaftor: Data from national US and UK registries. J Cyst Fibros 2020;19(1):68–79.

56. Ramos KJ, Quon BS, Heltshe SL, et al. Heterogeneity in Survival in Adult Patients With Cystic Fibrosis With FEV1 < 30% of Predicted in the United States. Chest 2017;151(6):1320–8.

57. Trimble AT, Donaldson SH. Ivacaftor withdrawal syndrome in cystic fibrosis patients with the G551D mutation. J Cyst Fibros 2018;17(2):e13–6.

58. Hassoun PM. Pulmonary Arterial Hypertension. N Engl J Med 2021;385(25):2361–76.

59. Kuntz CL, Hadjiliadis D, Ahya VN, et al. Risk factors for early primary graft dysfunction after lung transplantation: a registry study. Clin Transpl 2009; 23(6):819–30.

60. Diamond JM, Lee JC, Kawut SM, et al. Clinical risk factors for primary graft dysfunction after lung transplantation. Am J Respir Crit Care Med 2013;187(5): 527–34.

61. Baillie TJ, Granton JT. Lung Transplantation for Pulmonary Hypertension and Strategies to Bridge to Transplant. Semin Respir Crit Care Med 2017; 38(5):701–10.

62. Campo A, Mathai SC, Le Pavec J, et al. Outcomes of hospitalisation for right heart failure in pulmonary arterial hypertension. Eur Respir J 2011;38(2): 359–67.

63. Sandoval J, Gomez-Arroyo J, Gaspar J, et al. Interventional and surgical therapeutic strategies for pulmonary arterial hypertension: Beyond palliative treatments. J Cardiol 2015;66(4):304–14.

64. Goldstein JN, Refaai MA, Milling TJ Jr, et al. Four-factor prothrombin complex concentrate versus plasma for rapid vitamin K antagonist reversal in patients needing urgent surgical or invasive interventions: a phase 3b, open-label, non-inferiority, randomised trial. Lancet 2015;385(9982):2077–87.

65. Refaai MA, Goldstein JN, Lee ML, et al. Increased risk of volume overload with plasma compared with four-factor prothrombin complex concentrate for urgent vitamin K antagonist reversal. Transfusion 2015;55(11):2722–9.

66. Harano T, Rivosecchi RM, Morrell MR, et al. Dabigatran reversal with idarucizumab prior to lung transplantation. Clin Transpl 2021;35(1):e14142.

67. Crespo-Leiro MG, Lopez-Vilella R, Lopez Granados A, et al. Use of Idarucizumab to reverse the anticoagulant effect of dabigatran in cardiac transplant surgery. A multicentric experience in Spain. Clin Transpl 2019;33(12):e13748.

Inpatient Management of the Acutely Decompensating Lung Transplant Candidate

Stephan A. Soder, MD[a], Eduardo Fontena, MD[b], Juan C. Salgado, MD[c], Abbas Shahmohammadi, MD[d], Marcos N. Samano, MD, PhD[e,f], Tiago N. Machuca, MD, PhD[g,*]

KEYWORDS

- Critical illness • Lung transplant • Extracorporeal membrane oxygenation • Rehabilitation

KEY POINTS

- The urgency-based lung allocation has increased the complexity and acuity of candidates being listed and ultimately receiving a lung transplant.
- Frequently, transplant teams have to manage candidates with acute decompensation of their advanced lung disease.
- Careful patient selection by multidisciplinary teams is needed to avoid futile therapies and to provide support for patients who can benefit from lung transplantation (LTx) with favorable outcomes.
- Extracorporeal life support (ECLS) is an effective bridge to LTx, with equivalent long-term conditional survival in bridged and nonbridged recipients.
- Rehabilitation plays a fundamental role in the selection and preparation of patient bridged to transplantation.

INTRODUCTION

Lung allocation in the US changed nearly 15 years ago from time accrued on the waiting list to disease severity and likelihood of posttransplant survival, represented by the lung allocation score (LAS). Notably, the risk of death within a year plays a stronger role on the score calculation than posttransplant survival.[1] While this change was associated with the intended decrease in waitlist mortality (most recently reported at 14.6%), it was predictable that transplant teams would have to care for increasingly older and complex candidates and recipients.[2] This urgency-based allocation also led centers to routinely consider transplanting patients with higher acuity, often

[a] Division of Thoracic Surgery and Lung Transplant Program, Irmandade da Santa Casa de Misericordia de Porto Alegre. 295, Professor Annes Dias Street. Hospital Dom Vicente Scherer, 6th Floor. Centro Histórico. Porto Alegre, Rio Grande do Sul 90020-090, Brazil; [b] Lung Transplant Program, Hospital COPA D'Or, Rede D'Or Sao Luiz. 598, Figueiredo Magalhães Street. Room 39. Rio de Janeiro, Rio de Janeiro 22031-012, Brazil; [c] Division of Pulmonary, Allergy and Critical Care Medicine, Department of Medicine, Perelman School of Medicine, University of Pennsylvania, 3400 Spruce Street. Gates Pavilion 9036. Philadelphia, PA 19104, USA; [d] Lung Transplant and ECMO Program, University of Florida Division of Pulmonary, Critical Care and Sleep Medicine 1600 SW Archer Road, Room M452 Gainesville, FL 32610-0225, USA; [e] Lung Transplant Program, Hospital Israelita Albert Einstein, Sao Paulo, Brazil. Av. Albert Eintein, 627, Bloco A1, sala 418 Sao Paulo, Sao Paulo 05652-900, Brazil; [f] Division of Thoracic Surgery, University of Sao Paulo, Sao Paulo, Brazil. Av. Dr. Eneas Carvalho Aguiar, 44, Sao Paulo, São Paulo 05403-900, Brazil; [g] Division of Thoracic Surgery, UF Lung Transplant Program, Adult ECMO, University of Florida, PO Box 100129, Gainesville, FL 32610-0129, USA
* Corresponding author. Division of Thoracic Surgery, PO Box 100129, Gainesville, FL 32610-0129.
E-mail address: Tiago.NoguchiMachuca@surgery.ufl.edu

Thorac Surg Clin 32 (2022) 121–134
https://doi.org/10.1016/j.thorsurg.2022.02.001
1547-4127/22/© 2022 Elsevier Inc. All rights reserved.

hospitalized and, not infrequently, in the intensive care unit (ICU). According to the Scientific Registry for Transplant Recipients, from 2009 to 2019, the proportion of lung recipients hospitalized and those admitted to the ICU at the time of transplant increased from 18.9% to 26.8% and from 9.2% to 16.5%, respectively.[2,3]

Furthermore, as the implementation of an urgency-based allocation, more interstitial lung disease (ILD) than patients with chronic obstructive pulmonary disease (COPD) is being waitlisted and transplanted. From 2009 to 2019, the percentage of recipients transplanted for COPD declined from 33% to 22.9% while those transplanted for ILD increased from 44.5% to 63.5%.[2,3] The ILD group tends to be significantly more complex, unstable, and with less predictable trajectory of their advanced lung disease. Offering lung transplantation (LTx) to a growing population of complex candidates with increased disease severity requires that transplant teams become knowledgeable with the identification and management of acute decompensations of chronic lung disease.[4] Such patients often require hospital admission, escalation of care in the ICU, and ultimately, difficult discussions about continuing transplant candidacy or delisting (**Fig. 1**). Herein, we review the management of LTx candidates with acute decompensation, potential bridging strategies, patient rehabilitation, and triggers for delisting.

THE IMPACT OF DISEASE SEVERITY ON OUTCOMES AFTER LUNG TRANSPLANTATION

While waitlist mortality decreased as expected in the early years after the LAS implementation, the sickest patients derived the lowest transplant survival benefit. In an analysis of the United Network for Organ Sharing (UNOS) database including 6082 patients transplanted between May 2005 and May 2009, the net survival benefit was 3.44 years for patients with LAS 50 to 59 and 1.95 years for those with LAS greater than 90.[5] Analyzing UNOS data from 2006 to 2007, the same investigators found that the 1-year post-transplant survival was significantly worse as the LAS increased, being 83%, 79%, and 64% for patients with LAS less than 50, 50 to 74, and greater than 75, respectively.[6] The sickest group also had increased morbidity, including the need for renal replacement therapy and infections. With ongoing medical advances, improved bridging, and intraoperative management strategies, the outcomes of the sickest patients have significantly improved. Among 3548 adults in the upper LAS quartile, 1-year survival after lung transplant improved from 77% in the 2005 to 2008 era to 84% in the 2011

to 2014 era, despite an increase in mean LAS from 63 to 79.[7]

In 2007, France implemented a "High Emergency Lung Transplantation" system to prioritize the allocation of lungs to patients presenting with acute decompensation. The 1-year survival of this complex cohort was only 67% with 59% survival at 3 years.[8] One center with a large percentage of patients with cystic fibrosis (CF) (81% of 37) had more favorable outcomes, comparable to their non-high emergency cohort, with a time on the ventilator of 15.5 days versus 11 days and a 1-year survival of 81% versus 80% post-LTx, respectively.[9]

In the Scandinavian experience, with urgent allocation implemented in 2009, the prioritization of candidates based on disease severity considerably shortened the time to lung transplant. Among candidates listed as urgent, 81% were transplanted within 4 weeks versus only 4.3% of those listed as regular status. The 1-year survival was 81.3% in the urgent cohort versus 85.5% in the regular cohort, a nonstatistically significant difference. The deaths on the urgent listing group were mostly related to patients bridged with extracorporeal membrane oxygenation (ECMO).[10]

The group from Temple University reported their experience managing 37 patients with acute exacerbation of idiopathic pulmonary fibrosis compared with 52 stable patients.[11] Only 28 of the 37 patients presenting with an acute exacerbation underwent transplant (waitlist mortality 32%). The 1-year survival of those transplanted with acute exacerbation was 71% versus 94% for those with stable disease.

Similarly, the University of Florida reported the outcomes of 27 listed candidates admitted for acute decompensation from ILD compared to 69 with stable ILD.[12] Only 2 patients died on the waitlist for each group and the 1-year survival post-transplantation was comparable at 96% on the acute decompensation cohort versus 92.5% for stable patients. The authors speculate that the excellent survival in the acute exacerbation cohort may be related to the following factors: (1) listed acute exacerbation patients were cared for in a dedicated thoracic unit staffed by the LTx medical and surgical teams, (2) prompt access to donor lungs, with acute exacerbation patients being transplanted after a median of 10 days, (3) high utilization of intraoperative veno-arterial ECMO as opposed to cardiopulmonary bypass, and (4) a relatively younger population when compared with the Temple cohort (60 vs 67 years).

Further, patients urgently listed, defined as those listed and transplanted during the same hospitalization, can have acceptable outcomes. In a

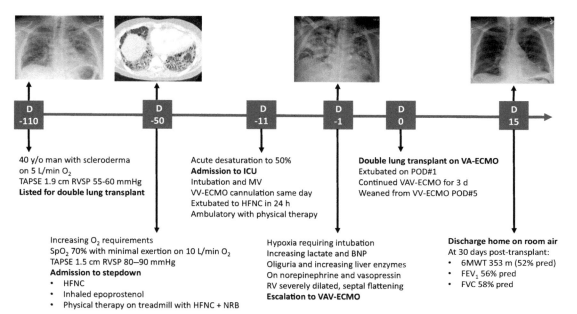

Fig. 1. Clinical picture detailing the evolution of an end-stage lung disease patient experiencing progressive worsening and acute deterioration.1: Hospital admission; 2: Stepdown unit admission; 3: ICU admission; 4 : Escalation of ECLS strategy; 5: Double lung transplant; 6: Hospital discharge. 6MWT, six-minutes walking test; BNP, brain natriuretic peptide; DC, discharge; ECMO, extracorporeal membrane oxygenation; FEV1, forced expiratory volume in one second; FVC, forced vital capacity; HFNC, high-flow nasal cannula; ICU, intensive care unit; MV, mechanical ventilation; NRB, nonrebreathing oxygen face mask; POD, postoperative day; PRED, predicted; RV, right ventricle; RVSP, right ventricular systolic pressure; TAPSE, tricuspid annular plane systolic excursion; VA-ECMO, Veno-arterial ECMO; VAV-ECMO, veno-arterial-venous ECMO; VV-ECMO, veno-venous ECMO.

cohort of 201 patients transplanted at the Cleveland Clinic from 2006 to 2017,[13] urgently listed patients were younger (54 vs 57 years), more often had ILD (76% vs 48%), and were more frequently on the ventilator (49% vs 1%) or on extracorporeal life support (ECLS) (22% vs 0.14%). With a 32% waitlist mortality in the urgently listed patients, they identified older age, higher bilirubin, and transfer from outside the hospital as significant predictors of early waitlist death. Interestingly, after LTx the reported overall morbidity was similar, as was the incidence of primary graft dysfunction (PGD) at 72 hours (17% for urgently listed vs 12% for selectively listed). Moreover, posttransplant survival was comparable (hospital mortality 13% vs 11%) as was allograft function up to 6 years after transplantation. This study highlights the possibility of favorable outcomes even with patients transferred in respiratory extremis when cared for in programs with robust experience.

There is an ongoing debate about the impact of center volume on outcomes for hospitalized candidates. A UNOS database analysis of 18,416 adults who underwent LTx from 2007 to 2017, found that 20% were hospitalized at the time of transplantation.[14] These patients were younger (55 vs

60 years), less likely to had COPD (10% vs 22%) and had higher LAS (70 vs 38). Expectedly, the wait time for these patients was shorter (27 vs 73 days); however, they experienced prolonged mechanical ventilation (MV) more often (56.7% vs 30%) and had a longer length of hospital stay (median 22 vs 15 days). Admission into higher volume centers (average 25 transplants/y during the study period) was associated with improved survival compared with low volume centers, and this difference was more pronounced in patients with CF. These results raise the potential benefit of identifying centers better suited to manage patients with higher acuity or even opening the window for possible second opinion consultations between transplant centers with different levels of expertise and risk-taking behavior.

Resource utilization considerations need to be made when considering transplantation for patients with higher acuity. Arnaoutakis *and colleagues* in 2011 reported that charges are significantly higher in patients in the highest LAS quartile not only for the index admission (Q4 $276,668 vs Q1-3 188,342) but also during the 1-year after transplantation (Q4 292,247 vs Q1-3 188,342).[15] More recently, the Mayo Clinic group reported a steady increase in hospital costs and posttransplant costs with the increase in LAS.[16] On a multivariate model, they were able to show a 12% increased index admission cost for every 10 points increase in the LAS at transplant.

The results from the studies above highlight the challenges lung transplant programs are facing worldwide and the need to: (1) develop strategies to better support listed patients with an acute decompensation, (2) expand the current donor pool, (3) improve perioperative management to extend posttransplant survival, and lastly, and (4) refine candidate selection to avoid futile listing/transplantation.

MEDICAL MANAGEMENT OF ACUTELY DECOMPENSATING LUNG TRANSPLANT CANDIDATES

The outpatient follow-up of lung transplant candidates varies according to disease severity. At our centers, stable patients are usually seen in the clinic every 1 to 2 months for health assessment and to update their LAS. Patients with LAS above 50 are seen every 2 weeks. While there are no absolute criteria for admitting those with acute exacerbation, we use a variety of indicators such as: a >50% sudden increase in oxygen requirement, need for > 8 to 10 L/min O2, inability to continue physical activity with conventional low-flow oxygen devices at home.[12]

Interstitial Lung Disease

ILD comprises a wide variety of parenchymal lung diseases with a clinical course that tends to be variable and unpredictable. A small subset of patients will develop acute exacerbations of ILD, with an in-hospital mortality reaching up to 90%.[17,18] This could either be due to rapidly progressive fibroproliferative process or triggered by factors such as infection.[17] These patients have progressive acute on chronic hypoxemic respiratory failure and, in more advanced stages, may also develop hypercapnia. In the absence of effective therapy for ILD exacerbations, management is strictly supportive; while commonly used, high-dose steroids have no proven efficacy.[19] The most important therapeutic pathway is expedited lung transplant evaluation for eligible patients.

Respiratory management can be escalated in a stepwise fashion from nasal cannula to face masks, high-flow nasal cannula (HFNC), noninvasive positive pressure ventilation (NPPV), MV and ECLS.[20] Compared with conventional low-flow oxygen, HFNC may provide the physiologic benefits of improved oxygenation, decreased anatomic dead space, decreased metabolic cost of breathing, generation of positive nasopharyngeal and tracheal airway pressure, improved work of breathing, preconditioning of inspired gas, better secretion clearance, and improved comfort.[21] In randomized clinical trials of patients with acute respiratory failure, HFNC has been associated with reduced need for intubation and lower mortality compared with conventional low-flow oxygen or NPPV.[22,23] While data to support HFNC for patients with ILD are scarce, it may function as a suitable alternative for those with need for higher oxygen flows and/or concentration requirement.[20] Similarly, NPPV may be attempted to stabilize the respiratory status before invasive MV. Given the mortality associated with MV, the American Thoracic Society recommends not offering intubation for these patients, except in select groups such as LTx candidates or those with a clear reversible cause for decompensation.[19]

Once respiratory failure progresses despite HFNC and NPPV, the addition of inhaled pulmonary vasodilators (ie, inhaled nitric oxide, epoprostenol) may be beneficial. Inhaled pulmonary vasodilators may improve oxygenation and support for right ventricular (RV) dysfunction/pulmonary hypertension (PH) often seen in patients with ILD, while avoiding ventilation/perfusion (V/Q) mismatch often seen in intravenous (IV) pulmonary vasodilators.[24]

Chronic Obstructive Pulmonary Disease

Since the implementation of the LAS, patients with COPD are waiting longer for transplant and consequently can present with acute decompensation. The BODE index (Body-mass index, airflow Obstruction, Dyspnea, and Exercise) is a useful resource for prognostication, showing transplant survival benefit in patients in the highest quartile. The 2021 Consensus Document for the Selection of Lung Transplant Candidates continues to rely on this score as a guide for referral and listing timing.[25] Patients with COPD waitlisted typically have a BODE score greater than 7 along with history of frequent exacerbations, a forced expiratory volume in 1 second (FEV1) ≤20% of predicted, PH, and/or hypercapnia.

As COPD progresses, it is imperative to adjust oxygen supplementation to maintain an acceptable level of physical conditioning and adequate nutritional status in waitlisted patients. Further, patient education on pursed-lip breathing and pacing are needed to prevent exercise-induced hyperinflation as much as possible.

Acute exacerbations in advanced COPD are typically triggered either by infections, inability to compensate for respiratory acidosis, PH, and gastroesophageal reflux disease. Pharmacologic therapies including bronchodilators, steroids, antimicrobials (including antivirals if needed), along with supportive care (including oxygen up-titration and noninvasive and invasive ventilation) have been the backbone strategies for transient support. HFNC, as well as NPPV, have become the preferred methods for support and avoidance of MV. Even though there is limited evidence regarding outcomes with the use of HFNC in COPD exacerbation, small prospective case series have shown a significant decrease in respiratory rate and a decrease in $Paco_2$.[26,27] Moreover, it may be better tolerated than NIV.[28] Nevertheless, given the limited data available, the European Respiratory Society has recently recommended a trial of NIV before HFNC in hypercapnic respiratory failure secondary to COPD exacerbation.[29]

Pulmonary Arterial Hypertension

Among patients with PH, those with pulmonary arterial hypertension (PAH) and chronic thromboembolic pulmonary hypertension (CTEPH) more commonly present with decompensated right heart failure, which carries a high risk of morbidity and mortality.[30] A recent report from a referral center in France, showed the 3-month and 1-year mortality after admission for decompensation from PAH as 31% and 41%, respectively. When LTx was not an option, the mortality was even higher at 46% and 56%, respectively.[31] With advances in PH therapy translating into improved quality of life (QoL) and lower disease-related morbidity and mortality, patients admitted to the ICU with decompensated PH with RV failure are those who have been on maximal medical therapy and often have exhausted all treatment options.[30] As the treatment of these patients is complicated, they should ideally be managed at an advanced lung failure center with expertise in PAH, ECLS, and LTx.

The triggers for decompensation are multiple, including infections, stressful conditions such as pregnancy and surgery, arrhythmia, and nonadherence, among others. Besides addressing the trigger, attention should be paid to the optimization of preload/fluid balance. RV afterload reduction is conducted with IV prostanoid such as epoprostenol, phosphodiesterase (PDE) inhibitors, and inhaled pulmonary vasodilators such as iNO or inhaled epoprostenol. For those not responding, inotropes such as dobutamine and inodilators such as milrinone, aiming to augment RV contractility, could be considered with the goal of a cardiac index greater than 2 L/min/m^2 and a venous oxygen saturation (SvO2) > 65%. Perfusion pressures are maintained with pressors with a

preference for vasopressin, which has demonstrated a pulmonary vasodilator effect, and norepinephrine, due to its beneficial effect on RV/pulmonary arterial circulation coupling and inotropic effects.

Respiratory failure with hypoxia is treated similar to ILD exacerbation with the use of supplemental oxygen, HFNC, and NPPV. However, every effort should be made to avoid intubation and MV. Endotracheal intubation and sedation can precipitate a hemodynamic collapse in those with advanced RV failure due to the depression of cardiac contractility and vasodilation. Awake fiberoptic intubation with cautious sedation and appropriate use of hemodynamic support and pressors are often needed.

When the above therapies have failed to show improvement of clinical status, ECLS should be considered. Before consideration for ECLS, 2 questions should be answered: (1) does the patient have a reversible cause of PAH decompensation and (2) is the patient a potential lung/heart–lung transplant candidate.

Cystic Fibrosis

CF continues to be a common indication for LTx in North America and Europe with a modest decline over the last decade as a result of CF transmembrane conductance regulator (CFTR) modulators, a new class of drugs that act by improving production, intracellular processing, and/or function of the defective CFTR protein.[32] They have been shown to improve FEV_1 and symptom-related QoL, and to reduce acute exacerbations mainly in patients with mild to moderate CF lung disease, including emerging data of its benefits in patients with advanced lung disease.[33] Of note, there is a significant proportion of patients who do not present any mutation approved for one of the available CFTR modulators. This category represents approximately 8% of non-Hispanic White patients, 25% of Hispanic patients, and 30% of Black/African American patients with CF.[34]

The management of CF-listed patients presenting with an exacerbation includes empiric antibiotic therapy against known lung microbiota and intense airway clearance. Common practice is to select at least one antibiotic to cover each bacterial isolate that is cultured from respiratory secretions and 2 antibiotics for *Pseudomonas aeruginosa* infections. Antibiotic duration is based on the initial response, and ranges from 10 days for those with rapid response, to 14 days or longer for those with slower response and those who require ICU level of care. In such patients, antibiotics are continued until symptoms and FEV_1

improvement have plateaued (typical duration is 14–21 days).[35] In regard to airway clearance strategies, continuation of outpatient treatments including inhaled agents, that is, hypertonic saline, as well as mechanical chest physiotherapy, such as percussive therapy or more novel intrapulmonary percussive ventilation devices, are recommended.[36] In patients with CF with severe parenchymal destruction, acute exacerbations can be complicated by massive hemoptysis. In such cases, emergent bronchoscopy may help identify and tamponade the bleeding lung segment, though systemic artery embolization may be ultimately needed.

BRIDGE TO TRANSPLANTATION

LTx candidates who become critically ill have a high risk of death while waiting for a suitable organ. A bridge therapy with a device may be needed in selected patients to avoid further deterioration and maintain LTx candidacy. Furthermore, an increased number of transplants are being performed for acute or subacute diseases with irreversible lung damage, such as COVID-19 ARDS, for whom a bridge therapy may be used along with the enlisting process.[37]

MV has been used for decades as a bridge. However, the need for sedation, physical deconditioning, failure to reach LTx, and poorer posttransplant survival,[38,39] along with increasing experience with ECLS has made this mode of bridging less appealing in the modern era.[40]

Experience with Extracorporeal Life Support as a Bridge to Lung Transplantation

The use of ECLS bridge to transplantation (BTT) relies on avoiding or reducing the need for MV, decreasing sedation, and facilitating ambulation while maintaining transplant eligibility. The occurrence of critical illness myopathy (CIM) in patients supported with ECLS is variable and ranges from 30% to 75%.[41,42] Reduced sedation protocols and early mobilization are associated with improved outcomes,[43,44] and active rehabilitation in such patients can shorten posttransplant MV duration, ICU and hospital length of stay.[45] Weaning from MV, mobilization, and ambulation were associated with a higher likelihood of successful BTT in several series.[46–48]

Successful bridging to LTx is achieved in 56%[49] to 89%[47,50] in most of the published series, with a reported 100% success in a 1-year time-lapsed single-center experience.[51] In a large cohort, Simplified Acute Physiologic Score II, unplanned intubation while on ECLS, renal replacement therapy, and cerebrovascular accident were identified

as independent predictors of unsuccessful BTT. On the other hand, ambulation was associated with successful BTT.[48] The median duration of the bridge ranged from 2[51] to 17 days,[52] and veno-venous extracorporeal membrane oxygenation (VV-ECMO) was the most used configuration.

PGD grade 3 at 72h in bridged patients is variably reported in the literature and can be as low as 5.6%.[50] Frequently, ECLS is maintained postoperatively, and PGD should be classified as "ungradable" in that situation. There is an expected longer in-hospital stay[51] and higher mortality for bridged patients in the early period following LTx[50,52] secondary to the clinical severity and potential deconditioning. However, for bridged patients who achieve LTx, conditional survival is shown to be equivalent to nonbridged transplanted patients,[46–48,53,54] especially in high-volume centers, with 1-year, 3-year, and 5-year survival ranging from 58%[52] to 100%,[51] from 63%[47] to 83%,[48] and from 55%[47] to 65%,[50] respectively. Furthermore, the real survival benefit attributed to ECLS bridged patients has to take into account the unequivocal mortality of this cohort *without* LTx.

Indication for Transplantation Versus Prognosis

The evaluation of relevant clinical aspects that may impact the outcomes of LTx candidates and patients on ECLS BTT is crucial for the decision-making process and management. Patients with CF seem to have a better prognosis with BTT.[47,55,56] A large series of patients with transplanted CF reported 1-year conditional survival after LTx of 81% in bridged patients, which was no statistically different compared with nonbridged patients.[56] Case reports of uncontrolled pulmonary infection treated with double pneumonectomy with successful ECLS BTT have been reported.[57] Conversely, patients with idiopathic PAH and RV dysfunction are associated with worse survivals.[47,58] Patients with ILD exhibit widely variable outcomes in different series.[47,55,58]

Bridge to retransplantation is another negative prognostic factor. A case series from the Toronto group revealed that the median survival of patients bridged to their first transplant was significantly superior to those bridged to retransplantation (60 vs 15 months, $P = 0.041$), with 5-year overall survival of 39% in the latter group.[47]

Initiation and Choice of Extracorporeal Life Support Configuration

ECLS can be instituted not only to better support patients on the ventilator but also to obviate the need for intubation in rapidly deteriorating patients. One of the main concepts of contemporary approaches is ambulatory bridging. ECLS must be instituted with the goal of keeping patients awake as much as possible and, preferentially, able to ambulate. In 2012, the Hannover group reported improved outcomes not only with ECMO compared with MV but even better outcomes when patients were cannulated awake without requiring intubation.[59] Subsequently, several reports demonstrated a growing experience associated with ever-improving outcomes.[47,48,60,61]

Cannulation sites are intimately related to mobilization, and cannulas must be installed and secured to avoid dislodgement and sustain blood flow while allowing for mobilization. Even though femoral cannulation has traditionally been associated with limited out-of-bed physical therapy,[62] trained teams have reported increasingly accomplished ambulation with these patients.[62–66] Pasrija *and colleagues* reported an experience with femoral veno-arterial ECMO (VA-ECMO) and possibility of ambulatory status in 14% of the patients. There was no flow compromise during or after ambulation, no major bleeding or vascular complications.[66] In a large series evaluating factors related to out-of-bed physical therapy in ECMO supported patients, there was an increased frequency of mobilization during the study timeframe, and 51% of femoral cannulated patients ambulated.[62]

To date, there is no consensus on the precise triggers to initiate the evaluation for ECLS BTT. Transplant candidates who were actively enrolled in rehabilitation and present with acute decompensation refractory to standard medical therapies or who develop progressive worsening exercise tolerance with the inability to ambulate despite maximal noninvasive ventilation support are eligible for ECLS BTT.[47] Progressive hypercapnia (Pco_2>70 mm Hg in the arterial blood) despite continuous positive airway pressure[50] and for those intubated, sedated and incapable of weaning off MV, with the possibility of physical rehabilitation, ECLS may be considered. Additionally, cardiogenic shock, RV failure, or excessively high pulmonary artery systolic pressure can also indicate the need for RV support.

Once a patient is deemed eligible for ECLS BTT, the configuration should address the patient's underlying pathophysiologic state and restore vital needs, enable optimal mobility with simplicity and safety for bedside management. Firstly, the respiratory impairment should be divided into predominantly hypercapnic failure or hypoxemic failure with or without hypercapnia. Secondly, it is important to identify significant RV strain with impending RV failure. Notably, most patients

presenting with an acute respiratory exacerbation may also be hemodynamically unstable. Nevertheless, significant improvement in the hemodynamic status is seen once the hypoxia and/or acidosis are addressed with VV-ECMO. Importantly, some patients may need to change the ECLS configuration during the bridge, depending on the clinical evolution. A proposed ECLS BTT diagram is presented in **Fig. 2**.

Anticoagulation

Patients undergoing ECLS support present impaired coagulation function due to the blood-circuit interface. Both major thrombotic and bleeding events can occur. Nevertheless, improvements in ECMO technology with biocompatible circuits are less likely to activate coagulation and innate immune responses, enabling longer ECMO runs, decreased blood product consumption, and reduced surface-triggered inflammation.[67]

With heparin-coated circuits, high-flow VV-ECMO can be safely maintained without mandatory anticoagulation thereby preventing bleeding complications, albeit at the theoretic cost of faster membrane deterioration secondary to fibrin formation and clotting. In a recent study, Kurihara *and colleagues* compared their institutional experience with 38 patients receiving anticoagulation (heparin or bivalirudin) versus 36 patients only receiving thromboprophylaxis. The former group presented with higher incidence of gastrointestinal bleeding and blood product transfusion requirement. Interestingly, there were no cases of circuit thrombosis in either group.[68] For patients supported by VA-ECMO, anticoagulation continues to be standard practice due to the high risk for and major morbidity related to arterial thromboembolism. Nevertheless, a recent report supports the feasibility and benefits of VA-ECMO without anticoagulation in 75 patients.[69]

REHABILITATION DURING ACUTE DECOMPENSATION

Active rehabilitation of transplant candidates presenting with an acute decompensation is crucial as debility/deconditioning is one of the main factors associated with delisting or transitioning to comfort-focused care. Although these patients are obvious targets for early rehabilitation to maintain their transplant candidacy, patients on ECLS have been, historically, considered too unstable for active physical therapy and managed with sedation and neuromuscular blockade. However, the ability to perform awake ECLS with early mobilization is evolving rapidly with advances in

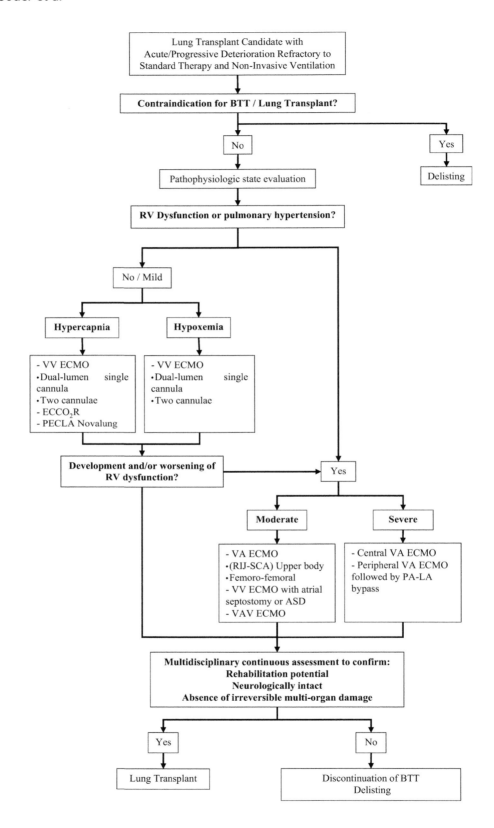

Table 1
Advantages, challenges, and management of the awake patient on ECLS support

Advantages of awake, Spontaneously Breathing Patient	Potential Challenges of Awake ECMO	Overcoming the Challenges
Improved tone of respiratory muscles and diaphragm	Increased oxygen demand and $Paco_2$ secondary to higher breathing work Elevated transpulmonary pressure may facilitate spontaneous induced lung injury.	Adjust sedation to prevent fatigue and avoid symptoms of respiratory distress Change from ETT to tracheostomy Sweep gas adjustment
Increased negative pressure during inspiration, leading to improved venous return and cardiac output and favoring lymphatic drainage	Intermittent IVC collapse around drainage cannula promoting circuit chattering	Correction of hypovolemia if contributing to the chattering Sedation and ECMO flow adjustments
Increased comfort	Decreased clearance of secretions	Preference for tracheostomy over extubation in tubed patients for secretions toileting.
Get patients actively involved in exercises and physical therapy	Cannula dislodgments Equipment failure	Readily available emergency equipment for intubation and resuscitation in catastrophic events Enough multidisciplinary staff to assist patients while in physical therapy/ambulation
Less ICU psychosis/delirium	Difficulty to withdraw care in awake patients if additional complications emerge	Keep family continuously involved throughout care

Abbreviations: ECMO, extracorporeal membrane oxygenation; ETT, endotracheal tube; ICU, intensive care unit; IVC, inferior vena cava.

extracorporeal technology and increasing expertise of multidisciplinary teams.[70]

Pretransplant exercise training is recommended throughout the waiting period to prevent inactivity and physical deconditioning. Rehabilitation guidelines can be modified taking into account disease severity. In case of disease progression and functional worsening, physical therapy goals, as well as oxygen titration, need to be constantly reevaluated. The program's intensity should be correlated with exertional oxygen saturation, heart rate, symptoms of dyspnea, and fatigue. LTx rehabilitation guidelines suggest maintaining oxygen saturation (SO2) of at least 88% during exercise. As patients with BTT are at risk for CIM, rehabilitation should focus to keep proximal muscle and lower limb strength.

The rationale of keeping these patients spontaneously breathing includes a reduction in a V/Q mismatch, and preservation of respiratory muscles and diaphragmatic tone. Additionally, spontaneous breathing improves venous return and cardiac filling.[71] The understanding of heart-lung-ECMO interactions in a spontaneously breathing patient is of paramount importance for the application of awake ECMO (**Table 1**).

Fig. 2. Summarized algorithm of the ECLS approach as a bridge to transplantation in decompensated lung transplant candidates. This diagram highlights the choice of ECLS modality and cannulation in potential candidates to BTT. This content provides a shortcut of highly complex clinical assessment and decision-making process, and procedural selection is subjected to resources availability, local expertise, and training of the multidisciplinary teams involved. ASD, atrial septal defect; $ECCO_2R$, extracorporeal CO_2 removal; ECLS BTT, extracorporeal life support as a bridge to transplantation; ECMO, extracorporeal membrane oxygenation; PA-LA bypass, pulmonary artery-to-left atrium bypass; PECLA, pumpless extracorporeal lung assist device; PH, pulmonary hypertension; RIJ-SCA, right internal jugular vein-subclavian artery configuration; RV, right ventricle; VA-ECMO, Veno-arterial ECMO; VAV-ECMO, veno-arterial-venous ECMO; VV-ECMO, veno-venous ECMO.

Table 2
Frailty assessment tools used currently to evaluate patients under clinical conditions

Assessment Tool	Characteristics
Fried Frailty Phenotype (Fried et al., 2001)[76]	• Weight loss (more than 10lbs) • Weakness (grip strength) • Exhaustion (self-report) • Walking Speed (15 feet) • Physical Activity (Kcals/wk)
Deficit Accumulation Frailty Index (Mitnitski et al. 2015)[78]	• Checklist of clinical conditions and disease based on 70 items. • Ratio of deficits presented in a person to the total number of deficits considered
Frail Scale (Van Kan et al. 2008)[79]	• Fatigue (are you fatigued?) • Resistance (can you climb a single flight of stairs?) • Ambulation (can you walk one block?) • Illnesses (more than 5) • Loss of weight (more than 5%)

Short Physical Performance Battery (Singer JP et al, 2018)[77]	• Three-component battery:
	  ○ Gait speed
	  ○ Chair stands
	  ○ Balance

Each method uses characteristics to score and categorize levels of frailty

Rehabilitation During Awake Extracorporeal Membrane Oxygenation

To avoid intubation and deep sedation in patients who are candidates for LTx, peripheral ECMO cannulation is preferred. Cannulation with conscious sedation and percutaneous techniques is feasible and is becoming the standard. In the first 24 to 48 hours, if patients are intubated, the goals are to reach respiratory and hemodynamic stability and wean any neuromuscular blockade. Once the patient stabilizes, sedation should be progressively reduced to obtain a smooth awakening and weaning off MV. Analgesia and delirium control with fentanyl or dexmedetomidine infusion maybe required to facilitate this process.

The use of NPPV or HFNC may facilitate successful extubation. Early tracheostomy is beneficial for patients that are too deconditioned to be weaned from MV or present with significant dyssynchrony.[72–74] Tracheostomy is associated with advantages such as decreased airway resistance, less sedation requirements, facilitating airway clearance, and so forth. Additionally, patients can be fed orally and mobilized more safely than those orally intubated.

The sedation plan should be guided by the patient's needs, pursuing early mobilization. A team-based approach for the rehabilitation of patients on ECLS BTT has been adopted by many centers. This includes collaborative work and combined rounds with physical and occupational therapy, bedside nurse, nurse practitioners, respiratory therapist, ECMO specialist, intensive care team, and the lung transplant team of surgeons, pulmonologists, and advanced practice providers.

TRIGGERS FOR DELISTING

There are different institutional protocols and multidisciplinary decision-making regarding bridged patients with progressive deterioration despite optimal support. The stringency of patient selection and the regular reevaluation of transplant candidacy is directly associated with the likelihood to successfully BTT and with posttransplant survival. More rigorous requirements of physical conditioning and multi-organ function can lead to more discontinuation of bridge therapy and higher conditional posttransplant survival.[48] Groups maintaining transplant eligibility for patients not capable of ambulating and with reversible renal dysfunction have high rates of BTT albeit at the cost of potentially higher perioperative mortality.[47,50]

As we continue to push boundaries for expanding access to LTx for critically ill patients, we need to remain cognizant of "bridging too far." For instance, frailty is prevalent in acutely decompensating lung transplant candidates and is associated with an increased risk of early mortality after lung transplant.[75] Frailty can be defined as a phenotypic condition which includes slowness, weakness, low physical activity, shrinking, and exhaustion and can be measured by tools such as the fried frailty phenotype (FFP)[76] and short physical performance battery (SPPB),[77] as shown in **Table 2**.[76–79] Frailty scores have been adapted to critical care scenario whereby patients are categorized as fit, vulnerable, frail and terminally ill.[80] Frail patients have increased risk for delisting or death compared with nonfrail patients by 1-year (36% vs 16%, using SPPB and 27% vs 13% with FFP).[81] The challenge is to determine how to incorporate these findings in daily clinical practice for the assessment of lung transplant candidates and optimize organ allocation.

Delisting may also occur in the event of additional organ failure. However, in selected "young" candidates, multi-organ transplants such as lung–kidney and heart–lung have been reported following COVID-19 infection.[82,83] Otherwise, lung–liver and heart–lung transplants are mostly reserved for chronic conditions. Pan-resistant organisms may also be considered a potential reason for delisting a decompensated patient.

Regardless of the circumstances noted above, in these difficult scenarios, palliative care/team has the potential to improve QoL, alleviate symptom burden and optimize health care utilization.[84] Furthermore, due to daily variability in the clinical condition of acutely deteriorating patients on or off ECLS, early involvement of palliative team can be paramount in supporting both the patient and the family.

SUMMARY

Despite the high complexity and the increasing number of acutely deteriorating patients with end-stage lung disease requiring admission and advanced support, satisfactory outcomes following LTx can be achieved in selected patients at experienced centers. Multidisciplinary teamwork plays a crucial role in the continuous transplant eligibility evaluation, optimal medical management focusing on underlying diseases peculiarities, and active rehabilitation. Stringent selection criteria are crucial for identifying suitable BTT candidates. Patient/disease-specific ECLS strategies can provide support for patients and allow rehabilitation as the candidate awaits lung transplantation.

CLINICS CARE POINTS

- The management of acutely decompensated lung transplant candidates should address underlying disease peculiarities while providing vital support as needed while in the waitlist.
- To enroll critically ill patients in an active rehabilitation program is of paramount importance and correlates with posttransplant survival.
- Conditional survival of ECLS bridged patients to lung transplantation is comparable to non-bridged patients.
- Prolonged ECMO runs are feasible and can provide support to critically ill patients while maintaining transplant eligibility and rehabilitation.

REFERENCES

1. Eberlein M, Garrity ER, Orens JB. Lung allocation in the united states. Clin Chest Med 2011;32(2): 213–22.
2. Valapour M, Lehr CJ, Skeans MA, et al. OPTN/SRTR 2019 annual data report: lung. Am J Transplant 2021;21(S2):441–520.
3. Organ procurement and transplantation network and scientific registry of transplant recipients 2010 data report. Am J Transplant 2012;12(SUPPL. 1): 1–156.
4. Shigemura N, Toyoda Y. Elderly patients with multiple comorbidities: insights from the bedside to the bench and programmatic directions for this new challenge in lung transplantation. Transpl Int 2020; 33(4):347–55.
5. Russo MJ, Worku B, Iribarne A, et al. Does lung allocation score maximize survival benefit from lung transplantation? J Thorac Cardiovasc Surg 2011; 141(5):1270–7.
6. Russo MJ, Iribarne A, Hong KN, et al. High lung allocation score is associated with increased morbidity and mortality following transplantation. Chest 2010; 137(3):651–7.
7. Crawford TC, Grimm JC, Magruder JT, et al. lung transplant mortality is improving in recipients with a lung allocation score in the upper quartile. Ann Thorac Surg 2017;103(5):1607–13.
8. Orsini B, Sage E, Olland A, et al. High-emergency waiting list for lung transplantation: early results of a nation-based study. Eur J Cardiothorac Surg. 2014;46(3):e41–7. discussion e47.
9. Roux A, Beaumont-Azuar L, Hamid AM, et al. high emergency lung transplantation: dramatic decrease of waiting list death rate without relevant higher posttransplant mortality. Transpl Int 2015;28(9): 1092–101.
10. Auråen H, Schultz HHL, Hämmäinen P, et al. Urgent lung allocation system in the Scandiatransplant countries. J Hear Lung Transplant 2018;37(12): 1403–9.
11. Dotan Y, Vaidy A, Shapiro WB, et al. Effect of acute exacerbation of idiopathic pulmonary fibrosis on lung transplantation outcome. Chest 2018;154(4): 818–26.
12. Chizinga M, Machuca TN, Shahmohammadi A, et al. Lung transplantation for acute exacerbation of interstitial lung disease. Thorax 2021.
13. Tang A, Thuita L, Siddiqui HU, et al. Urgently listed lung transplant patients have outcomes similar to those of electively listed patients. J Thorac Cardiovasc Surg 2021;161(1):306–17. e8.
14. Ranganath NK, Malas J, Chen S, et al. high lung transplant center volume is associated with increased survival in hospitalized patients. Ann Thorac Surg 2021;111(5):1652–8.

15. Arnaoutakis GJ, Allen JG, Merlo CA, et al. Impact of the lung allocation score on resource utilization after lung transplantation in the United States. J Hear Lung Transplant 2011;30(1):14–21.

16. Keller CA, Gonwa TA, White LJ, et al. Utilization and cost analysis of lung transplantation and survival after 10 years of adapting the lung allocation score. Transplantation 2019;103(3):638–46.

17. Collard HR, Ryerson CJ, Corte TJ, et al. Acute exacerbation of idiopathic pulmonary fibrosis an international working group report. Am J Respir Crit Care Med 2016;194(3):265–75.

18. Leuschner G, Behr J. Acute exacerbation in interstitial lung disease. Front Med 2017;4(OCT).

19. Raghu G, Collard HR, Egan JJ, et al. An Official ATS/ERS/JRS/ALAT Statement: Idiopathic pulmonary fibrosis: Evidence-based guidelines for diagnosis and management. Am J Respir Crit Care Med 2011;183(6):788–824.

20. Faverio P, De Giacomi F, Sardella L, et al. Management of acute respiratory failure in interstitial lung diseases: Overview and clinical insights. BMC Pulm Med 2018;18(1):70.

21. Drake MG. High-flow nasal cannula oxygen in adults: An evidence-based assessment. Ann Am Thorac Soc 2018;15(2):145–55.

22. Frat J-P, Thille AW, Mercat A, et al. High-flow oxygen through nasal cannula in acute hypoxemic respiratory failure. N Engl J Med 2015;372(23):2185–96.

23. Jones PG, Kamona S, Doran O, Sawtell F, Wilsher M. Randomized controlled trial of humidified high-flow nasal oxygen for acute respiratory distress in the emergency department: the HOT-ER study. Respir Care 2016;61(3):291–9.

24. Ventetuolo CE, Klinger JR. Management of acute right ventricular failure in the intensive care unit. Ann Am Thorac Soc 2014;11(5):811–22.

25. Leard LE, Holm AM, Valapour M, et al. Consensus document for the selection of lung transplant candidates: an update from the international society for heart and lung transplantation. J Hear Lung Transplant 2021;40(11):1349–79.

26. Plotnikow GA, Accoce M, Fredes S, et al. High-flow oxygen therapy application in chronic obstructive pulmonary disease patients with acute hypercapnic respiratory failure: a multicenter study. Crit Care Explor 2021;3(2):e0337.

27. Pisani L, Betti S, Biglia C, et al. Effects of high-flow nasal cannula in patients with persistent hypercapnia after an acute COPD exacerbation: a prospective pilot study. BMC Pulm Med 2020;20(1):12.

28. Pisani L, Astuto M, Prediletto I, Longhini F. High flow through nasal cannula in exacerbated COPD patients: a systematic review. Pulmonology 2019; 25(6):348–54.

29. Oczkowski S, Ergan B, Bos L, et al. ERS clinical practice guidelines: high-flow nasal cannula in acute respiratory failure. Eur Respir J 2021;2101574.

30. Hoeper MM, Granton J. Intensive care unit management of patients with severe pulmonary hypertension and right heart failure. Am J Respir Crit Care Med 2011;184(10):1114–24.

31. Savale L, Vuillard C, Pichon J, et al. Five-year survival after an acute episode of decompensated pulmonary arterial hypertension in the modern management era of right heart failure. Eur Respir J 2021;58(3).

32. Davis PB. Therapy for cystic fibrosis — the end of the beginning? N Engl J Med 2011;365(18):1734–5.

33. Shteinberg M, Taylor-Cousar JL. Impact of cftr modulator use on outcomes in people with severe cystic fibrosis lung disease. Eur Respir Rev 2020; 29(155).

34. McGarry ME, McColley SA. Cystic fibrosis patients of minority race and ethnicity less likely eligible for CFTR modulators based on CFTR genotype. Pediatr Pulmonol 2021;56(6):1496–503.

35. Wagener JS, Williams MJ, Millar SJ, Morgan WJ, Pasta DJ, Konstan MW. Pulmonary exacerbations and acute declines in lung function in patients with cystic fibrosis. J Cyst Fibros 2018;17(4):496–502.

36. Hassan A, Milross M, Lai W, Shetty D, Alison J, Huang S. Feasibility and safety of intrapulmonary percussive ventilation in spontaneously breathing, non-ventilated patients in critical care: a retrospective pilot study. J Intensive Care Soc 2021;22(2):111–9.

37. Bharat A, Machuca TN, Querrey M, et al. Early outcomes after lung transplantation for severe COVID-19: a series of the first consecutive cases from four countries. Lancet Respir Med 2021;9(5):487–97.

38. Elizur A, Sweet SC, Huddleston CB, et al. Pre-transplant mechanical ventilation increases short-term morbidity and mortality in pediatric patients with cystic fibrosis. J Hear Lung Transplant 2007;26(2):127–31.

39. Mason DP, Thuita L, Nowicki ER, Murthy SC, Pettersson GB, Blackstone EH. Should lung transplantation be performed for patients on mechanical respiratory support? The US experience. J Thorac Cardiovasc Surg 2010;139(3):765–73.

40. Hayanga JWA, Hayanga HK, Holmes SD, et al. Mechanical ventilation and extracorporeal membrane oxygenation as a bridge to lung transplantation: closing the gap. J Hear Lung Transplant 2019; 38(10):1104–11.

41. Dellgren G, Riise GC, Swärd K, et al. Extracorporeal membrane oxygenation as a bridge to lung transplantation: a long-term study. Eur J Cardiothorac Surg 2015;47(1):95–100.

42. Crotti S, Iotti GA, Lissoni A, et al. Organ allocation waiting time during extracorporeal bridge to lung transplant affects outcomes. Chest 2013;144(3):1018–25.

43. Brahmbhatt N, Murugan R, Milbrandt EB. Early mobilization improves functional outcomes in critically ill patients. Crit Care 2010;14(5):321.

44. Polastri M, Loforte A, Dell'Amore A, Nava S. Physiotherapy for patients on awake extracorporeal membrane oxygenation: a systematic review. Physiother Res Int 2016;21(4):203–9.

45. Rehder KJ, Turner DA, Hartwig MG, et al. Active rehabilitation during extracorporeal membrane oxygenation as a bridge to lung transplantation. Respir Care 2013;58(8):1291–8.

46. Hoopes CW, Kukreja J, Golden J, Davenport DL, Diaz-Guzman E, Zwischenberger JB. Extracorporeal membrane oxygenation as a bridge to pulmonary transplantation. J Thorac Cardiovasc Surg 2013;145(3):862–8.

47. Hoetzenecker K, Donahoe L, Yeung JC, et al. Extracorporeal life support as a bridge to lung transplantation–experience of a high-volume transplant center. J Thorac Cardiovasc Surg 2018;155(3):1316–28. e1.

48. Tipograf Y, Salna M, Minko E, et al. Outcomes of extracorporeal membrane oxygenation as a bridge to lung transplantation. Ann Thorac Surg 2019;107(5):1456–63.

49. Biscotti M, Gannon WD, Agerstrand C, et al. Awake extracorporeal membrane oxygenation as bridge to lung transplantation: a 9-year experience. Ann Thorac Surg 2017;104(2):412–9.

50. Benazzo A, Schwarz S, Frommlet F, et al. Twenty-year experience with extracorporeal life support as bridge to lung transplantation. J Thorac Cardiovasc Surg 2019;157(6):2515–25. e10.

51. Todd EM, Biswas Roy S, Hashimi AS, et al. Extracorporeal membrane oxygenation as a bridge to lung transplantation: A single-center experience in the present era. J Thorac Cardiovasc Surg 2017;154(5):1798–809.

52. Yeo HJ, Lee S, Yoon SH, et al. Extracorporeal life support as a bridge to lung transplantation in patients with acute respiratory failure. Transplant Proc 2017;49(6):1430–5.

53. Toyoda Y, Bhama JK, Shigemura N, et al. Efficacy of extracorporeal membrane oxygenation as a bridge to lung transplantation. J Thorac Cardiovasc Surg 2013;145(4):1065–71.

54. Langer F, Aliyev P, Schäfers HJ, et al. Improving outcomes in bridge-to-transplant: Extended extracorporeal membrane oxygenation support to obtain optimal donor lungs for marginal recipients. ASAIO J 2019;65(5):516–21.

55. Lafarge M, Mordant P, Thabut G, et al. Experience of extracorporeal membrane oxygenation as a bridge to lung transplantation in France. J Hear Lung Transplant 2013;32(9):905–13.

56. Yeung JC, Machuca TN, Chaparro C, et al. Lung transplantation for cystic fibrosis. J Hear Lung Transplant 2020;39(6):553–60.

57. Cypel M, Waddell T, Singer LG, et al. Bilateral pneumonectomy to treat uncontrolled sepsis in a patient awaiting lung transplantation. J Thorac Cardiovasc Surg 2017;153(4):e67–9.

58. Kukreja J, Tsou S, Chen J, et al. risk factors and outcomes of extracorporeal membrane oxygenation as a bridge to lung transplantation. Semin Thorac Cardiovasc Surg 2020;32(4):772–85.

59. Fuehner T, Kuehn C, Hadem J, et al. Extracorporeal membrane oxygenation in awake patients as bridge to lung transplantation. Am J Respir Crit Care Med 2012;185(7):763–8.

60. Lang G, Kim D, Aigner C, et al. Awake extracorporeal membrane oxygenation bridging for pulmonary retransplantation provides comparable results to elective retransplantation. J Hear Lung Transplant 2014;33(12):1264–72.

61. Schechter MA, Ganapathi AM, Englum BR, et al. spontaneously breathing extracorporeal membrane oxygenation support provides the optimal bridge to lung transplantation. Transplantation 2016;00(00):1.

62. Abrams D, Madahar P, Eckhardt CM, et al. Early mobilization during extracorporeal membrane oxygenation for cardiopulmonary failure in adults: factors associated with intensity of treatment. Ann Am Thorac Soc 2022;19(1):90–8.

63. Schmidt F, Jack T, Sasse M, et al. Back to the roots? dual cannulation strategy for ambulatory ECMO in adolescent lung transplant candidates: an alternative? Pediatr Transplant 2017;21(4):e12907.

64. Wells CL, Forrester J, Vogel J, Rector R, Tabatabai A, Herr D. Safety and feasibility of early physical therapy for patients on extracorporeal membrane oxygenator: university of maryland medical center experience. Crit Care Med 2018;46(1):53–9.

65. Shudo Y, Kasinpila P, Lee AM, Rao VK, Woo YJ. Ambulating femoral venoarterial extracorporeal membrane oxygenation bridge to heart-lung transplant. J Thorac Cardiovasc Surg 2018;156(3):e135–7.

66. Pasrija C, Mackowick KM, Raithel M, et al. ambulation with femoral arterial cannulation can be safely performed on venoarterial extracorporeal membrane oxygenation. Ann Thorac Surg 2019;107(5):1389–94.

67. Thomas J, Kostousov V, Teruya J. Bleeding and thrombotic complications in the use of extracorporeal membrane oxygenation. Semin Thromb Hemost 2018;44(01):020–9.

68. Kurihara C, Walter JM, Karim A, et al. Feasibility of venovenous extracorporeal membrane oxygenation

without systemic anticoagulation. Ann Thorac Surg 2020;110(4):1209–15.

69. Wood KL, Ayers B, Gosev I, et al. venoarterial-extracorporeal membrane oxygenation without routine systemic anticoagulation decreases adverse events. Ann Thorac Surg 2020;109(5):1458–66.

70. Abrams D, Javidfar J, Farrand E, et al. Early mobilization of patients receiving extracorporeal membrane oxygenation: a retrospective cohort study. Crit Care 2014;18(1):R38.

71. Langer T, Vecchi V, Belenkiy SM, et al. Extracorporeal gas exchange and spontaneous breathing for the treatment of acute respiratory distress syndrome: an alternative to mechanical ventilation? Crit Care Med 2014;42(3).

72. DiChiacchio L, Boulos FM, Brigante F, et al. Early tracheostomy after initiation of venovenous extracorporeal membrane oxygenation is associated with decreased duration of extracorporeal membrane oxygenation support. Perfusion 2020;35(6):509–14.

73. Swol J, Strauch JT, Schildhauer TA. Tracheostomy as a bridge to spontaneous breathing and awake-ECMO in non-transplant surgical patients. Eur J Heart Fail 2017;19:120–3.

74. Salna M, Tipograf Y, Liou P, et al. Tracheostomy is safe during extracorporeal membrane oxygenation support. ASAIO J 2020;66(6):652–6.

75. Schaenman JM, Diamond JM, Greenland JR, et al. Frailty and aging-associated syndromes in lung transplant candidates and recipients. Am J Transplant 2021;21(6):2018–24.

76. Fried LP, Tangen CM, Walston J, et al. Frailty in older adults: evidence for a phenotype. J Gerontol A Biol Sci Med Sci 2001;56(3):M146–57.

77. Singer JP, Diamond JM, Anderson MR, et al. Frailty phenotypes and mortality after lung transplantation: a prospective cohort study. Am J Transplant 2018; 18(8):1995–2004.

78. Mitnitski A, Rockwood K. Aging as a process of deficit accumulation: Its utility and origin. Interdiscip Top Gerontol 2014;40:85–98.

79. van Kan GA, Rolland YM, Morley JE, Vellas B. Frailty: toward a clinical definition. J Am Med Dir Assoc 2008;9(2):71–2.

80. De Biasio JC, Mittel AM, Mueller AL, Ferrante LE, Kim DH, Shaefi S. Frailty in critical care medicine: a review. Anesth Analg 2020;130(6):1462–73.

81. Singer JP, Diamond JM, Gries CJ, et al. Frailty phenotypes, disability, and outcomes in adult candidates for lung transplantation. Am J Respir Crit Care Med 2015;192(11):1325–34.

82. Guenthart BA, Krishnan A, Alassar A, et al. First lung and kidney multi-organ transplant following COVID-19 infection. J Heart Lung Transplant 2021;40(8): 856–9.

83. COVID patient's heart-lung transplant is world's first. Available at. https://news.vumc.org/2020/10/08/covid-patients-heart-lung-transplant-is-worlds-first/.

84. Wentlandt K, Weiss A, O'Connor E, Kaya E. Palliative and end of life care in solid organ transplantation. Am J Transplant 2017;17(12):3008–19.

Lung Transplantation for Acute Respiratory Distress Syndrome

Ankit Bharat, MD[a],*, Konrad Hoetzenecker, MD[b]

KEYWORDS

- Acute respiratory distress syndrome • Lung transplantation • Acute lung injury • Lung failure

KEY POINTS

- Despite optimized medical treatment, the mortality in patients with severe acute respiratory distress syndrome (ARDS) remains high
- Lung transplant is a life-saving treatment in carefully selected patients with ARDS
- Despite the complex medical course before transplantation, posttransplant survival in patients with ARDS is excellent

INTRODUCTION

The World Health Organization reports that respiratory illnesses are one of the top 5 causes of global deaths). For example, influenza alone causes 40 to 60 million new infections each year in the United States alone with 40 to 60,000 deaths; a large majority due to the development of lung injury and the acute respiratory distress syndrome (ARDS). Both infectious and noninfectious etiologies cause ARDS. While the global population-based estimate of the incidence of ARDS is mere approximations, it can vary from about 3.65 to 86.0 cases per 100,000 person-years.[1,2] The incidence in the United States is one of the highest, ranging from 64.2 to 86.0 cases/100,000 person-years or about 200,000 cases annually.[3] It is estimated that about 10% to 15% of patients admitted to the intensive care unit (ICU) and up to 23% of mechanically ventilated patients meet the definition of ARDS.[4–7] In an international study of nearly 30,000 ICU patients, 10% of admissions to the ICU were due to ARDS.[8] Accordingly to the Berlin definition, ARDS is classified as mild, moderate, or severe, based on the ratio of arterial partial pressure of oxygen (Pa$_{O2}$) and fraction of inspired oxygen (Fi$_{O2}$) of

300, 200, and 100 mm.[9] Only about 25% of ARDS cases are initially classified as mild while 75% are moderate to severe. A third of the mild cases go on to progress to moderate or severe disease. The mortality associated with mild, moderate, and severe disease is 27%, 32%, and 45%, respectively, with a pooled mortality of about 43%.[10,11] Hence, the burden of disease from ARDS is tremendous.

Pathophysiology of Acute Respiratory Distress Syndrome Resulting in End-stage Lung Disease

ARDS represents a common terminal pathway of lung injury that spans highly variable phases in response to a variety of etiologies. It starts with alveolar-capillary damage leading to a proliferative phase, usually associated with lung healing and improvement in pulmonary function, and ultimately resulting in a fibrotic phase, which marks the end of the acute injury. The key histologic changes include alveolar edema, endothelial and epithelial injury, and leakage of proteinaceous fluid and blood into the alveolar space. Patients with ARDS are susceptible to nosocomial infections, multiorgan dysfunction, and baro- or volutrauma, which along with their underlying health

a Division of Thoracic Surgery, Northwestern University Feinberg School of Medicine, Chicago, USA;
b Department of Thoracic Surgery, Medical University of Vienna, Vienna, Austria
* Corresponding author.
E-mail address: abharat@nm.org
Twitter: @AnkitbharatMD (A.B.); @khoetzenecker (K.H.)

Thorac Surg Clin 32 (2022) 135–142
https://doi.org/10.1016/j.thorsurg.2022.01.005

status and comorbidities can influence the outcomes, which range from spontaneous recovery to severe lung parenchymal necrosis, bronchiectasis, or fibroproliferation. With advances in ICU care, the mortality in patients with severe ARDS has decreased but still remains substantial.[12] Death early in the course of severe ARDS is related to complications such as pneumonia, sepsis, and multiorgan dysfunction. However, in those who survive the early infectious complications, the development of fibroproliferation can predispose to nosocomial complications with the inability to wean the mechanical life support, ultimately leading to the redirection of care to comfort measures in a large proportion of patients.[13]

Studies indicate that substantial fibroproliferation resulting in insufficient pulmonary function is common in patients with ARDS.[14–16] Evidence of extensive collagen deposition has been described as early as the first 72 hours following the onset of ARDS[17,18] and presence of collagen products, such as procollagen peptide III, correlate with fatal outcomes.[19] The release of profibrotic chemicals such as TGF-β_1 and insulin-like growth factor-I have been shown to be released and proposed to contribute to the fibroproliferative response in patients with ARDS.[20] Clinically evident fibroproliferation is common even with the low tidal volume ventilation.[21] Pulmonary fibrosis is characterized by aberrant and disorganized collagen deposition in the lung parenchyma, particularly affecting the alveolar spaces, similar to that observed in some chronic end-stage lung diseases.

We recently compared the three-dimensional matrix organization of normal human lungs with those obtained from either patients with severe COVID-19 ARDS or those with end-stage idiopathic pulmonary fibrosis necessitating transplantation. While normal human lungs showed a well-formed intricate matrix, those obtained from COVID-19 ARDS showed a complete absence of matrix organization with punctate islands of cells surrounding fibrotic airway regions. This pattern was similar to that observed in lungs from patients with end-stage idiopathic pulmonary fibrosis.[22,23] Transcriptional atlases created using single-cell RNA-sequencing (RNA-Seq)[24–27] have identified unique cell populations in the fibrotic lung that could be causally implicated in the development of fibrosis.[28–31] Using a transfer learning approach[32] to compare single-cell RNA-Seq data from lung tissue of patients with end-stage pulmonary fibrosis[26] and COVID-19 ARDS, we found striking homology between the 2 across many cell populations. We additionally found that a population of cells, expressing TP63, KRT5, KRT17, LAMB3, LAMC2, VIM, CHD2, FN1, COL1A1, TNC, HMGA2, and

several senescence markers (CDKN1A, CDKN2A, CCND1, CCND2, MDM2, SERPINE1), accumulate during fibrosis, potentially contributing to disease pathogenesis through the expression of TGFB1, ITGAV and ITGB6.[26,27] In the normal lung, expression of KRT17 is restricted to basal, club, and ciliated cells in the proximal airways but they are absent in distal airways.[24,26] In contrast to the normal lungs, these cells were readily observed in patients with end-stage COVID-19 and pulmonary fibrosis in distal airways. Furthermore, direct comparison of differential gene expression in KRT17+ cells between patients with pulmonary fibrosis and COVID-19 did not identify genes uniquely present in one condition, further highlighting similarities between these conditions. Additionally, comparison of differential gene expression in macrophages between patients with pulmonary fibrosis and COVID-19 ARDS also demonstrated considerable similarities between these 2 conditions. Our analysis also identified a small group of cells observed in patients with COVID-19 ARDS characterized by either expression of genes involved in calcium (AK5, SIGLEC15, CKB, and SLC9B2), iron (SLC40A1, CD163), and lipid (MERTK, PLTP, ABCA1) metabolism, as well as motility and immune signaling (MARCKS, TLR2, CCL20), likely reflecting superinfection and ongoing inflammation in patients with ARDS.[22,23] Profibrotic macrophages stimulate fibroblasts by forming self-sustaining circuits promoted by the autogenous release of growth factors.[33,34] Our data indicated that fibroblasts from patients with pulmonary fibrosis and those from patients with severe COVID-19 were largely similar. Collectively, these data suggest that some patients with COVID-19 ARDS develop end-stage lung disease, which is similar to other conditions such as pulmonary fibrosis.

Unfortunately, no medical or pharmacologic therapies targeting fibroproliferation have been effective. Steroids have also failed to show improvement in outcomes in patients with ARDS-associated fibroproliferation.[35] Other agents such as tyrosine kinase inhibitors,[36] compounds that target extracellular matrix proteins,[37] and TGF-β directed therapies[38] are in the exploratory phase and their role in preventing fibroproliferation remains unknown. As such, lung transplantation is the only possible solution for selected patients with ARDS who develop end-stage pulmonary fibrosis.

Clinical Considerations for Lung Transplantation

The medical debate about the use of lung transplantation for patients with ARDS is centered around the topics of "benefit" and "candidacy." Concerns include the potential for recurrence of the inciting infections in the allograft, technical challenges imposed by the acute injury to the native lung, and potential risk for allograft infection by pathogens associated with ventilator-associated pneumonia in the native lung. More importantly, the native lung might recover, resulting in long-term outcomes preferable to transplant. We believe that the following 2 broad criteria could be considered to determine the need for transplantation in patients with ARDS. First, the lung damage is sufficient to prevent weaning from the mechanical life support, both the mechanical ventilator and/or extracorporeal membrane oxygenation (ECMO) support, after sufficient time from the onset of ARDS has elapsed and optimized medical treatment has been administered. Second, there is a development of pulmonary or pleural complications which are refractory to medical treatment. Some common scenarios associated with these criteria include the development of fibroproliferative ARDS, lung necrosis with cavitation or pneumatoceles, or severe bronchiectasis. How to accurately identify patients who would not recover spontaneously and benefit from lung transplantation remains unclear. The preferred approach in our experience has been to continue to provide medical management in patients as long as lung recovery is deemed possible as patients have been reported to spontaneously recover after an extended duration of extracorporeal life support (ECLS).[22,23] Lung transplant should be considered when sufficient time has elapsed as the onset of ARDS and lung recovery is deemed unlikely. Consideration of lung transplantation too early in the course could result in the deviation of the care pathway away from spontaneous recovery, reducing its likelihood. While the duration of time necessary to determine irreversibility is unclear at this time, we suggest that at least 4 to 6 weeks be allowed following the onset of ARDS before considering lung transplantation. However, exception could be made when severe pulmonary complications such as pulmonary hypertension with concomitant right ventricular failure, refractory nosocomial pneumonia, or recurrent pneumothoraces, develop that cannot be medically managed with or without ECMO. For COVID-19-associated ARDS, following the stipulated time, we have found the following indicators to be helpful in the medical decision-making for lung transplant consideration: (1) development of pulmonary sequelae as described above, (2) presence of lung necrosis with cavitation especially if associated with sepsis, (3) presence of significant pulmonary hypertension, (4)

lung compliance less than 20 mL/cm H2O, and (5) evidence of diffuse pulmonary fibrosis. Transplantation should be deferred in patients who show signs of lung recovery, as suggested by improvement in lung compliance, chest radiographs, and gas exchange. We have previously proposed an approach to transplant consideration for patients with severe COVID-19-associated ARDS.[22,39] Given the similarities between COVID-19 and non–COVID-19 ARDS, we believe that the same principles can be used for all patients with ARDS.

Review of Available Literature and Reported Outcome of Lung Transplantation for Acute Respiratory Distress Syndrome

While posttransplant outcomes for chronic lung diseases are established, the benefit of lung transplantation for ARDS is still emerging.[40] Patients with severe ARDS are critically ill and develop considerable ICU-related comorbidities by the time lung recovery is deemed unlikely and transplant is considered. The medical course of severe ARDS is also often complicated by pulmonary complications such as pneumothorax, hemothorax, empyema, lung necrosis, and nosocomial pneumonia.[41] Hence, there are concerns related to the technical feasibility of lung transplantation in these patients, potentially inferior posttransplant outcomes due to frailty, and recurrence of nosocomial pathogens following transplantation. Besides a handful of case reports, 3 larger case series on lung transplantation for ARDS have been published to date (**Table 1**). The first series reported the experience of this practice in a cohort of Korean patients. A total of 14 patients were evaluated and 9 ultimately received a transplantation between 2008 and 2013.[40] Importantly, 3 of the transplants were in fact combined heart–lung transplantation due to left ventricular failure, right-sided heart insufficiency, or severe pulmonary hypertension. In 2021, Harano and colleagues performed a retrospective UNOS registry analysis. This represents the largest case series to date, including 65 patients listed for lung transplantation between 2005 and 2018.[42] Sixty-one percent (n = 39) reached transplantation. The remaining patients were delisted either due to further deterioration or because their native lungs ultimately recovered. Recently, Frick and colleagues presented a combined report from 3 European high-volume lung transplant centers (Vienna-Austria; Leuven- Belgium; Groningen-Netherlands).[43] Between 1998 and 2018, 13 patients were transplanted for ARDS. While all published patient series included patients with

Table 1
Studies reporting lung transplantation for ARDS

Authors	Chang et al. (Korean Single-Center)	Harano et al. (UNOS Database)	Frick et al. (European Multi-Center)
Inclusion period	October 2008–October 2013	May 2005–December 2018	August 1998–May 2020
Pts transplanted/ listed (N)	9/14	39/63	13/-[a]
Cause of ARDS (N)	Disinfectant inhalation (4) Pneumonia (4) Near drowning (1)	n/a	Viral (7) Bacterial (5) Postoperative (1)
Median recipient age	39	35	29
Median duration of MV (days)[b]	11	n/a	33
Median hospital stay (days)	56	33	54
In-hospital mortality	11.1%	10.3%	7.7%
1-y survival	78%	82.1%	71.6%
3-y survival	78%	69.2%	n/a
5-y survival	n/a	n/a	54.2%

n/a; not available.
[a] Not reported.
[b] MV; mechanical ventilation.

severe ARDS, the underlying cause of ARDS largely differed between the published cohorts. In the Korean study, half of the patients developed lung failure due to the inhalation of humidifier disinfectant (n = 7) while the second most frequent cause was pneumonia (n = 5). In the European series, viral (n = 7) and bacterial (n = 5) infections were the predominant causes of ARDS.[43] The UNOS database study could not provide detailed data on ARDS cause.

There is general agreement that lung transplantation for ARDS is complex and the intra- and postoperative management is challenging. Thus, an outcome similar to other indications (ILD, CF, COPD) may not be expected. In fact, the data from the 3 above-mentioned cohort studies confirmed this assumption. All 3 series report prolonged mechanical ventilation after lung transplantation with a median length of mechanical ventilation (LMV) of 11 to 33 days[40,43] and a prolonged hospital stay with a median of 33 to 56 days (see **Table 1**).[40,42,43] However, these results are comparable to other complex patient groups, especially those with acute on chronic lung disease who require ECLS bridging to lung transplant.[44–48] Long-term survival following lung transplantation for ARDS was also lower compared with contemporary benchmarks. The Korean group reported 1- and 3-year survival rates

of 78%. One patient out of 9 (11.1%) died in the immediate postoperative course.[40] The UNOS series by Harano and colleagues reported survival rates of 82.1% at one, and 69.2% at 3 years, respectively. The authors also provided a propensity-score matched analysis comparing patients with ARDS with a control group of 79 patients with restrictive lung disease. A 2:1 matching included lung allocation score, sex, age, and transplant type ensuring a control group of equal complexity. The propensity-matched cohort showed similar long-term outcomes to the ARDS cohort with a 1-year survival of 85.9% and a 3-year survival of 65.4%. A further comparison of bridged versus nonbridged patients regardless of ARDS/non-ARDS diagnosis also showed no significant difference.[42] In the European series reported by Frick and colleagues, one out of 13 patients died early postoperatively, resulting in an in-hospital mortality rate of 7.7%. Survival rates were 71.6% at 1 year and 54.2% at 5 years. As these studies included patients going back as far as 1993, the possibility of an era effect on outcomes should be considered, especially as the European group reported improved outcomes for patients with ARDS transplanted after 2016.[43] Nevertheless, patients bridged with ECMO to transplant reach comparable survival rates of 76% to 88% at 1 year, 61% to 83% at 3 years and 55% to

68% at 5 years.[44–50] Indeed, our recent study from an international cohort of patients with COVID-19 ARDS supports that lung transplantation may be a viable life-saving treatment option for severe COVID-19-associated ARDS even those being supported on ECMO. Collectively, currently available evidence leads to the conclusion that carefully selected patients with ARDS can achieve lung transplantation outcomes comparable to other patients in similarly severe condition.

Lung Transplantation Workup

It is self-evident that in the acute setting of an ARDS, some routine examinations performed to determine lung transplant candidacy have to be waived. For instance, as most of the patients with ARDS who are considered for transplantation are young, the likelihood of an undetected malignancy or significant cardiovascular comorbidity is low. We suggest the following examinations are important:

- a computed tomography (CT) scan of the chest and abdomen
- virology (Ebstein–Barr virus, Cytomegalovirus, Hepatitis A/B, Human immunodeficiency virus)
- panel reactive antibody (PRA) test and unacceptable HLA antigens in case of presensitized patients
- an ultrasound examination of the peripheral vessels to evaluate for venous thrombosis
- in case of nonawake bridging a CT scan of the brain to exclude major bleeding/ischemia (though we acknowledge this may be a relative contraindication for some centers)
- echocardiography
- in patients aged greater than 50 years, CT coronary angiogram or left heart catheterization
- ultrasound of the liver/fibroscan
- no mammography, no coronary angiography, no colonoscopy, no gastroscopy

Bridging a Patient with Acute Respiratory Distress Syndrome While Awake or Sedated

Bridging patients awake has become an increasingly used practice in lung transplantation. In some centers, an awake patient is even considered a prerequisite for transplantation. In our opinion, there are mainly 2 reasons for this: (1) several studies have shown that the outcome of patients who can be bridged awake is significantly better compared with patients who are bridged sedated to.[45,51,52] (2) The decision for lung transplantation is of such importance that a first-person consent is considered necessary.

In our opinion, both arguments are only valid for patients suffering from chronic lung disease who require ECLS bridging—in ARDS they may not apply. Waking up patients with ARDS is often impossible, as unlike fibrosis patients who require ECLS bridging, patients with ARDS are usually severely sick.[43] Their lung compliance is extremely poor with tidal volumes less than 100 mL. These unique challenges often result in severe stress and episodes of desaturation.

Our perspective is that given the severity of the disease and the lack of alternative therapies in transplant candidates a personal consent can be waived in many European countries. This requires the consent of a health care proxy or adult representative. However, in cases whereby the implementation of such a representative (designated by a court) takes too long, the presumed will of the sedated patient has to be followed and a next-of-kin consent for transplantation is acceptable—under the assumption that the patient wants medically indicated treatment to save his/her life. When considering lung transplantation in patients with ARDS, the "right timing" is essential. Once the irreversibility of lung damage is confirmed, we recommend no attempts at weaning sedation to obtain personal consent. In critically ill patients, a longer ECLS time directly translates into higher complication rates, threating the success of a transplantation.[53] This "window of opportunity" has to be considered when discussing the optimal time for listing patients with ARDS.

Considerations for Delisting in Case of Deterioration

As published evidence is limited to a few case reports and only 3 small case series, no clear recommendation can be given about when and under what conditions to delist a deteriorating patient. Ideally, ARDS transplant candidates should be in a stable condition with a single-system organ failure. However, dysfunction of other organs is frequently seen. A temporary kidney failure in a patient with a previous normal kidney function is generally not considered a contraindication for lung transplantation in our centers. Therefore, patients who require kidney replacement therapy during their wait time should not be delisted. However, cholestatic liver dysfunction can pose a significant challenge. Secondary sclerosing cholangitis (SCC) is a dreadful complication in patients requiring prolonged ECLS for ARDS.[54,55] As therapeutic options in patients who develop SSC are limited and mortality is extremely high, we consider rising cholestasis parameters a contraindication to lung transplantation in patients with

ARDS. The other 2 major contra-indications for ARDS lung transplantation are the development of uncontrolled diffuse bleeding during ECLS or a septic shock. However, if the reason for the septic shock is clearly the lung and the patient fails to stabilize, a bilateral pneumonectomy with a central Novalung/VA ECMO bridging concept can be considered.[56]

SUMMARY

Although the number of transplants for ARDS remains low compared with other indications, lung transplantation has become an established treatment of the subgroup of patients who do not recover. However, sufficient time on ECLS has to be given to determine the regenerative potential of the native lung. Patient selection is crucial and transplantation should be reserved for those without a prospect of recovery. This usually limits the option of lung transplantation to those who were relatively healthy before the onset of ARDS. Good long-term results have been described after lung transplant in the carefully selected cohort of patients with ARDS.

CLINICS CARE POINTS

- Mortality in patients with severe acute respiratory distress syndrome (ARDS) remains high
- A significant proportion of patients with severe ARDS develops irrecoverable lung damage and remains unweanable from mechanical life support
- Life transplantation may be a life-saving treatment in some of the patients that develop irrecoverable lung damage from severe ARDS

DISCLOSURE

AB was supported by the National Institutes of Health (NIH HL145478, HL147290, and HL147575).

REFERENCES

1. Pham T, Rubenfeld GD. Fifty Years of Research in ARDS. The Epidemiology of Acute Respiratory Distress Syndrome. A 50th Birthday Review. Am J Respir Crit Care Med 2017;195(7):860–70.

2. Rubenfeld GD, Caldwell E, Peabody E, et al. Incidence and outcomes of acute lung injury. N Engl J Med 2005;353(16):1685–93.

3. Diamond M, Peniston Feliciano HL, Sanghavi D, et al. Acute Respiratory Distress Syndrome. StatPearls, Treasure Island: FL); 2021.

4. Frutos-Vivar F, Nin N, Esteban A. Epidemiology of acute lung injury and acute respiratory distress syndrome. Curr Opin Crit Care 2004;10(1):1–6.

5. Estenssoro E, Dubin A, Laffaire E, et al. Incidence, clinical course, and outcome in 217 patients with acute respiratory distress syndrome. Crit Care Med 2002;30(11):2450–6.

6. Esteban A, Anzueto A, Frutos F, et al. Mechanical Ventilation International Study, G., Characteristics and outcomes in adult patients receiving mechanical ventilation: a 28-day international study. JAMA 2002;287(3):345–55.

7. Zaccardelli DS, Pattishall EN. Clinical diagnostic criteria of the adult respiratory distress syndrome in the intensive care unit. Crit Care Med 1996; 24(2):247–51.

8. Bellani G, Laffey JG, Pham T, et al. Epidemiology, Patterns of Care, and Mortality for Patients With Acute Respiratory Distress Syndrome in Intensive Care Units in 50 Countries. JAMA 2016;315(8): 788–800.

9. Force ADT, Ranieri VM, Rubenfeld GD, et al. Acute respiratory distress syndrome: the Berlin Definition. JAMA 2012;307(23):2526–33.

10. Sedhai YR, Yuan M, Ketcham SW, et al. Validating Measures of Disease Severity in Acute Respiratory Distress Syndrome. Ann Am Thorac Soc 2021; 18(7):1211–8.

11. Zambon M, Vincent JL. Mortality rates for patients with acute lung injury/ARDS have decreased over time. Chest 2008;133(5):1120–7.

12. Burnham EL, Janssen WJ, Riches DW, et al. The fibroproliferative response in acute respiratory distress syndrome: mechanisms and clinical significance. Eur Respir J 2014;43(1):276–85.

13. Ketcham SW, Sedhai YR, Miller HC, et al. Causes and characteristics of death in patients with acute hypoxemic respiratory failure and acute respiratory distress syndrome: a retrospective cohort study. Crit Care 2020;24(1):391.

14. Bulpa PA, Dive AM, Mertens L, et al. Combined bronchoalveolar lavage and transbronchial lung biopsy: safety and yield in ventilated patients. Eur Respir J 2003;21(3):489–94.

15. Patel SR, Karmpaliotis D, Ayas NT, et al. The role of open-lung biopsy in ARDS. Chest 2004;125(1): 197–202.

16. Papazian L, Doddoli C, Chetaille B, et al. A contributive result of open-lung biopsy improves survival in acute respiratory distress syndrome patients. Crit Care Med 2007;35(3):755–62.

17. Farjanel J, Hartmann DJ, Guidet B, et al. Four markers of collagen metabolism as possible indicators of disease in the adult respiratory distress syndrome. Am Rev Respir Dis 1993;147(5):1091–9.

18. Meduri GU, Tolley EA, Chinn A, et al. Procollagen types I and III aminoterminal propeptide levels during acute respiratory distress syndrome and in response to methylprednisolone treatment. Am J Respir Crit Care Med 1998;158(5 Pt 1):1432–41.

19. Clark JG, Milberg JA, Steinberg KP, et al. Type III procollagen peptide in the adult respiratory distress syndrome. Association of increased peptide levels in bronchoalveolar lavage fluid with increased risk for death. Ann Intern Med 1995;122(1):17–23.

20. Krein PM, Sabatini PJ, Tinmouth W, et al. Localization of insulin-like growth factor-I in lung tissues of patients with fibroproliferative acute respiratory distress syndrome. Am J Respir Crit Care Med 2003;167(1):83–90.

21. Marshall RP, Bellingan G, Webb S, et al. Fibroproliferation occurs early in the acute respiratory distress syndrome and impacts on outcome. Am J Respir Crit Care Med 2000;162(5):1783–8.

22. Bharat A, Machuca TN, Querrey M, et al. Early outcomes after lung transplantation for severe COVID-19: a series of the first consecutive cases from four countries. Lancet Respir Med 2021;9(5):487–97.

23. Bharat A, Querrey M, Markov NS, et al. Lung transplantation for patients with severe COVID-19. Sci Transl Med 2020;12(574).

24. Reyfman PA, Walter JM, Joshi N, et al. Single-Cell Transcriptomic Analysis of Human Lung Provides Insights into the Pathobiology of Pulmonary Fibrosis. Am J Respir Crit Care Med 2019;199(12):1517–36.

25. Valenzi E, Bulik M, Tabib T, et al. Single-cell analysis reveals fibroblast heterogeneity and myofibroblasts in systemic sclerosis-associated interstitial lung disease. Ann Rheum Dis 2019;78(10):1379–87.

26. Habermann AC, Gutierrez AJ, Bui LT, et al. Single-cell RNA sequencing reveals profibrotic roles of distinct epithelial and mesenchymal lineages in pulmonary fibrosis. Sci Adv 2020;6(28):eaba1972.

27. Adams TS, Schupp JC, Poli S, et al. Single-cell RNA-seq reveals ectopic and aberrant lung-resident cell populations in idiopathic pulmonary fibrosis. Sci Adv 2020;6(28):eaba1983.

28. Strunz M, Simon LM, Ansari M, et al. Alveolar regeneration through a Krt8+ transitional stem cell state that persists in human lung fibrosis. Nat Commun 2020;11(1):3559.

29. Kobayashi Y, Tata A, Konkimalla A, et al. Persistence of a regeneration-associated, transitional alveolar epithelial cell state in pulmonary fibrosis. Nat Cell Biol 2020;22(8):934–46.

30. Jiang P, Gil de Rubio R, Hrycaj SM, et al. Ineffectual Type 2-to-Type 1 Alveolar Epithelial Cell Differentiation in Idiopathic Pulmonary Fibrosis: Persistence of the KRT8(hi) Transitional State. Am J Respir Crit Care Med 2020;201(11):1443–7.

31. Wu H, Yu Y, Huang H, et al. Progressive Pulmonary Fibrosis Is Caused by Elevated Mechanical Tension on Alveolar Stem Cells. Cell 2020;180(1):107–21.e17.

32. Lotfollahi M, Naghipourfar M, Luecken MD, et al. Query to reference single-cell integration with transfer learning. bioRxiv 2020;2020.

33. Joshi N, Watanabe S, Verma R, et al. A spatially restricted fibrotic niche in pulmonary fibrosis is sustained by M-CSF/M-CSFR signalling in monocyte-derived alveolar macrophages. Eur Respir J 2020;55(1).

34. Zhou X, Franklin RA, Adler M, et al. Circuit Design Features of a Stable Two-Cell System. Cell 2018;172(4):744–57.e17.

35. Steinberg KP, Hudson LD, Goodman RB, et al. Blood Institute Acute Respiratory Distress Syndrome Clinical Trials, N., Efficacy and safety of corticosteroids for persistent acute respiratory distress syndrome. N Engl J Med 2006;354(16):1671–84.

36. Beyer C, Distler JH. Tyrosine kinase signaling in fibrotic disorders: Translation of basic research to human disease. Biochim Biophys Acta 2013;1832(7):897–904.

37. Yamaguchi Y, Takihara T, Chambers RA, et al. A peptide derived from endostatin ameliorates organ fibrosis. Sci Transl Med 2012;4(136):136ra71.

38. Wrighton KH, Lin X, Feng XH. Phospho-control of TGF-beta superfamily signaling. Cell Res 2009;19(1):8–20.

39. Machuca TN, Cypel M, Bharat A. Comment on Let's Build Bridges to Recovery in COVID-19 ARDS, not Burn Them! Ann Surg 2020;274(6):e870–1.

40. Chang Y, Lee SO, Shim TS, et al. Lung Transplantation as a Therapeutic Option in Acute Respiratory Distress Syndrome. Transplantation 2018;102(5):829–37.

41. Botta M, Tsonas AM, Pillay J, et al. Ventilation management and clinical outcomes in invasively ventilated patients with COVID-19 (PRoVENT-COVID): a national, multicentre, observational cohort study. Lancet Respir Med 2020;9(2):139–48.

42. Harano T, Ryan JP, Chan EG, et al. Lung transplantation for the treatment of irreversible acute respiratory distress syndrome. Clin Transplant 2021;35(2):e14182.

43. Frick AE, Gan CT, Vos R, et al. Lung transplantation for acute respiratory distress syndrome: A multicenter experience. Am J Transplant 2021;22(1):144–53.

44. Abdelnour-Berchtold E, Federici S, Wurlod DA, et al. Outcome after extracorporeal membrane oxygenation-bridged lung retransplants: a single-centre experience. Interact Cardiovasc Thorac Surg 2019;28(6):922–8.

45. Benazzo A, Schwarz S, Frommlet F, et al. Twenty-year experience with extracorporeal life support as bridge to lung transplantation. J Thorac Cardiovasc Surg 2019;157(6):2515–2525 e10.

46. Hoetzenecker K, Donahoe L, Yeung JC, et al. Extra-corporeal life support as a bridge to lung transplantation-experience of a high-volume transplant center. J Thorac Cardiovasc Surg 2018; 155(3):1316–1328 e1.

47. Ius F, Natanov R, Salman J, et al. Extracorporeal membrane oxygenation as a bridge to lung transplantation may not impact overall mortality risk after transplantation: results from a 7-year single-centre experience. Eur J Cardiothorac Surg 2018;54(2): 334–40.

48. Langer F, Aliyev P, Schafers HJ, et al. Improving Outcomes in Bridge-to-Transplant: Extended Extracorporeal Membrane Oxygenation Support to Obtain Optimal Donor Lungs for Marginal Recipients. ASAIO J 2019;65(5):516–21.

49. Hayanga JWA, Hayanga HK, Holmes SD, et al. Mechanical ventilation and extracorporeal membrane oxygenation as a bridge to lung transplantation: Closing the gap. J Heart Lung Transplant 2019; 38(10):1104–11.

50. Tipograf Y, Salna M, Minko E, et al. Outcomes of Extracorporeal Membrane Oxygenation as a Bridge to Lung Transplantation. Ann Thorac Surg 2019; 107(5):1456–63.

51. Biscotti M, Gannon WD, Agerstrand C, et al. Awake Extracorporeal Membrane Oxygenation as Bridge to Lung Transplantation: A 9-Year Experience. Ann Thorac Surg 2017;104(2):412–9.

52. Fuehner T, Kuehn C, Hadem J, et al. Extracorporeal membrane oxygenation in awake patients as bridge to lung transplantation. Am J Respir Crit Care Med 2012;185(7):763–8.

53. Oh DK, Hong SB, Shim TS, et al. Effects of the duration of bridge to lung transplantation with extracorporeal membrane oxygenation. PLoS One 2021; 16(7):e0253520.

54. Patel KV, Zaman S, Chang F, et al. Rare case of severe cholangiopathy following critical illness. BMJ Case Rep 2014;2014.

55. Tunney R, Scott J, Rudralingam V, et al. Secondary sclerosing cholangitis following extracorporeal membrane oxygenation for acute respiratory distress in polytrauma. Clin Case Rep 2018;6(9): 1849–53.

56. Cypel M, Waddell T, Singer LG, et al. Bilateral pneumonectomy to treat uncontrolled sepsis in a patient awaiting lung transplantation. J Thorac Cardiovasc Surg 2017;153(4):e67–9.

Management of the Potential Lung Donor

Ashwini Arjuna, MD[a,b],*, Anna Teresa Mazzeo, MD[c], Tommaso Tonetti, MD[d,e], Rajat Walia, MD[a,b], Luciana Mascia, MD[f]

KEYWORDS

- Lung donor management • Donation after neurologic determination of death
- Donation after circulatory determination of death • Organ donation • Lung-protective ventilation
- COVID donor screening • Deceased donor evaluation for SARS-CoV-2
- Intensive care management of donor

KEY POINTS

- Potential donor lung management involves optimizing patient- and organ-related factors leading to successful graft survival.
- Optimizing marginal organ donors can expand the donor pool with successful lung transplantation.
- Donor lung management should involve protocol-based strategies for improving pulmonary and extrapulmonary physiology.
- The COVID-19 pandemic has added a new dimension to donor pool selection, screening, and management strategies.

INTRODUCTION

Lung transplantation can be a life-extending treatment for patients with end-stage respiratory failure; however, despite continuous improvement in donor management, donor organ shortages remain a major concern. Optimization and protection of organ function are pillars of intensive care medicine. This concept applies also to care of the potential organ donor; when a patient with irreversible brain injury evolves to brain death, the clinical priority shifts from cerebral protection to care of the potential organ donor. The window of opportunity to improve organ function starts at the moment of intensive care unit (ICU) admission and covers all phases of ICU care until brain death diagnosis. Among solid organs, lungs are the most difficult to maintain and therefore are retrieved in only 15% to 20% of multiorgan donors.[1] Although factors such as age or smoking history cannot be changed, other modifiable factors should be considered in a bedside management strategy, as proposed by Miñambres and colleagues.[2,3] A large proportion of transplanted lungs comes from donors after neurologic determination of death (DNDD, previously termed brain death). Long-term survival rates achieved with the use of donor organs after circulatory determination of death (DCDD) compare favorably to those with conventional DNDD donors.[4] The implementation of bundles of care is the mainstay of donor management in the ICU: DNDD donors experience peculiar pathophysiologic changes due to neurogenic pulmonary edema, and protective

[a] Norton Thoracic Institute, St. Joseph's Hospital and Medical Center, 500 West Thomas Road, Suite 500, Phoenix, AZ 85013, USA; [b] Creighton University School of Medicine–Phoenix Campus, Phoenix, AZ, USA; [c] Department of Adult and Pediatric Pathology, University of Messina, Messina, Italy; [d] University of Bologna, Bologna, Italy; [e] Department of Medical and Surgical Sciences, Anesthesia and Intensive Care Medicine, Sant'Orsola Research Hospital - Bologna, Bologna, Italy; [f] Dipartimento di Scienze Biomediche e Neuromotorie, University of Bologna, Bologna, Italy
* Corresponding author. Norton Thoracic Institute, St. Joseph's Hospital and Medical Center, 500 West Thomas Road, Suite 500, Phoenix, AZ 85013.
E-mail address: ashwini.arjuna@commonspirit.org
Twitter: @tomton87 (T.T.)

Thorac Surg Clin 32 (2022) 143–151
https://doi.org/10.1016/j.thorsurg.2021.11.005
1547-4127/22/© 2021 Elsevier Inc. All rights reserved.

mechanical ventilation is the cornerstone of managing this condition. Additional management strategies are directed at preserving organ function through meticulous and aggressive care in collaboration with the organ procurement organization and transplant teams, and include diuresis, therapeutic bronchoscopy, chest physiotherapy, aspiration prevention, lung-protective ventilation, and regular recruitment maneuvers to potentially improve oxygenation and enhance recovery (also referred to as procurement) rates in general. A new dimension being explored to expand the donor pool is the utilization of COVID-positive donors. In this section, we discuss lung donor management strategies to preserve candidacy for donation and optimize physiologic parameters before recovery.

VENTILATORY MANAGEMENT AND BLOOD GAS EXCHANGE

Recommendations about ventilatory management of the potential DNDD donor have drastically changed over the past 20 years, focusing on both avoiding ventilator-induced lung injury to preserve lung function and minimizing multiorgan dysfunction. The pathophysiology of DNDD donors involves a complex systemic derangement, mainly driven by intracranial hypertension and a massive endogenous catecholamine release with loss of autonomic vascular tone and hypotension. Consequently, brain death is characterized by cardiovascular collapse due to myocardial injury and multiorgan ischemia together with neurogenic pulmonary edema (NPE). NPE is characterized by catecholamine storm, increased pulmonary capillary permeability, and cytokine release. Indeed, NPE is similar to acute respiratory distress syndrome (ARDS) in terms of radiologic and clinical features, such as arterial hypoxemia and bilateral chest radiograph infiltrates.[5]

A *double hit* model, which has been validated by experimental and clinical data, explains the development of lung failure after devastating brain injury that evolves to brain death.[5–7] The *first hit* is a consequence of the sympathetic storm and the proinflammatory cascade triggered by brain injury. Once primed, the respiratory system is then vulnerable to further inflammatory insults caused by the mechanical stress of ventilation.[8] The deterioration of respiratory function further damages the central nervous system in a vicious circle.[7] Lungs primed by an inflammatory response elicited by brain injury can be further injured by sequential noxious stimuli. Because the first hit is related to the severity of the injury, clinical interventions are limited and unlikely to be successful.

On the other hand, appropriate ventilatory settings are likely to influence *secondary hits* that may impair distal organ function.

Indeed, traumatic brain injury has been identified as a predisposing factor for ARDS.[9] Recently, Rincon and colleagues[10] reported that this complication carried a higher risk of in-hospital death after brain injury. In a prospective observational study in patients with severe brain injury, injurious mechanical ventilation was a contributing factor to the development of ARDS, which was associated with longer ventilator dependency and longer ICU stay.[11]

In the case of severe brain injury evolving to brain death, critical care management of the potential organ donors shifts from a "cerebral protective" to an "organ protective" strategy to optimize organ donation. The lungs are responsible for maintaining systemic homeostasis: optimal oxygenation and optimal acid-base balance (pH); whereas, the heart is responsible for optimal perfusion of peripheral organs. Traditionally, clinical management of a potential organ donor was oriented to guarantee optimal oxygenation and perfusion rather than to primarily protect the cardiothoracic organs. From this perspective, the cardiothoracic organs play a 2-sided role in organ donation as they are needed to protect the peripheral organs, but both are also potential donor organs (**Fig. 1**). A sequential reevaluation of organ function during the donation process is therefore crucial to combine clinical priorities of the different organs while keeping in mind that parameters of suitability may change over time.

In a multicenter, randomized, controlled trial of potential organ donors, the use of a lung-protective strategy doubled the lung recovery rate (54% vs 27%; $P<.005$) compared with the use of a conventional ventilator protocol.[12] The protocol applied was a tidal volume of 6 to 8 mL/kg predicted body weight (PBW), 8 to 10 cm positive end-expiratory pressure (PEEP), a closed circuit for suctioning, continuous positive airway pressure equal to previous PEEP for apnea test, and recruitment maneuvers after any disconnection from the ventilator. In line with this evidence, Rech and colleagues[13] concluded that the best evidence in the management of organ donors supports protective mechanical ventilation, whereas evidence for other strategies such as hormonal replacement is weak. Similar conclusions were recently reached by Slutsky and Ranieri,[8] who recommended the use of a protective lung strategy in heart-beating organ donors.

Consequently, the most recent consensus statement on donor management[14] recommends a protective ventilatory strategy obtained by

The Two-Sided Role of Cardiothoracic Organs

Protection of peripheral organs for donation

- **Optimal perfusion**
  - Neutral fluid balance
  - Moderate catecholamine level
  - Low PEEP

- **Optimal oxygenation and pH**
  - No specific strategies

Protection of heart-lung for donation

- **Cardiac protection**
  - Optimal fluid balance
  - Low catecholamine level
  - Low PEEP

- **Lung protection**
  - Low FiO_2
  - Moderate PEEP
  - Low tidal volume
  - Negative fluid balance

Fig. 1. Cardiothoracic organs play a 2-sided role in organ donation: the lungs guarantee optimal oxygenation and acid-base balance, and the heart guarantees optimal perfusion of peripheral organs, but both are potential donor organs.

applying tidal volumes between 6 and 8 mL/kg PBW, lowering driving pressures, and optimizing PEEP between 8 and 10 cmH$_2$O with peak airway pressure less than 35 mm Hg.[2,4,14,15] Recruitment maneuvers should be performed after tracheal suctioning or any disconnection of the ventilator circuit, and circuit humidification should always be provided.[16] If the patient requires high PEEP, tracheal suctioning should be performed only to clear secretions to avoid derecruitment.[6] The endotracheal tube cuff should be inflated to a pressure high enough to prevent aspiration and the head-of-bed elevation should be 30°.[17] Pao$_2$ should be maintained between 80 and 100 mm Hg using the minimal fraction of inspired oxygen (Fio$_2$) to not only guarantee oxygen delivery but also avoid damage induced by hyperoxia in lung recipients. Normocapnia (Paco$_2$ between 35 and 45 mm Hg) should guarantee correction of acidosis. Judicious use of diuretics may be required to further reduce ventilation-perfusion mismatching and diffusion abnormalities increasing the Paco$_2$/Fio$_2$ ratio.[18] This intensive lung donor protocol is associated with an increase in lung recovery rates, without a negative impact on early survival of lung recipients or primary graft dysfunction.

In conclusion, a strong line of evidence suggests that (1) brain injury evolving to brain death is a predisposing factor for ARDS, (2) an injurious

mechanical ventilation strategy enhances the risk of ventilator-induced lung injury in vulnerable lungs of potential organ donors, and (3) a protective ventilation strategy significantly increases the number of donor lungs without affecting function of other organs. It is important to note that the available guidelines from organ procurement organizations no longer suggest the use of high tidal volume and low level of PEEP in concurrence with the strong line of evidence supporting protective mechanical ventilation in potential organ donors.[19]

FLUID MANAGEMENT

A critical point in the chain of organ recovery is the early identification of patients with devastating brain injury. Indeed, timely diagnosis and referral of potential organ donors are the keys of recovery. Autonomic dysfunction, loss of peripheral vascular tone, and release of inflammatory mediators together with altered fluid balance contribute to impairment in preload, contractility, and afterload. Identifying causative factors of hemodynamic instability is particularly important in terms of fluid management.[20]

Progressive brainstem ischemia occurs when a rise of intracranial pressure threatens cerebral perfusion, causing rapid changes in cardiovascular function, termed *autonomic storm*. Generalized inflammatory responses are expected with several effects at the pulmonary level. The intense lung-heart cross-talk after acute brain injury culminates at the moment of brain death. When cerebral perfusion ceases, profound peripheral vasodilation follows and relative hypovolemia occurs. Diabetes insipidus frequently develops as a consequence of loss of vasopressin, causing inappropriate diuresis, hypernatremia, and worsening hypovolemia. Close monitoring, early detection, and prompt treatment are imperative when these changes begin. Hypotonic polyuria, hypernatremia, serum osmolality greater than 295 mmol/kg H_2O, and urine osmolality less than 200 mmol/kg H_2O are diagnostic criteria for diabetes insipidus and, together with clinical suspicion, dictate prompt fluid replacement and missing hormone administration.

Euvolemia is therefore the primary therapeutic goal when caring for a potential organ donor, and prompt correction of hypovolemia should be the target. The recent consensus statement on donor heart and lung procurement[14] suggests that in donors with decreased preload, isotonic crystalloid solutions are the preferred choice for fluid repletion and maintenance. In those who remain hypernatremic after hypovolemia correction, dextrose-containing fluids or hypotonic solutions, such as 0.45% sodium chloride, should be used.

Potential donors at the time of DNDD may have very similar physiology to patients with ARDS.[21] Traditional hemodynamic targets such as mean arterial pressure (MAP), central venous pressure (CVP), and urine output are easily measured at the bedside. More recently, echocardiography has been introduced in critical care to assess the hemodynamic status at the bedside and can be especially helpful when myocardial stunning, NPE, or cardiac or pulmonary contusions may hamper thoracic organ donation.[14]

Transpulmonary thermodilution-derived, real-time pulse wave results, such as an increase (>10%) in cardiac output induced by a passive leg raising test or an increase (>5%) by an end-expiratory occlusion test, and respiratory measurements of continuous pulse pressure variation and stroke volume variation are the more recently introduced dynamic indices of fluid responsiveness available at the bedside and can guide clinicians to optimize fluid management to guarantee oxygen delivery while avoiding an increase in lung edema. In a small single-center study, fluid responsiveness assessed by pulse pressure variation was detected in 48% of donors, and the number of transplanted organs was higher in preload responsive donors.[22] More recently, the first large multicenter randomized (MOnIToR) trial in brain-dead donors tested the hypothesis that a "protocol-guided fluid therapy" algorithm targeting cardiac index, MAP, and pulse pressure variation would increase the number of organs transplanted. However, no significant difference was found, underscoring the need for larger studies to assess the efficacy of donor management based on fluid responsiveness.[23]

The importance of preventing lung edema while maintaining adequate systemic perfusion of peripheral organs through a tight modulation of fluid status is another critical point in the management of a potential lung donor. Restrictive versus liberal fluid strategies are a classic example of these competing interests and represent a challenge in the care of both patients with ARDS and the potential organ donor. Nevertheless, Miñambres and colleagues[24] showed that a strict fluid balance could prevent NPE and increase the number of lungs suitable for transplantation while also preserving kidney graft survival. The same research group also showed in a larger study that the use of an intensive lung donor treatment strategy does not negatively affect heart, liver, kidney, and pancreas retrieval rates.[3] The concept of meeting donor management goals[25] applies to all organs and should be pursued also for lungs; the main goals are MAP 60 to 80 mm Hg, CVP 6 to 10 mm Hg, Pao_2 80 to 100 mm Hg on the lowest Fio_2, temp 36 to 37.5 C°, urine output 0.5 to 2 mL/kg per hour, and serum Na 135 to 150 mMol/L. If vasopressors are needed, the minimum dose should be infused. A consensus on the vasopressor of choice has not been reached, but norepinephrine or phenylephrine may be preferred to treat distributive shock; vasopressin in the case of refractory shock; and dopamine, dobutamine, or epinephrine in primary cardiac pump dysfunction.[14,19] Recent studies found that meeting donor management goals was an independent predictor of more than 4 organs transplanted per donor[25] and was associated with a 90% higher chance of transplanting 3 or more organs when expanded donor criteria (older and with comorbidities) were considered.[26]

CAUSE OF DEATH AND ITS IMPLICATIONS

The acceptance rate of offered donor lungs is 15% to 20% (the lowest of all solid organs).[1] DNDD requires a clinical evaluation including the systemic and neurologic systems and documentation of the presence of coma, the absence of brain stem reflexes, and apnea testing (as performed via guidelines).[19] Ancillary testing (eg, electroencephalography, computed tomography [CT] angiography, and MRI/angiography) may be needed if clinical testing is nonconfirmatory. Trauma and cerebrovascular accident (CVA) remain the most common causes of brain death.[14] The cause of brain death is associated with specific complications of the thoracic organs, for example, NPE, cardiac and pulmonary contusions, or myocardial injury in trauma donors. A variety of systemic diseases should be considered in CVA donors, including left ventricular hypertrophy, vascular arterial disease, and hypertension. Drug-related deaths may have certain implications for cardiac contractility. Organs from DCDD donors are increasingly being used, especially after the introduction of ex vivo conditioning techniques. The most common concerns are warm ischemic injury and the ethical dilemma associated with this type of donation. Warm ischemia time is defined as the time from cardiac arrest to organ in situ perfusion and should be lower than 150 minutes.[27] Cardiopulmonary criteria for the absence of circulation must be met. Time from withdrawal of life support to death can be extended up to 90 minutes, or even further from 120 to 180 minutes in some programs, given the relative tolerance of the lungs to warm ischemia time.[28] A recent United Network of Organ Sharing study[4] did not reveal significant differences in perioperative mortality, airway dehiscence, dialysis requirement, postoperative length of stay, or overall survival between DNDD and DCDD recipients.

BRONCHOSCOPY

Bronchoscopy is a therapeutic and diagnostic tool and should be performed in all potential lung donors, including donors with normal radiographs and Pao$_2$. Early bronchoscopy during the beginning of donor lung recruitment can help document endobronchial anatomy and assess for aspirated gastric contents or blood, infection, inflammation, and purulent secretions. Bronchoalveolar lavage samples can help guide antimicrobial treatment for lower respiratory tract infections.[29] In our experience, it is important to reassess the bronchial tree if copious secretions are noted on the first inspection to help clear secretions and reduce pathogen load. The frequency of repeat inspection is informed by findings from the initial bronchoscopy and the quality of the inspection as well as changes in subsequent chest imaging or concern for a new infection. Initial bronchoscopy can guide the need for repeated suctioning, physiotherapy, revision of antibiotic therapy, or lung recruitment strategies if atelectasis is suspected.

At least one inspection of the bronchial tree is recommended before donor lung retrieval in DNDD donors.[19] The presence of airway erythema or secretions alone should not preclude organ retrieval. In DCDD donors, airway inspection before withdrawal of support is based on center-specific protocols; anecdotally, more organ procurement organizations are beginning to request bronchoscopy before organ allocation to maximize organ placement.

THORACIC RADIOGRAPHIC IMAGING

A clear chest radiograph is often listed as a prerequisite for donor lung acceptability; however, an abnormal chest radiograph alone should not preclude suitability for lung recovery.[4] A chest radiograph can help estimate total lung capacity[30] and identify vascular congestion, edema, infiltrates, and contusions while also indicating the need for dedicated imaging, such as CT, or further workup for infection, such as sampling of sputum or tracheal aspirate or bronchoscopy and lavage. Daily portable chest radiographs are the norm until plans for donor organ recovery are in place, and current practices in both the United States and Europe use at least one chest CT to assess donor lungs and identify nodules or infiltrates missed on chest radiographs, screen for structural lung diseases and anatomic abnormalities, and estimate lung volumes.[31]

MICROBIOLOGICAL CULTURE RESULTS AND ANTIBIOTICS

The incidence of donor lung allograft infection is high (up to 50%),[32] and increased duration of intubation is correlated with greater rates of bronchial tree colonization.[29] However, donor lung colonization rates do not correlate with rates of posttransplant pneumonia or graft outcomes.[33] Infection with multidrug-resistant organisms and invasive fungal or mycobacterial organisms continues to be a relative contraindication to lung transplantation, whereas active *Mycobacterium tuberculosis* infection remains an absolute contraindication. In the era of empiric broad-spectrum antibiotics, most donor lungs with active bacterial infection are salvageable with aggressive antibiotic treatment.[34] An infectious disease consultation should be sought for atypical infections. In donor lungs with heavy candida growth, antifungal prophylaxis can play a role in reducing rates of invasive candidiasis; however, recent studies have not shown an association with prophylactic antifungal use and reduced rates of posttransplant allograft infections or colonization rates. Instead, the degree of hypoxemia secondary to infection may be a more accurate indicator of donor lung salvageability. Furthermore, donor bacteremia or sepsis is generally not considered an absolute contraindication to organ donation unless strongly supported by infectious nodules seen on imaging and microbiology data.

EFFECT OF BLOOD TRANSFUSION IN DONOR LUNG MANAGEMENT

Massive blood transfusion (defined as >10 units of blood products) has been associated with both 30-day and 90-day mortality after lung transplantation,[35] even in low-risk recipients. Specifically, donor blood transfusion has been identified as a potential risk factor for primary graft dysfunction. Although the mechanisms remain unclear, biomarkers such as soluble receptor for advanced glycation end products (sRAGE) have been identified in patients with both primary graft dysfunction and transfusion-related acute lung injury (TRALI),[36] providing some correlation between acute lung injury and TRALI, thus reflecting transfusion-related mortality risk. Massive transfusions are needed in the early stabilization of young trauma patients who are major contributors to the donor pool. As trauma and damaged blood products increase the risk of primary graft dysfunction, center-specific risk tolerance and experience in aggressively managing primary graft dysfunction should inform the decision to select donor lungs subjected to a massive blood transfusion.

CORONAVIRUS DISEASE 2019 SCREENING GUIDELINES

The International Society for Heart and Lung Transplantation (ISHLT)[37] recommends avoiding transplantation from donors with a positive severe acute respiratory syndrome coronavirus 2 (SARS-CoV-2) polymerase chain reaction (PCR) test, donors currently suffering from coronavirus disease 2019 (COVID-19) clinical syndrome,[38] or donors with COVID-19 pneumonia on thoracic imaging even in the absence of symptoms, but donors with known exposure to a confirmed or probable case of COVID-19 within the past 14 days without a clinical syndrome consistent with COVID-19 may be considered. There are limited data on antigen testing for lung donor evaluation at this time.[38] All potential donors must be screened for SARS-CoV-2 infection risk before organ recovery given that the virus can cause severe infection in recipients on potent immunosuppression medication after transplantation. This entails taking a careful history to stratify donor SARS-CoV-2 exposure risk and obtaining chest imaging as well as microbiology sampling in potential lung donors. Reverse transcription (RT)-PCR remains the gold standard

for the detection of active infection.[39] COVID-19 vaccination status of the donor does not alter these recommendations.[38] For DCDD donors, a minimum of one respiratory tract sample is needed. The European guidelines mirror that of the ISHLT recommendations.

Deceased Donor Evaluation and Testing for Coronavirus Disease 2019

Three SARS-CoV-2 transmissions to lung recipients have been reported by the Centers for Disease Control and Prevention despite a negative SARS-CoV-2 result in the donor upper respiratory tract sample; in all 3 events, lower respiratory tract samples from the donor tested positive retrospectively.[38,40–42] To minimize the risk of donor-derived SARS-CoV-2 infection while maximizing donor utilization, the Organ Procurement and Transplantation Network (OPTN) recommends testing all deceased donors for SARS-CoV-2 by nucleic acid test (NAT) from upper or lower respiratory tract specimen (nasopharyngeal [NP] swab, NP wash, NP aspirate, nasal wash, nasal aspirate, mid-turbinate swab, oropharyngeal swab, tracheal aspirate, bronchial suction or wash, bronchoalveolar lavage, or lung biopsy) within 72 hours, but ideally closest to the time of organ recovery. OPTN policy further warrants prospective testing of a lower respiratory tract sample when donor lungs are recovered for transplantation. A negative NAT test in a respiratory sample decreases the risk of transmission of an unrecognized infection; however, the safety and potential transmission risk with the use of SARS-CoV-2 antibody testing, NAT testing of a nonrespiratory sample, and radiographic imaging as the sole diagnostic method have not been established. Furthermore, the impact of resolved versus active COVID-19 and donor SARS-CoV-2 vaccination status on transmission risk is unclear at present.

Deceased Donors with Resolved Coronavirus Disease 2019

Resolved COVID-19 is defined as an immunocompetent donor with a history of confirmed COVID-19 who is more than 21 days from the date of disease onset with resolution of symptoms. Such donors with a negative SARS-CoV-2 NAT test at the time of donor evaluation are unlikely to transmit infection as per OPTN.[42] However, data on allograft quality and long-term outcomes are limited. The decision in such cases is driven by the candidates' risk of remaining on the waitlist. It is also believed that deceased donors with a history of mild COVID-19 (who did not require oxygen supplementation or inpatient stabilization) who are 10 to

21 days from date of disease onset with resolution of symptoms as well as deceased donors with resolved COVID-19 and a positive SARS-CoV-2 NAT test 21 to 90 days from date of disease onset are unlikely to transmit infection to the recipient.[43]

Deceased Donors with Active Coronavirus Disease 2019

Active COVID-19 is defined as an immunocompetent donor with a history of confirmed COVID-19 and a positive SARS-CoV-2 NAT of a respiratory sample who is less than 21 days from disease onset.[42,44] The transmission risk from these donors to organ recipients and transplant teams is unclear; however, it has been observed that transmission risk to lung recipients is higher than the transmission risk to other solid organ recipients.[44] In Europe, organs from a donor with a positive SARS-CoV-2 test result are being offered only to recipients who are positive for SARS-CoV-2 or had a previous SARS-CoV-2 infection, are in severe clinical condition, and have a higher risk of death from remaining on the waitlist than from potential infective disease transmission. Antibody titers in recipients are recommended, even if available only after transplantation, and adequate informed consent is required. As an exception to this rule, in June 2021, an Italian transplant center gave permission for a cardiac transplantation in 2 recipients, a 64-year-old and a 15-year-old, who were negative for SARS-CoV-2 and without antibodies and who received organs from donors who tested positive for SARS-CoV-2.[45] This was authorized given the recipients' high risk of death while on the waitlist. Neither recipient developed a SARS-CoV-2 infection.

Living Donor Evaluation and Testing

Infection control practices, self-quarantine during the 14 days before organ recovery, and testing a respiratory sample for SARS-CoV-2 with a NAT close to the time of organ recovery (but within 72 hours prior) are recommended for living donors to reduce transmission risk to the recipient. However, long-term outcome data are lacking.

SUMMARY

Transplantation is the result of a multidisciplinary team working inside and outside the hospital, and the goal of multiple organ transplants can be reached by the combined efforts of a collaborating team. The ultimate target of donor management is in fact to preserve the donation opportunity and to maximize the number and quality of donor organs for transplantation.

FUTURE DIRECTIONS

Despite an increase in the number of organ donors worldwide, organ utilization remains suboptimal given multiple challenges. Optimal critical care management is the natural background for a successful organ donation program. Managing marginal donors will help increase the number of organs available for transplantation while maintaining recipient safety and acceptable allograft outcomes and recipient survival. Successful organ recovery involves an effective team approach, aggressive resuscitative strategies, standardized donor management protocols, clear communication, family support, community awareness, and ongoing education and training.[46] Moving forward, routine chest CT and lower respiratory tract RT-PCR SARS-CoV-2 testing will remain the standard of care. The use of ex vivo lung perfusion will expand the donor pool and help bridge the supply and demand gap in lung transplantation. Our understanding of the impact of the COVID-19 pandemic on lung transplantation will continue to evolve.

CLINICS CARE POINTS

- Every critically ill patient in the ICU acts as a potential donor with a multidisciplinary approach and closed loop communication to make lungs and other organs salvageable.

- Comparable short-term and long-term survival rates between donation after neurological determination of death and donation after circulatory determination of death should encourage centers to embrace both modes of donation to meet the demand and supply gap in lung transplantation.

- Early protective ventilator strategies, ongoing lung recruitment maneuvers as needed, and fine fluid balance remain cornerstones of therapy in managing a potential lung for donation.

- Chest imaging and bronchoscopy results should further help medical management of the donor including need for diuresis, broadening antibiotics, and therapeutic aspiration of secretions.

- With the pandemic adding a new dimension to the donor pool, adequately screening donors for COVID infection with good history taking, lower respiratory tract sample testing, imaging, and clinical judgment will help procure more lungs.

ACKNOWLEDGMENTS

The authors thank Dr Deepika Razia for help with writing this article.

DISCLOSURE

The authors have nothing to disclose.

REFERENCES

1. Wey A, Valapour M, Skeans MA, et al. Heart and lung organ offer acceptance practices of transplant programs are associated with waitlist mortality and organ yield. Am J Transplant 2018;18(8):2061–7.
2. Miñambres E, Pérez-Villares JM, Chico-Fernández M, et al. Lung donor treatment protocol in brain dead-donors: a multicenter study. J Heart Lung Transplant 2015;34(6):773–80.
3. Miñambres E, Pérez-Villares JM, Terceros-Almanza L, et al. An intensive lung donor treatment protocol does not have negative influence on other grafts: a multicentre study. Eur J Cardiothorac Surg 2016;49(6):1719–24.
4. Van Raemdonck D, Neyrinck A, Verleden GM, et al. Lung donor selection and management. Proc Am Thorac Soc 2009;6(1):28–38.
5. Busl KM, Bleck TP. Neurogenic pulmonary edema. Crit Care Med 2015;43(8):1710–5.
6. Mascia L, Mastromauro I, Viberti S, et al. Management to optimize organ procurement in brain dead donors. Minerva Anestesiol 2009;75(3):125–33.
7. Pelosi P, Rocco PR. The lung and the brain: a dangerous cross-talk. Crit Care 2011;15(3):168.
8. Slutsky AS, Ranieri VM. Ventilator-induced lung injury. N Engl J Med 2013;369(22):2126–36.
9. Gajic O, Dabbagh O, Park PK, et al. Early identification of patients at risk of acute lung injury: evaluation of lung injury prediction score in a multicenter cohort study. Am J Respir Crit Care Med 2011;183(4):462–70.
10. Rincon F, Ghosh S, Dey S, et al. Impact of acute lung injury and acute respiratory distress syndrome after traumatic brain injury in the United States. Neurosurgery 2012;71(4):795–803.
11. Mascia L, Zavala E, Bosma K, et al. High tidal volume is associated with the development of acute lung injury after severe brain injury: an international observational study. Crit Care Med 2007;35(8):1815–20.
12. Mascia L, Pasero D, Slutsky AS, et al. Effect of a lung protective strategy for organ donors on eligibility and availability of lungs for transplantation: a randomized controlled trial. JAMA 2010;304(23):2620–7.
13. Rech TH, Moraes RB, Crispim D, et al. Management of the brain-dead organ donor: a systematic review and meta-analysis. Transplantation 2013;95(7):966–74.
14. Copeland H, Hayanga JWA, Neyrinck A, et al. Donor heart and lung procurement: a consensus statement. J Heart Lung Transplant 2020;39(6):501–17.
15. Botha P, Rostron AJ, Fisher AJ, et al. Current strategies in donor selection and management. Semin Thorac Cardiovasc Surg 2008;20(2):143–51.
16. Philpot SJ, Pilcher DV, Graham SM, et al. Lung recruitment manoeuvres should be considered when assessing suitability for lung donation. Crit Care Resusc 2012;14(3):244–5.
17. Lorente L, Blot S, Rello J. New issues and controversies in the prevention of ventilator-associated pneumonia. Am J Respir Crit Care Med 2010;182(7):870–6.
18. Powner DJ, Hewitt MJ, Levine RL. Interventions during donor care before lung transplantation. Prog Transplant 2005;15(2):141–8.
19. Kotloff RM, Blosser S, Fulda GJ, et al. Management of the potential organ donor in the ICU: Society of Critical Care Medicine/American College of Chest Physicians/Association of Organ Procurement Organizations Consensus Statement. Crit Care Med 2015;43(6):1291–325.
20. Meyfroidt G, Gunst J, Martin-Loeches I, et al. Management of the brain-dead donor in the ICU: general and specific therapy to improve transplantable organ quality. Intensive Care Med 2019;45(3):343–53.
21. Keddissi JI, Youness HA, Jones KR, et al. Fluid management in acute respiratory distress syndrome: a narrative review. Can J Respir Ther 2019;55:1–8.
22. Murugan R, Venkataraman R, Wahed AS, et al. Preload responsiveness is associated with increased interleukin-6 and lower organ yield from brain-dead donors. Crit Care Med 2009;37(8):2387–93.
23. Al-Khafaji A, Elder M, Lebovitz DJ, et al. Protocolized fluid therapy in brain-dead donors: the multicenter randomized MOnIToR trial. Intensive Care Med 2015;41(3):418–26.
24. Miñambres E, Rodrigo E, Ballesteros MA, et al. Impact of restrictive fluid balance focused to increase lung procurement on renal function after kidney transplantation. Nephrol Dial Transplant 2010;25(7):2352–6.
25. Malinoski DJ, Patel MS, Daly MC, et al. The impact of meeting donor management goals on the number of organs transplanted per donor: results from the United Network for Organ Sharing Region 5 prospective donor management goals study. Crit Care Med 2012;40(10):2773–80.
26. Patel MS, Zatarain J, De La Cruz S, et al. The impact of meeting donor management goals on the number of organs transplanted per expanded criteria donor: a prospective study from the UNOS Region 5 Donor Management Goals Workgroup. JAMA Surg 2014;149(9):969–75.

27. Domínguez-Gil B, Duranteau J, Mateos A, et al. Uncontrolled donation after circulatory death: European practices and recommendations for the development and optimization of an effective programme. Transpl Int 2016;29(8):842–59.

28. Levvey B, Keshavjee S, Cypel M, et al. Influence of lung donor agonal and warm ischemic times on early mortality: analyses from the ISHLT DCD Lung Transplant Registry. J Heart Lung Transplant 2019; 38(1):26–34.

29. Avlonitis VS, Krause A, Luzzi L, et al. Bacterial colonization of the donor lower airways is a predictor of poor outcome in lung transplantation. Eur J Cardiothorac Surg 2003;24(4):601–7.

30. Schlesinger AE, White DK, Mallory GB, et al. Estimation of total lung capacity from chest radiography and chest CT in children: comparison with body plethysmography. AJR Am J Roentgenol 1995; 165(1):151–4.

31. Gauthier JM, Bierhals AJ, Liu J, et al. Chest computed tomography imaging improves potential lung donor assessment. The J Thorac Cardiovasc Surg 2019;157(4):1711–8.e1.

32. Ruiz I, Gavaldà J, Monforte V, et al. Donor-to-host transmission of bacterial and fungal infections in lung transplantation. Am J Transplant 2006;6(1): 178–82.

33. Weill D, Dey GC, Hicks RA, et al. A positive donor gram stain does not predict outcome following lung transplantation. J Heart Lung Transplant 2002; 21(5):555–8.

34. Bonde PN, Patel ND, Borja MC, et al. Impact of donor lung organisms on post-lung transplant pneumonia. J Heart Lung Transplant 2006;25(1):99–105.

35. Borders CF, Suzuki Y, Lasky J, et al. Massive donor transfusion potentially increases recipient mortality after lung transplantation. J Thorac Cardiovasc Surg 2017;153(5):1197–203.e2.

36. Shah RJ, Bellamy SL, Localio AR, et al. A panel of lung injury biomarkers enhances the definition of primary graft dysfunction (PGD) after lung transplantation. J Heart Lung Transplant 2012;31(9):942–9.

37. International Society of Heart and Lung Transplantation. Guidance from the International Society of Heart and Lung Transplantation regarding the SARS CoV-2 pandemic. 2021. Available at: https://ishlt.org/ishlt/media/documents/SARS-CoV-2_Guidance-for-Cardiothoracic-Transplant-and-VAD-center.pdf. Accessed June 18, 2021.

38. International Society of Heart and Lung Transplantation. Deceased donor and recipient selection for cardiothoracic transplantation during the COVID-19 pandemic. April 12, 2021. Available at: https://ishlt.org/ishlt/media/documents/COVID-19_Guidance Document_Deceased-donor-and-recipient-selection-for-cardiothoracic-transplantation.pdf. Accessed June 18, 2021.

39. Halpern SE, Olaso DG, Krischak MK, et al. Lung transplantation during the COVID-19 pandemic: safely navigating the new "normal. Am J Transplant 2020;20(11):3094–105.

40. Kaul DR, Valesano AL, Petrie JG, et al. Donor to recipient transmission of SARS-CoV-2 by lung transplantation despite negative donor upper respiratory tract testing. Am J Transplant 2021;21(8):2885–9.

41. Kumar D, Humar A, Keshavjee S, et al. A call to routinely test lower respiratory tract samples for SARS-CoV-2 in lung donors. Am J Transplant 2021; 21:2623–4.

42. Organ Procurement and Transplantation Network. Summary of current evidence and information–donor SARS-CoV-2 testing & organ recovery from donors with a history of COVID-19. Version release date: April 26, 2021. Available at: https://optn.transplant.hrsa.gov/media/4424/sars-cov-2-summary-of-evidence.pdf. Accessed June 30, 2021.

43. American Society of Transplantation. COVID-19 information. Available at: https://www.myast.org/covid-19-information. Accessed August 12, 2021.

44. Michaels MG, La Hoz RM, Danziger-Isakov L, et al. Coronavirus disease 2019: Implications of emerging infections for transplantation. Am J Transplant 2020; 20(7):1768–72.

45. World's 1st transplants from COVID-positive donors performed in Italy. Available at: https://www.ansa.it/english/news/2021/06/10/worlds-1st-transplants-from-covid-positive-donors_9079492d-1f77-468d-b61a-9af28a8bfaf8.html. Accessed 8/23/2021. ANSAit. June 10, 2021.

46. Wojda TR, Stawicki SP, Yandle KP, et al. Keys to successful organ procurement: an experience-based review of clinical practices at a high-performing health-care organization. Int J Crit Illn Inj Sci 2017; 7(2):91–100.

Donation After Circulatory Death in lung transplantation

Dirk Van Raemdonck, MD, PhD[a,b,*], Laurens J. Ceulemans, MD, PhD[a,b],
Arne Neyrinck, MD, PhD[c,d], Bronwyn Levvey, RN[e], Gregory I. Snell, MBBS, MD[e]

KEYWORDS

- Donation after brain death • Donation after circulatory death • End-of-life care
- Lung transplantation • Normothermic regional perfusion • Primary graft dysfunction
- Withdrawal from life-sustaining therapy

KEY POINTS

- Lung transplantation from controlled donors after circulatory death results in similar short-term and long-term outcomes as donors after brain death.
- Lung transplantation from selected uncontrolled donors after circulatory death is feasible, but larger experience by more transplant centers is further awaited.
- Ex-vivo lung perfusion is optional to assess the pretransplant quality of lungs from controlled donors after withdrawal from life-sustaining therapy but mandatory for lungs from uncontrolled donors and controlled donors with long functional warm ischemic times.
- Rapid procurement following a no-touch period is the simplest technique to recover lungs from controlled donors after circulatory death and can be combined with normothermic regional perfusion of abdominal organs.
- Thoracoabdominal normothermic regional perfusion turns the procurement into a postmortem heart-beating procedure, thereby eliminating the need for ex-situ lung evaluation with machine perfusion before transplantation.

INTRODUCTION

Lung transplantation (LTx) has become a standard therapy with growing activity over the years that improves the quantity and the quality of life for selected patients suffering from end-stage lung disease.[1] Unfortunately, not all lung transplant candidates can benefit because of the lack of acceptable organs. Optimizing the lung donor pool should get utmost priority. Besides improvement in current practices with better donor registration, detection, reporting, and management, the use of alternative donors not matching the standard donor lung criteria should be explored.[2]

Historically, the largest source of transplantable organs arises in the setting where donation after a neurologic determination of brain death occurs (DBD donors). Unfortunately, the average lung yield from these donors remains low at around 20% to 40% even after extending lung criteria. Many transplant programs worldwide have more recently explored the use of organs coming from an additional pool where donation after a circulatory determination of death occurs (DCD donors).

[a] Department of Thoracic Surgery, University Hospitals Leuven, UZ Gasthuisberg, Herestraat 49, Leuven B-3000, Belgium; [b] Department of Chronic Diseases and Metabolism, KU Leuven University, Leuven, Belgium; [c] Department of Anesthesiology, University Hospitals Leuven, UZ Gasthuisberg, Herestraat 49, Leuven B-3000, Belgium; [d] Department of Cardiovascular Sciences, KU Leuven University, Leuven, Belgium; [e] Lung Transplant Service, The Alfred Hospital and Monash University, 55 Commercial Road, Melbourne, Victoria 3004, Australia
* Corresponding author. Department of Thoracic Surgery, University Hospital Gasthuisberg, Herestraat 49, Leuven B-3000, Belgium.
E-mail address: dirk.vanraemdonck@uzleuven.be

Thorac Surg Clin 32 (2022) 153–165
https://doi.org/10.1016/j.thorsurg.2021.11.002
1547-4127/22/© 2021 Elsevier Inc. All rights reserved.

Reports of successful DCD LTx have now emerged from the United Kingdom, the Netherlands, Belgium, Spain, Switzerland, Australia, Canada, and the United States.[3]

CATEGORIES OF DCD DONATION

To indicate the amount of ischemia and thus the risk for primary nonfunction or dysfunction of the transplanted organ, the Maastricht Classification[4] with 4 categories of DCD were described: category I represented death at arrival to hospital, category II an unsuccessful resuscitation, category III an expected cardiac arrest, and category IV an unexpected cardiac arrest in a DBD donor. Categories I and II were grouped as "uncontrolled" DCDs (uDCD), whereas categories III and IV represented "controlled" DCDs (cDCD). Based on evolving experience, modified classifications with additional subcategories have since been formulated[5,6] and are described in **Table 1**.

EVALUATION OF THE DCD DONOR

The same standard and extended DBD lung selection criteria apply for cDCD.[7] Clinical criteria for uDCD lung donation are scarce and experience is based on small case series from Spain[8–10] and Canada[11] and single case reports from Italy.[12,13] Important to notice is that because of the unexpected circulatory arrest (CA), no donor information and history are available and donor lung quality cannot be assessed in advance via standard imaging, bronchoscopy, and oxygenation challenge tools.

In contrast to DBD donation whereby brain death may precipitate a systemic inflammation and neurogenic lung edema resulting in donor lung injury, this is absent in a potential DCD donor. Nevertheless, both DBD and DCD lungs are at risk to injuries such as aspiration and infection related to intubation and ventilation similar to any patient admitted to the intensive care unit (ICU).

TOLERATED WARM ISCHEMIA

Organs retrieved from DCDs are vulnerable to the effects of warm ischemia with potential important consequences on post-transplant outcomes. The main concern is the duration of the agonal phase before and the asystolic phase after the moment of (un)foreseen CA and extending until pulmonary arterial cold flush preservation. Compared with other solid organs transplanted from DCD, lungs are privileged to sustain ischemia as the alveoli remain filled with oxygen in the absence of perfusion.[14] cDCD lung retrieval, therefore, can be facilitated in a more relaxed way when compared with abdominal organs such as kidney[15] and liver.[16]

The agonal phase is generally considered the most important trigger for lung injury as blood flow cessation induces an endothelial response

Table 1
Modified Maastricht classification of DCD

Category	Description	Details
Category I. Uncontrolled	Found dead IA. Out-of-hospital IB. In-hospital	Sudden unexpected CA without any attempt of resuscitation
Category II. Uncontrolled	Witnessed cardiac arrest IIA. Out-of-hospital IIB. In-hospital	Sudden unexpected irreversible CA with unsuccessful resuscitation
Category III. Controlled	Withdrawal of life-sustaining therapy	Planned withdrawal of life-sustaining therapy[a]; expected CA
Category IV. Uncontrolled	Cardiac arrest in a brain-dead donor	Sudden CA after brain death diagnosis during donor life-management but before planned organ recovery
Category V. Controlled	Cardiac arrest after medical assistance in dying or euthanasia VA. Out-of-hospital VB. In-hospital	Sudden expected CA following lethal injection[b]

Abbreviations: CA, circulatory arrest; DCD, donation after circulatory death.
[a] This category mainly refers to the decision to withdraw life-sustaining therapies.
[b] Legislation in some countries allows euthanasia or medical assistance in dying and subsequent organ donation described as the fifth category.
Data from Refs.[4–6]

by a change in shear stress rather than by hypoxia.[17] Different time points and intervals after withdrawal from life-sustaining therapy (WLST) in cDCD have been defined by the International Society for Heart and Lung Transplantation (ISHLT) (**Table 2**).[18]

Most centers will accept a waiting time for lungs after WLST of up to 60 to 120 minutes. However, more important is the length of the hypotensive period defining the functional warm ischemia time (WIT; ie, T2-T5). In a multicenter multivariable ISHLT DCD Registry analysis of 507 cDCD LTx, no association of agonal time or functional WIT on 1-year recipient mortality was found.[19] Similarly, in a single-center series, the duration of documented agonal phase was assessed in 180 cDCD LTx and no significant differences were found in short-term and long-term recipient survival, primary graft dysfunction (PGD), ICU stay, mechanical ventilation days, or total hospital stay.[20] These authors concluded that lungs with an agonal phase greater than 60 minutes can be safely used in their hands. In addition, the Toronto group also reported good outcomes in cases with periods longer than 120 min from WLST to CA (ie, T0-T3).[21] They also described a case of lungs procured 12 hours after WLST using a technique of static lung inflation upon CA in the ICU before retrieval with cold flush in the operating room (OR) nearly 2 hours later.[22] Notably, the donor's systemic blood pressure did not fall less than 50 mm Hg until 10 hours 54 minutes after WLST, with CA 25 minutes later. The functional WIT was therefore within the usual range as previously reported in the ISHLT DCD Registry.[19] The group from Melbourne recently reported on an audit of their lung donor pool. They concluded that a time-extended DCD lung donation pathway (>90 minutes–24 hours postwithdrawal) could substantially expand their lung donor pool.[23]

WLST, INCLUDING COMFORT THERAPY, IN CONTROLLED DCD

Practices to stop medical therapy may well vary across communities and continents. This might be especially true in decision-making for critically ill patients with no further treatment options for recovery from their underlying condition. WLST after informed consent from the next of kin is an option for these patients when all attempts to improve the medical situation have failed. The decision to stop therapy is reached when continued treatments are not anticipated to enable the patient's survival with an acceptable quality of life.[24] When conducted expertly, WLST is a shared human experience that can be fulfilling especially in the context of organ donation, although difficult for all concerned.[25] Clearly, transplant physicians taking care of recipients on their waiting list carry a conflict of interest and therefore must have no role or responsibility in the WLST decision and its practice.[26]

The percentage of aborted procedures may depend on criteria used for the selection of potential donors and comfort therapy given during end-of-life care. The number of donors who do not develop CA within a time window of 120 minutes after WLST is estimated to be around 40%. Therefore, many LTx teams are reluctant to travel long distances because of the financial risk for a futile donor run. Algorithms have been developed in an attempt to predict the likelihood of progression,[27,28] but usefulness is lacking because of their inaccuracy. In our own experience with cDCDs in Belgium, less than 1% of procedures are aborted (Belgian Transplantation Society, unpublished data, 2021).

Comfort therapy given to the donor during WLST could indirectly affect the duration of the agonal phase, although evidence is equivocal. Concerns have been raised about potential physical and psychological suffering imposed on the donor after WLST. Therefore, during end-of-life care and the withdrawal phase, titrated comfort therapy should be considered for the dying patient (according to local legal and clinical practice

Table 2
Time points, intervals, and phases after withdrawal from life-sustaining therapy in cDCD defined by ISHLT

Time Point	Description
T0	Withdrawal of life-sustaining therapies or euthanasia.
T1	Oxygen saturation <80%.
T2	Systolic blood pressure <50 mm Hg.
T3	Cessation of cardiac output/ asystole.
T4	Resumed lung inflation/ ventilation.
T5	Start of pulmonary flush.

Abbreviations: cDCD, controlled donation after circulatory death; ISHLT, International Society for Heart and Lung Transplantation; T0-T5, total warm ischemic time; T2-T5, functional warm ischemic time phases; T0-T3, agonal phase; T3-T5, asystolic phase.

Data from Cypel M, Levvey B, Van Raemdonck D, et al. International Society for Heart and Lung Transplantation donation after circulatory death registry report. J Heart Lung Transplant 2015;34:1278-82.

constraints). At the same time, organ protective measures could also be taken. Currently, there are no useful guidelines to assist the method of withdrawal of therapy and only general principles are provided. Although poorly documented, no association could be demonstrated between quantities of sedatives and analgesics and time to death.[28–30]

Overall, there is no consensus and the issue of comfort therapy creates an ethical debate on whether this practice indirectly results in shortening the life of consented donors.[31] Arguably, titrated comfort therapy could be given to a potential donor after WLST recognizing the same therapy is administered daily in other suffering terminally ill ICU patients without further treatment options. Shortening of suffering does not mean shortening of life. The development of International guidelines on end-of-life care in cDCD would be beneficial.

SURGICAL TECHNIQUE FOR DCD LUNG RECOVERY

The surgical technique for DCD lung preservation and recovery does not differ substantially compared with DBD except that the heart has already arrested. An ISHLT consensus statement on donor's heart and lung procurement was recently published describing the technique for both DBD and DCD.[32] Gastric decompression with nasogastric tube is recommended to avoid airway aspiration after extubation at the time of WLST. In accordance with country-specific legislation, a certain period of no-touch (3-5-20 min) following CA is mandated to comply with the dead-donor rule and to exclude the possibility of autoresuscitation. Following median sternotomy, the anterior pericardium and both pleura are opened widely. Lungs will collapse and cold saline solution can be used for topical cooling. The congested right heart is vented by transecting the right atrial appendage or the inferior vena cava. A large sump is needed to drain the venous blood and to vent the liver. The pneumoplegia cannula is then inserted into the main pulmonary artery (PA) and secured by a purse-string or ligature around the PA. Alternatively, the cannula can be inserted by incising the right ventricular outflow tract and cannulating the PA through the pulmonary valve in case the heart is not banked for the valves. The cannula is then de-aired and connected to the pneumoplegia flush line. A large bolus of a prostaglandin solution can be injected directly into the PA via a 3-way tap. Antegrade flush with 60 mL/kg cold low-potassium dextran solution is started and the left atrial appendage is transected to vent the left heart while both lungs are re-ventilated to ensure uniform distribution of the preservation solution. A

bronchoscopy at this time ensures full expansion of all lobes. The lungs can then be inspected and palpated carefully at the end of the flush while deflated. The heart is excised and a retrograde flush can be administered via the 4 pulmonary veins with lungs being re-ventilated. Alternatively, the heart-lung bloc is excised first, split on the back-table followed by retrograde lung flush.

Typically, pulmonary grafts are approved and accepted for transplantation at a later stage during the DCD retrieval process compared with the DBD donor where lungs can already be grossly evaluated and accepted before CA. In case of doubt, lung donor quality can be further assessed with ex-vivo lung perfusion (EVLP) as further described.

Practices for cDCD and uDCD lung recovery largely vary between institutions and always need to be in accordance with existing ethical and legal frameworks.

Controlled Donors

Lung criteria in cDCD can usually be checked hours in advance before the planned procedure. Practice differs between countries and institutions with regards to the location of WLST (ICU vs OR), premortem administration of heparin, withdrawal of the endotracheal tube, administration of comfort therapy, monitoring of cardiac activity, length of no-touch period, timing of death declaration, and legal requirements for death certification.[33]

In many countries, WLST is practiced in the ICU where death is certified. In contrast, in Belgium, WLST takes place in the OR under the supervision of an intensivist or anesthesiologist (**Fig. 1**). The relatives of the donor can be present in the OR whenever requested. Death is certified by 3 independent physicians not being involved in the transplant process. This practice decreases the total length of the asystolic phase as additional transport and donor draping times are avoided.

In the largest study from the ISHLT DCD Registry reporting on 1090 DCD lung transplants, practices related to the DCD process varied widely across the 22 participating institutions in Europe, North America, and Australia with administration of heparin (53%), corticosteroids (58%), or fibrinolytics (0.2%), extubation (91%), presence of nasogastric tube (62%), and use of EVLP (15%) after graft retrieval.[34] So far, no large studies are available comparing the impact of different cDCD protocols on post-LTx outcomes.

Uncontrolled Donors

In contrast to cDCD, the asystolic phase between CA after failed cardiac resuscitation and preservation by cold flush perfusion in uDCD will be much

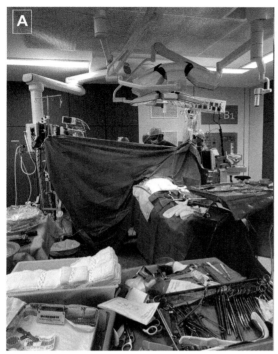
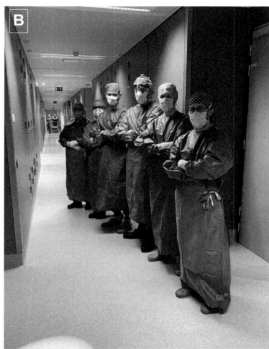

Fig. 1. The scene in the operating room for multiorgan retrieval from a cDCD in Leuven, Belgium. The donor is completely prepped and draped. An anesthesiologist ensures titrating comfort therapy. (*A*) The scrubbed procurement team is waiting outside the operating room for circulatory arrest to occur after WLST. (*B*) A 5-minute no-touch period is mandated. Surgery is not started until death is certified by 3 independent physicians.

longer as no OR and staff will be readily available. Different measures to protect the lung from warm ischemic injury inside the deceased body following death declaration until lung recovery have been described, varying from topical lung cooling with a cold solution inserted via chest drains by the Lund[35] and Madrid[8] groups, postmortem alveolar recruitment maneuvers by the Milan[36] group and lung inflation using continuous positive airway pressure by the Toronto[11] group. The worldwide experience with uDCD LTx is still limited and further studies are awaited to evaluate the impact of these different techniques on outcome.

ROLE OF POSTMORTEM PRETRANSPLANT EVALUATION OF LUNG QUALITY
Ex-situ Lung Evaluation and Preservation with EVLP

The exact usefulness of pretransplant EVLP for standard cDCD LTx is still unclear. In the largest report by the ISHLT DCD Registry, EVLP was used in only 15% of all cases, mainly by 1 institution.[34] In cases with a short agonal phase and total WIT, the need for pre-LTx assessment of pulmonary function with EVLP is not necessarily indicated if donor lungs grossly appear normal upon retrieval. Machuca and colleagues from Toronto compared outcomes after LTx from 55 cDCDs with (n = 28) or without EVLP (n = 27) between 2007 and 2013. No significant differences in survival were found. However, cDCD + EVLP cases presented shorter hospital stay (median 18 vs 23 days, $P = .047$) and a trend toward shorter length of mechanical ventilation (2 vs 3 days, $P = .059$).[37] In a recently updated series from Toronto with 372 EVLP cases, the use and lung utilization rates were compared between standard cDCD and high-risk cDCD over the years.[38] Utilization rates were 82% (40/49) versus 63% (69/109), respectively. The authors concluded that the use of EVLP in DCD lungs that otherwise have no obvious concerns at the time of organ assessment has not been routine and remains at the surgeon's discretion. In contrast, for extended-criteria DCD, including donors that do not arrest within 1 hour after WLST, and uncontrolled DCDs, EVLP may be a useful requirement for safe transplantation. Bozso and colleagues published an algorithm with selected EVLP use arguing that it would safely increase DCD lung use.[39] Although EVLP to increase the confidence in the use of DCD lungs appears reasonable, there is an associated increase in cost and resource utilization that may make EVLP prohibitive for many transplant centers.

In contrast to cDCD, assessment of uDCD lungs with EVLP is mandatory before transplantation, as no information on pulmonary graft function and performance is available before recovery. Moreover, serious lung injury may occur during prolonged donor resuscitation and the long asystolic phase. The Madrid group described a technique for in-situ evaluation of gas exchange with a single pulmonary blood flush.[8] Meanwhile, the group has reported the use of a lung device for ex-situ assessment and reconditioning of the pulmonary graft before transplantation.[9,40]

In-situ Lung Evaluation and Preservation During Normothermic Regional Perfusion

Rapid recovery with simple cold storage as the gold standard in DBD has proven to be less optimal to preserve abdominal organs from DCD donors.[15,16] Organ recovery and preservation of DCD organs using in-situ normothermic regional perfusion (NRP) with extracorporeal membrane oxygenation (ECMO) technology is slowly being adopted across Europe.[41] Current practice for cDCD organ retrieval after WLST, therefore, is likely to change considerably in the coming years.

In case NRP is limited to the abdominal organs (A-NRP), lungs will remain in a warm pleural cavity and should be preserved until recovery. Two methods to protect the lungs during this interval have been described. First, lungs can be rapidly flushed and removed with meticulous care for hemostasis in the chest during continued abdominal NRP.[42] Good outcome after LTx with this technique has been reported in a series by the Santander[43] and Madrid[44] groups. Alternatively, while waiting for abdominal NRP to be finished, lungs can be topically cooled via chest drains inserted in the pleural cavity. Second, lungs can be preserved in the deceased body by in-situ protective ventilation during abdominal NRP as reported by the Milan group.[45,46]

In the case of thoracoabdominal NRP (TA-NRP), the aim is to restart the arrested heart for DCD heart transplantation.[47] Once the heart has regained sufficient cardiac output, ECMO can be disconnected and the donor will turn into a heart-beating donor. Organs can now be resuscitated from the initial warm ischemic insult after WLST and their function can be reassessed in the standard way similar to DBD. Lungs will be preserved in the standard way with antegrade cold flush perfusion. Reports on the use of lungs after TA-NRP donors have been anecdotal so far.[48,49]

Concerns and ethical questions have been raised with the use of NRP including potential violation of the dead-donor-rule principle, the definition of circulatory death by permanent versus irreversible cessation of circulatory and respiratory functions, and the deliberate occlusion of cerebral circulation creating brain death.[50,51] It is very important that methods to accomplish in-situ NRP of organs must preclude the restoration of brain perfusion to not invalidate the determination of death. The unifying concept of death for organ donation requires brain circulation to have ceased indefinitely, resulting in the permanent cessation of brain function.[52] Monitoring the absence of brain perfusion or function during NRP is therefore an essential component of such protocols. Techniques used for isolating the brain from the circulation during A-NRP and TA-NRP have been described.[53]

OUTCOMES OF DCD LTx
Controlled Donors

Over the last decade, many groups have reported their single-center cDCD experience. In most studies, the outcome was compared with LTx from DBD. A summary of the largest studies published up to 2019 was tabulated by Ceulemans and colleagues in a previous review paper.[3] Generally speaking, results were excellent with most studies confirming that outcome after LTx from cDCD is comparable to DBD in terms of PGD, overall survival, and chronic lung allograft dysfunction (CLAD)-free survival.

The largest study comes from the ISHLT Thoracic Transplant Registry published in 2019 analyzing DCD data submitted by 22 participating centers from Europe, North America, and Australia.[34] The study cohort included 11,516 LTx, of which 1090 (9.5%) were from DCD-LTx with complete data. Maastricht category III DCD comprised 94.1% of the DCD cohort. Among the participating centers, the proportion of DCD-LTx performed each year increased from 0.6% in 2003 to 13.5% in 2016. The median time interval from WLST to CA was 15 min (interquartile range [IQR], 11–22 min) and to cold flush was 32 min (IQR, 26–41 min) (**Fig. 2**). Compared with DBD, donor age was higher in DCD (46 years [IQR, 34–55 years] vs 40 years [IQR, 24–52 years]), bilateral LTx was performed more often (88.3% vs 76.6%), and more recipients had chronic obstructive pulmonary disease or emphysema as their transplant indication. Five-year survival rates were comparable (63% vs 61%; $P = .72$) (**Fig. 3**). In multivariable analysis, recipient and donor ages, indication diagnosis, procedure type (single vs bilateral/double LTx), and transplant era (2003–2009 vs 2010/

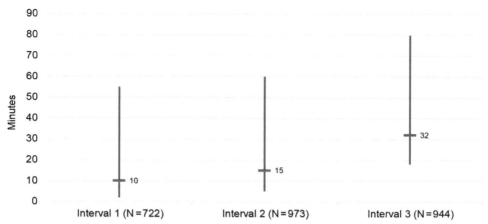

Fig. 2. The distribution of time intervals in the DCD process among DCD lung transplants between January 1, 2003, and June 30, 2017. Interval 1 = time from WLST to start of agonal phase (determined by systolic blood pressure <50 mm Hg); interval 2 = time from WLST to cessation of cardiac output/asystole; interval 3 = time from WLST to start of cold flush perfusion. Horizontal line = median; vertical bars = 5th to 95th percentile. (*From Van Raemdonck D, Keshavjee S, Levvey B, et al. Donation after circulatory death in lung transplantation - five-year follow-up from ISHLT Registry. J Heart Lung Transplant 2019;38:1235-45; with permission.*)

2016) were independently associated with survival (all *P*<.001); but donor type (DCD vs DBD) was not (hazard ratio [HR], 1.04 [0.90–1.19]; *P* = .61). In the 2019 ISHLT Registry analysis of risk factors for 10-year mortality, receiving a DCD donor was significantly associated with an improved 10-year outcome (HR, 0.65; *P*<.01).[1]

So far, 2 systematic reviews and meta-analysis of published data have been reported. In the first study by Krutsinger and colleagues published in 2015, 11 observational cohort studies were reviewed and 6 met the inclusion criteria for meta-analysis.[54] No differences in 1-year mortality were found between cDCD (n = 271) and DBD (n = 2369) cohorts with a relative risk (RR) of 0.88 ([95% confidence interval, 0.59–1.31]; *P* = .52; heterogeneity I² = 0%). There was also no difference between DCD and DBD in a pooled analysis of 5 studies reporting on PGD (RR, 1.09 [0.68–1.73]; *P* = .7; I² = 0%) and 4 studies reporting on acute rejection (RR, 0.72 [0.49–1.05]; *P* = .09; I² = 0%). In the second study by Palleschi and colleagues published in 2020, 9 observational cohort studies were reviewed with 403 cDCDs and 2570 DBDs.[55] Reported odds ratio for DBD versus DCD were: for 1-year (n = 8 studies) and 5-year (n = 5 studies) survival: 1.00 [0.70–1.44]; *P* = .973; I² = 19.2% and 0.57 [0.43–0.76]; *P*<.001; I² = 0%, respectively; for PGD grades 2 to 3 (n = 7 studies): 1.03 [0.74–1.44]; *P* = .867; I² = 0%; for 1-year CLAD-free survival (n = 6 studies): 0.57 [0.19–1.72]; *P* = .321: I² = 34.1%. Interestingly, more airway complications (n = 6 studies) were observed after cDCD-LTx (2.07 [1.09–3.94]; *P* = .026: I² = 0%).

In summary, survival after LTx from cDCD is comparable to survival after LTx from DBD in observational cohort studies. Further research is needed in terms of bronchial complications. cDCD appears to be a safe and effective method to expand the donor pool.

Uncontrolled Donors

Outcome data after uDCD-LTx are much smaller. In the early Madrid experience, higher PGD-3 incidence (38%) and lower survival rates than expected were observed (78% at 3 months, 68% at 1 year, and 51% at 5 years).[8] In their more recent paper outcome between 2002 and 2012 was compared between DBD (n = 292) versus uDCD (n = 38).[9] Both groups were comparable except for sex mismatch (male recipient-female donor was 17.8% in DBD vs 0% in uDCD, *P*<.002), total ischemic time (309 and 425 minutes vs 657 and 822 minutes for the first and second lung, respectively; *P*<.001), and ex-vivo evaluation (1.4% vs 21.1%, respectively; *P*<.001). Early and late outcomes were not different (ICU stay [9 vs 10.5 days], hospital stay [33.5 vs 35 days], PGD-3 [24% vs 34.2%], and CLAD (HR, 1.19 [0.61–2.32]), but overall survival was significantly lower for patients transplanted from uDCD (HR, 1.67 [1.06–2.64]). The authors concluded that uDCD-LTx offers poorer survival.

The group from Santander published their experience with 8 LTx from 9 uDCDs in 2019.[10] Mean no-flow time was 9.8 ± 8.6 minutes. Time from CA to topical cooling was 96.8 ± 16.8 minutes. Preservation time was 159 ± 31 minutes. EVLP

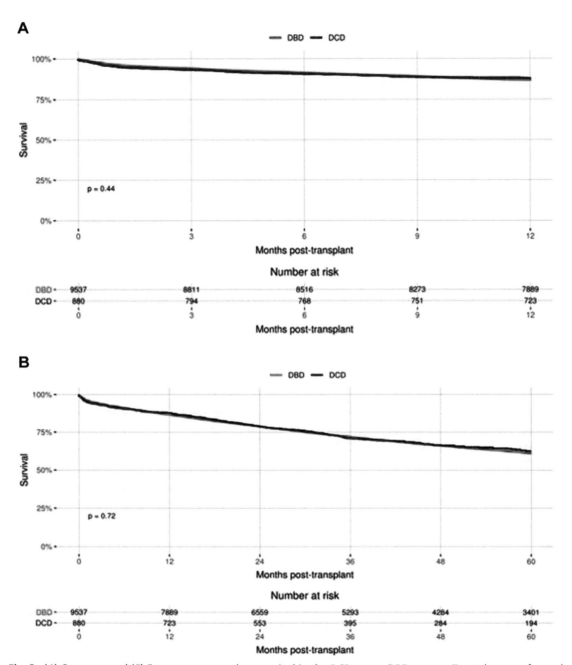

Fig. 3. (*A*) One-year and (*B*) 5-year post-transplant survival in the DCD versus DBD groups. Transplants performed between January 2003 and June 2016 are used for survival calculations and only Maastricht category III were included in the DCD group. (*From* Van Raemdonck D, Keshavjee S, Levvey B, et al. Donation after circulatory death in lung transplantation - five-year follow-up from ISHLT Registry. J Heart Lung Transplant 2019;38:1235-45; with permission.)

to assess lung function before LTx was done in 2 cases only. Total ischemic time was 678 ± 132 minutes. PGD grade 3 was observed in 2 cases (25%). One-month, 1-year, and 5-year survival rates were 100%, 87.5%, and 87.5%, respectively.

The Toronto group reported in 2020 the first North American series with 5 uDCD LTx.[11] Of 44 potential donors, family consent was obtained in 30 cases (68%) while 16 donors were evaluated on-site and 14 were considered for transplantation pending EVLP assessment with a utilization rate of

35.7%. A simple method of in-situ lung inflation was used for protection from warm ischemic injury with a mean time of 2.8 hours. No PGD-3 was observed at 24, 48, or 72 hours after transplant. Median ICU stay was 5 days (2–78 days), and median hospital stay was 17 days (8–100 days). The 30-day mortality was 0%. Four of 5 patients are alive at a median of 651 days (121–1254 days) with preserved lung function. This study demonstrates the proof of concept and the potential for uDCD lung donation using a simple donor intervention.

In summary, logistics for organ recovery from uDCD are challenging. Simple donor intervention with in-situ lung inflation is effective to protect the lungs during the asystolic interval. Survival after uDCD-LTx appears somewhat lower compared with cDCD and DBD. However, with improved in-situ preservation techniques and ex-situ evaluation of the pulmonary graft before transplantation, survival is expected to improve with more experience in years to come.

BARRIERS TO DCD LTx

Organ donation after circulatory death still has a large potential in many regions.[56,57] However, several barriers have been recognized that impact the use of DCD organs including the absence of national ethical, professional, and legal frameworks to address both public and professional concerns with all aspects of the DCD pathway. Recently, an International Collaborative Statement was published with the aim to expand the use of cDCD organs worldwide.[52] The statement addresses 3 fundamental aspects: (1) the process is described of determining a prognosis that justifies the WLST, a decision that should be made before and independent of any consideration of organ donation and in which transplant professionals must not participate; (2) the permanent cessation of circulation to the brain is the standard to determine death by circulatory criteria. Death may be declared after an elapsed observation period of 5 min without circulation to the brain, which confirms that the absence of circulation to the brain is permanent; and (3) the statement highlights the value of perfusion repair for increasing the success of cDCD organ transplantation, either by using cDCD protocols for in-situ or ex-situ perfusion consistent with the practice of each country.

In addition, organ yield from cDCD in countries with existing DCD legislation is substantially lower compared with DBD. Several factors may explain this difference: the belief until recently that the heart from a DCD cannot be successfully transplanted, feared lower organ quality related to the additional warm ischemic insult, and the uncertainty that cDCD may not arrest within the foreseen period after WLST. Donor scoring systems that reliably predict progression to asystole or that prognosticate early graft function based on measures of lung quality, ischemic time, and so forth, would be invaluable to increase confidence in successful recovery and transplantation.[58]

Large audits suggest there remains a large untapped pool of DCD lungs that may yet further dramatically increase lung transplant numbers. In a retrospective chart review, Chancellor and colleagues from the University of Virginia analyzed the potential for lung DCD in a rural referral hospital identifying all in-hospital mortalities from August 2014 to June 2015. Of a total of 857 deaths, 85 patients qualified for DCD lung donation.[59] Wide differences in lung yield also exist between different continents and countries. Although the overall utilization of lungs for transplant in the United States is relatively high (in 2018: 7.8 lung donors per million population [PMP] compared with 8.9 in Australia, 2.8 in the United Kingdom, 5.2 in the Netherlands, 8.0 in Spain, and 10.1 in Belgium), the contribution of DCD lungs in the United States, however, is poor (in 2018: 0.4 compared with 2.3 in Australia, 0.6 in the United Kingdom, 1.8 in the Netherlands, 1.4 in Spain, and 2.6 in Belgium).[60] A recent study investigated predictors of nonuse of DCD lungs based on data from the United Network for Organ Sharing in the United States between 2005 and 2019.[61] Of 30,916 DCD lungs, only 3.7% (1158) were used for transplantation and 72.8% were discarded primarily due to poor organ function. Consent was not requested in 8.4% with DCD being the leading reason (73.4%). The authors concluded that the discard rate was associated with potentially modifiable predonation factors, including organ procurement organizations' consenting behavior, and donor factors, including hypoxemia. Interventions to increase consent and standardize DCD donor management, including selective use of EVLP in the setting of hypoxemia, may increase the use of available lungs.

DCD lung donor management issues are equally important. EVLP as an assessment and lung resuscitation tool and donor lung quality biomarkers all have future promise for the clinical field.[62]

Barriers to uDCD are of a logistical and ethical-legal nature, as well as arising from the lack of confidence in the outcomes of transplants from uDCD donors. The procedure needs to be designed to reduce and limit the impact of the prolonged warm ischemia inherent to the uDCD process, and to deal with the ethical issues that this practice poses: termination of advanced life-saving cardiopulmonary resuscitation versus the extension of support solely for organ preservation, optimal timing for family donation discussions, criteria for the determination of death, or the use of NRP for in-situ preservation of organs.

SUMMARY

The continuing shortage of pulmonary grafts from potential DBDs has led to a resurgence of interest in lungs from DCDs. The largest experience worldwide comes with LTx from controlled DCDs while the use of lungs from uncontrolled DCDs is currently limited to small series. No apparent differences in outcome between DBD versus cDCD-LTx have been found in the large ISHLT DCD Registry and in 2 systematic reviews and meta-analyses.

Donor lungs are less vulnerable to the processes of combined warm and cold ischemia that threatens the viability of other DCD organs. New techniques for in-situ lung preservation with NRP in cDCD or alveolar recruitment in uDCD and ex-situ resuscitation and assessment with EVLP have become available to select donor lungs of good quality before transplantation.

There is still a large untapped pool of DCD lungs that may yet further dramatically increase LTx numbers. Several potentially modifiable barriers have been recognized that impact the use of organs from DCDs, including the absence of national ethical, professional, and legal frameworks to address both public and professional concerns. Further efforts are needed in many countries to address all these aspects of the DCD pathway if we want to increase the potential of this underutilized lung donor pool.

CLINICS CARE POINTS

- Donor lungs from DCDs should be selected according to the same standard and extended criteria as currently used for DBDs.

- Lungs from cDCDs should always be offered by the organ procurement organization and maximally evaluated by the procurement team on site.

- In contrast to retrieval of abdominal organs from cDCDs, there is no need to rush with lung procurement. A good suction device and scissors are the only instruments needed by the surgeon to safely introduce the pulmonary artery cannula and to vent the left heart upon the start of pulmoplegia. Lungs can be thoroughly inspected on the backtable following retrieval.

- In case of doubt, lung quality can be further assessed with EVLP to increase the confidence before acceptance.

- Cross-clamp times of DCD lungs are expected to be somewhat longer as final acceptance for transplantation with or without EVLP occurs at a later stage during the retrieval process.

DISCLOSURE

D. Van Raemdonck was supported by the Broere Charitable Foundation. L.J. Ceulemans was supported by a named chair at the KU Leuven University funded by Medtronic and a postdoctoral research fellowship granted by the University Hospitals Leuven (KOOR). A. Neyrinck was supported by a C2 research grant from KU Leuven University.

D. Van Raemdonck and G. Snell developed the design of the article and wrote the original draft. L.J. Ceulemans, A. Neyrinck, and B. Levvey reviewed the original manuscript as experts in the field. All authors approved the final version to be published.

REFERENCES

1. Chambers DC, Zuckermann A, Cherikh WS, et al. The International Thoracic Organ Transplant Registry of the International Society for Heart and Lung Transplantation: 37th adult lung transplantation report - 2020; focus on deceased donor characteristics. J Heart Lung Transplant 2020;39:1016–27.
2. Van Raemdonck D, Ceulemans LJ, Neyrinck A. Donor selection and management. In: Christie JD, editor. Chapter 11. Lung Transplant. 2nd edition. In: Janes S, editor. Encyclopedia of respiratory medicine. 2nd edition. Academic Press; 2021.
3. Ceulemans LJ, Inci I, Van Raemdonck D. Lung donation after circulatory death. Curr Opin Organ Transpl 2019;24:288–96.
4. Kootstra G, Daemen JH, Oomen AP. Categories of non-heart-beating donors. Transpl Proc 1995;27: 2893–4.
5. Evrard, Belgian Working Group on DCD National Protocol. Belgian modified classification of Maastricht for donors after circulatory death. Transpl Proc 2014;46:3138–42.
6. Thuong M, Ruiz A, Evrard P, et al. New classification of donation after circulatory death donors definitions and terminology. Transpl Int 2016;29:749–59.

7. Orens J, Boehler A, de Perrot M, et al. A review of lung transplant donor acceptability criteria. J Heart Lung Transpl 2003;22:1183–200.

8. Gomez-de-Antonio D, Campo-Canaveral JL, Crowley S, et al. Clinical lung transplantation from uncontrolled nonheart-beating donors revisited. J Heart Lung Transpl 2012;31:349–53.

9. Valdivia D, Gomez de Antonio D, Hoyoz L, et al. Expanding the horizons: uncontrolled donors after circulatory death for lung transplantation – first comparison with brain death donors. Clin Transplant 2019;33:e13561.

10. Suberviola B, Mons R, Ballesteros MA, et al. Excellent long-term outcome with lungs obtained from uncontrolled donation after circulatory death. Am J Transplant 2019;19:1195–201.

11. Healey A, Watanabe Y, Milis C, et al. Initial lung transplantation experience with uncontrolled donation after cardiac death in North America. Am J Transplant 2020;20:1574–81.

12. Musso V, Mendogni P, Scaravilli V, et al. Extended-criteria uncontrolled DCD donor for a fragile recipient: a case report about a challenging yet successful lung transplantation. Int J Surg Case Rep 2020;77S-(Suppl):S67–71.

13. Palleschi A, Rosso L, Ruggeri GM, et al. Overcoming the limits of reconditioning: seventeen hours of ex-vivo lung perfusion (EVLP) with successful transplantation from uncontrolled circulatory death donor. Transplantation 2021;105(12):2620–4.

14. Egan TM, Lambert CJ Jr, Reddick R, et al. A strategy to increase the donor pool: use of cadaver lungs for transplantation. Ann Thorac Surg 1991;52:1113–20.

15. Heylen L, Jochmans I, Samuel U, et al. The duration of asystolic ischemia determines the risk of graft failure after circulatory-dead donor kidney transplantation: a Eurotransplant cohort study. Am J Transplant 2018;18:881–9.

16. Coffey JC, Wanis KN, Monbaliu D, et al. The influence of functional warm ischemia time on DCD liver transplant recipients' outcomes. Clin Transplant 2017;31.

17. Song C, Al-Mehdi AB, Fisher AB. An immediate endothelial cell signaling response to lung ischemia. Am J Physiol Lung Cell Mol Physiol 2001;281:L993–1000.

18. Cypel M, Levvey B, Van Raemdonck D, et al. International Society for Heart and Lung Transplantation donation after circulatory death registry report. J Heart Lung Transpl 2015;34:1278–82.

19. Levvey B, Keshavjee S, Cypel M, et al. Influence of lung donor agonal and warm ischemic times on early mortality: analyses from the ISHLT DCD Lung Transplant Registry. J Heart Lung Transpl 2019;38:26–34.

20. Qaqish R, Watanabe Y, Hoetzenecker K, et al. Impact of donor time to cardiac arrest in lung donation after circulatory death. J Thorac Cardiovasc Surg 2021;161:1546–55.

21. Reeb J, Keshavjee S, Cypel M. Successful lung transplantation from a donation after cardiocirculatory death donor taking more than 120 min to cardiac arrest after withdrawal of life support therapies. J Heart Lung Transpl 2016;35:258–9.

22. Donahoe LL, Kato T, Healey A, et al. Successful lung transplantation from lungs procured 12 hours after withdrawal of life-sustaining therapy: changing the paradigm of controlled DCD donors? J Heart Lung Transpl 2021;40:1021.

23. Okahara S, Levvey B, McDonald M, et al. An audit of lung donor pool: optimal current donation strategies and the potential of novel time-extended donation after circulatory death donation. Heart Lung Circ 2021.

24. Kon AA, Shepard EK, Sederstrom NO, et al. Defining futile and potentially inappropriate interventions: a policy statement from the society of critical care medicine ethics committee. Crit Care Med 2016;44:1769–74.

25. Reynolds S, Cooper AB, McKneally M. Withdrawing life-sustaining treatment: ethical considerations. Thorac Surg Clin 2005;15:469–80.

26. Manara A. Bespoke end-of-life decision making in ICU: has the tailor got the right measurements? Crit Care Med 2015;43:909–10.

27. Munshi L, Dhanani S, Shemie SD, et al. Predicting time to death after withdrawal of life-sustaining treatment in potential donors after cardiac death. Crit Care Med 2012;40:1014–28.

28. Wind J, Snoeijs MGJ, Brugman CA, et al. Prediction of time of death after withdrawal of life-sustaining treatment in potential donors after cardiac death. Crit Care Med 2012;40:766–9.

29. Chan JD, Treece PD, Engelbergh RA, et al. Narcotic and benzodiazepine use after withdrawal of life support: association with time to death. Chest 2004;126:286–93.

30. Epker JL, Bakker J, Kompanje EJ. The use of opioids and sedatives and time until death after withdrawing mechanical ventilation and vasoactive drugs in a dutch intensive care unit. Anesth Analg 2011;112:628–34.

31. Ledoux D, Delbouille MH, Deroover A, et al. Does comfort therapy during controlled donation after circulatory death shorten the life of potential donors? Clin Transpl 2014;28:47–51.

32. Copeland H, Hayanga JWA, Neyrinck A, et al. Donor heart and lung procurement: a consensus statement. J Heart Lung Transpl 2020;39:501–17.

33. Gardiner D, Wind T, Cole B, et al. European vignettes in donation after circulatory death. Prog Transpl 2017;27:286–90.

34. Van Raemdonck D, Keshavjee S, Levvey B, et al. Donation after circulatory death in lung transplantation - five-year follow-up from ISHLT registry. J Heart Lung Transpl 2019;38:1235–45.

35. Steen S, Sjöberg T, Pierre L, et al. Transplantation of lungs from a nonheart-beating donor. Lancet 2001; 357:825–9.

36. Valenza F, Citerio G, Palleschi A, et al. Successful transplantation of lungs from an uncontrolled donor after circulatory death preserved in situ by alveolar recruitment maneuvers and assessed by ex vivo lung perfusion. Am J Transplant 2016;16:1312–8.

37. Machuca TN, Mercier O, Collaud S, et al. Lung transplantation with donation after circulatory determination of death donors and the impact of ex vivo lung perfusion. Am J Transplant 2015;15:993–1002.

38. Cypel M, Yeung JC, Donahoe L, et al. Normothermic ex vivo lung perfusion: does the indication impact organ utilization and patient outcomes after transplantation? J Thorac Cardiovasc Surg 2020;159: 346–55.

39. Bozso SJ, Nagendran J. Life after death: breathing life into lung transplantation from donation after circulatory death donors. Am J Transplant 2017;17: 2507–8.

40. Moradiellos J, Naranjo JM, Cordoba M, et al. Clinical lung transplantation after ex vivo evaluation of uncontrolled non heart-beating donor lungs: initial experience. J Heart Lung Transpl 2011;30:S38.

41. O'Neill S, Srinivasa S, Callaghan CJ, et al. Novel organ perfusion and preservation strategies in transplantation - where are we going in the UK? Transplantation 2020;104:1813–24.

42. Oniscu GC, Siddique A, Dark J. Dual temperature multi-organ recovery from a Maastricht category III donor after circulatory death. Am J Transplant 2014;14:2181.

43. Miñambres E, Ruiz P, Ballesteros MA, et al. Combined lung and liver procurement in controlled donation after circulatory death using normothermic abdominal perfusion. Initial experience in two Spanish centers. Am J Transplant 2020;20:231–40.

44. Tanaka S, Luis Campo-Cañaveral de la Cruz J, Crowley Carrasco S, et al. Effect on the donor lungs of using abdominal normothermic regional perfusion in controlled donation after circulatory death. Eur J Cardiothorac Surg 2021;60:590–7.

45. Palleschi A, Tosi D, Rosso L, et al. Successful preservation and transplant of warm ischemic lungs from donors after circulatory death by prolonged in situ ventilation during normothermic regional perfusion of abdominal organs. Interact Cardiovasc Surg 2019;29:699–705.

46. Zanierato M, Dondossola P, Palleschi A, et al. Donation after circulatory death: possible strategies for in-situ organ preservation. Minerva Anesthesiol 2020; 86:984–91.

47. Tsui SSL, Oniscu GC. Extending normothermic regional perfusion to the thorax in donors after circulatory death. Curr Opin Organ Transpl 2017;22: 245–50.

48. Vandendriessche K, Tchana-Sato V, Ledoux D, et al. Transplantation of donor hearts after circulatory death using normothermic regional perfusion and cold storage preservation. Eur J Cardiothorac Surg 2021; 60(4):813–9.

49. Urban M, Castleberry AW, Markin NW, et al. Successful lung transplantation with graft recovered after thoracoabdominal normothermic perfusion from donor after circulatory death. Am J Transplant 2021. https://doi.org/10.1111/ajt.16806.

50. American College of Physicians. Ethics, determination of death, and organ transplantation in normothermic regional perfusion (NRP) with controlled donation after circulatory determination of death (cDCD): American College of Physicians statement of concern. Available at: https://www.acponline.org/acp_policy/policies/ethics_determination_of_death_and_organ_transplantation_in_nrp_2021.pdf. Accessed July 21, 2021.

51. McGee A, Gardiner D, Murphy P. Determination of death in donation after circulatory death: an ethical propriety. Curr Opin Organ Transpl 2018;23:114–9.

52. Dominguez-Gil B, Ascher N, Capron AM, et al. Expanding controlled donation after the circulatory determination of death: statement from an international collaborative. Intensive Care Med 2021;47: 265–81.

53. Manara A, Shemie SD, Large S, et al. Maintaining the permanence principle for death during in situ normothermic regional perfusion for donation after circulatory death organ recovery: a United Kingdom and Canadian proposal. Am J Transplant 2020;20: 2017–25.

54. Krutsinger D, Reed RM, Blevins A, et al. Lung transplantation from donation after cardiocirculatory death: a systematic review and meta-analysis. J Heart Lung Transpl 2015;34:675–84.

55. Palleschi A, Rosso L, Musso V, et al. Lung transplantation from donation after controlled cardiocirculatory death. Systematic review and meta-analysis. Transpl Rev (Orlando) 2020;34:100513.

56. Smith M, Dominguez-Gil B, Greer DM, et al. Organ donation after circulatory death: current status and future potential. Intensive Care Med 2019;45: 310–21.

57. Rakhra SS, Opdam HI, Gladkis L, et al. Untapped potential in Australian hospitals for organ donation after circulatory death. Med J Aust 2017;207: 294–301.

58. Okahara S, Levvey B, McDonald M, et al. Improving the predictability of time to death in controlled donation after circulatory death lung donors. Transpl Int 2021;34:906–15.

59. Chancellor WZ, Charles EJ, Mehaffey JH, et al. Expanding the donor lung pool: how many donations after circulatory death organs are we missing? J Surg Res 2018;223:58–63.

60. European Directorate for the Quality of Medicines & Health Care. Newsletter Transplant. International figures on donation and transplantation 2018, vol. 24, 2019. Available at: https://www.edqm.eu/en/news/just-released-newsletter-transplant-2019. Accessed July 21, 2021.

61. Choi AY, Jawitz OK, Raman V, et al. Predictors of nonuse of donation after circulatory death lung allografts. J Thorac Cardiovasc Surg 2021;161:458–66.

62. Snell GI, Levvey BJ, Levin K, et al. Donation after brain death versus donation after circulatory death: lung donor management issues. Semin Respir Crit Care Med 2018;39:138–47.

Centralized Organ Recovery and Reconditioning Centers

Amit Bery, MD[a],*, Aadil Ali, PhD[b], Marcelo Cypel, MD, MSc, FRCSC[b],
Daniel Kreisel, MD, PhD[c,d]

KEYWORDS

- Lung transplantation • Organ donation • Specialized donor care facility • *Ex vivo* lung perfusion

KEY POINTS

- Compared with the traditional model, the SDCF model provides highly efficient and cost-effective donor management and organ recovery, resulting in improved organ yield and shorter ischemic times.
- The SDCF model results in decreased travel and more daytime transplant operations improving the safety of the organ recovery process and reducing surgeon burnout.
- EVLP allows for increased utilization of extended criteria donor lungs, and the ability of this modality to better prepare donor lungs with interventions such as anti-inflammatory, anticell death, and antiviral therapies before transplantation is currently under investigation.
- Centralized EVLP facilities have the potential to increase transplant volumes and utilization of extended criteria donor organs for smaller transplant programs in specified geographic regions.

INTRODUCTION

Lung transplantation is the only treatment option for end-stage pulmonary disease. Over the last decade, there has been a 50% increase in the volume of lung transplants and a 60% increase in lung donors.[1] Waitlist mortality remains high despite improvements in donor management and changes in organ allocation systems.[1] These challenges have resulted in increased attention to improving efficiency and decreasing the cost of donor management. This increased focus has resulted in the creation of 2 separate models of donor management and organ recovery: the traditional and the specialized donor care facility (SDCF) models.[2–4]

Donors are traditionally managed in the hospital where brain death is declared with the help of coordinators from the regional organ procurement organization (OPO).[3–5] In this model, brain-dead donors are frequently given lower priority, resulting in delays in evaluation, management, and operating room (OR) access.[3,4,6] Donor organ recovery scheduling requires coordination with surgical teams from multiple recipient hospitals, which can also lead to delays.[3] At the time of recovery, transplant surgeons must travel from recipient to donor hospitals to carry out organ recovery operations in unfamiliar facilities with inexperienced staff.[3,5,7] Challenges such as these have resulted in suboptimal donor organ recovery.[3,4]

[a] Division of Pulmonary and Critical Care Medicine, Department of Medicine, Washington University School of Medicine, 660 South Euclid Avenue, Campus Box 8052, St Louis, MO 63110, USA; [b] Toronto Lung Transplant Program, Division of Thoracic Surgery, Department of Surgery, University Health Network, University of Toronto, Toronto General Hospital, 200 Elizabeth Street, 9N969, Toronto, Ontario M5G 2C4, Canada; [c] Department of Surgery, Washington University School of Medicine, Campus Box 8234, 660 South Euclid Avenue, St Louis, MO 63110, USA; [d] Department of Pathology & Immunology, Washington University School of Medicine, Campus Box 8234, 660 South Euclid Avenue, St Louis, MO 63110, USA
* Corresponding author.
E-mail address: amit.bery@wustl.edu

Thorac Surg Clin 32 (2022) 167–174
https://doi.org/10.1016/j.thorsurg.2021.11.003
1547-4127/22/© 2021 Elsevier Inc. All rights reserved.

One OPO (Mid-America Transplant [MTS], St. Louis, MO), supported by its transplant centers, founded the first SDCF in the United States in 2001.[4,8] Evaluation of the initial experience, which included the transfer of 25 hemodynamically stable donors within a 20-mile radius to ORs in the MTS corporate headquarters, showed comparable mean organ yields and graft outcomes with a significant reduction in cost.[8] In 2008, a free-standing, 2-bed intensive care unit (ICU) was built and equipped with its own OR, tissue recovery room, cardiac catheterization suite, laboratory, and computed tomography (CT) scanner. Owing to a significant increase in the number of brain-dead donors, a sophisticated 6-bed ICU was built in 2018.

In the SDCF model, a high-volume center delivers efficient, timely, and cost-effective donor management and organ recovery. Donors are transferred to the SDCF early after authorization (mean 7 hours) with a median ICU care of 36 hours at the SDCF. Transportation has proven to be safe with only 2 cardiac arrests occurring in transit during the transfer of more than 2000 brain-dead donors. As of 2021, 12 OPOs in the United States along with centers in Spain and Canada have used some form of an SDCF to provide donor care.[9,10] Since 2001, multiple studies have highlighted the benefits of the SDCF model.[4,5,11–14]

COMPARISON OF ORGAN RECOVERY MODELS
Medical Expertise Required

In the traditional model, donors are managed by providers at the acute care hospital where brain death occurs. These providers care for a wide variety of critically ill patients simultaneously and generally lack experience with optimal donor management. This model also requires the presence of OR staff and anesthesia providers who may be inexperienced with donor organ recovery. In the SDCF model, specialized donor coordinators provide ICU-level care under the supervision of a physician medical director, who is trained in critical care.[3,4] These donor coordinators are nurses who have a minimum of 2 years of ICU experience and singularly provide donor care.[4] By using a team experienced in donor management, the SDCF can use protocolized care to optimize donors before organ recovery without the delays and variabilities in care experienced in large ICUs that look after many critically ill patients.[4,6] Donor coordinators perform bronchoscopies, lung ultrasounds, central/arterial line insertions, and liver biopsies at the SDCF. In addition, these coordinators continue to manage the donor in the OR during organ recovery, thereby eliminating the need for physician anesthesia care.[3]

Evaluation, Management, and Recovery

In the traditional model, donor evaluation requires utilization of hospital resources in competition for scheduling with other critically ill patients. The SDCF is equipped to perform cardiac catheterizations, bronchoscopies, echocardiographies, radiological studies (roentgenogram, CT), blood bank evaluations, and other laboratory studies.[3] In addition, the SDCF uses expert consultants (pathologists, radiologists, cardiologists, etc) in the form of independent contractors to complete the diagnostic evaluation of donors. Generally, these independent contractors can be present on-site to complete urgent evaluations, though in some cases, studies performed at the SDCF can be interpreted by the contracting physicians remotely. Thus, the SDCF can streamline donor evaluation by concentrating all investigations on-site, eliminating the competition for limited resources that exists at acute care hospitals.[3,9]

After brain death, physiologic changes in the donor can result in mucus plugging, atelectasis, neurogenic pulmonary edema, aspiration, and ventilator-induced lung injury.[15–20] Indeed, a significant proportion of brain-dead donors can develop acute lung injury that precludes lung utilization.[5,17,19,21] Several studies have suggested that protocolized management of donors can improve lung utilization rates.[5,11,14,19,21–23] The SDCF model is particularly suited for the development and implementation of protocolized donor management.[5,11,14,24–26] Donor coordinators use protocolized care to optimize donors without the inconsistency in care experienced in the traditional model at acute care hospitals. Prior investigations have shown higher mean organ yields and increased use of extended criteria donors and drug overdose donors in the SDCF model compared with the traditional model.[4,27] In addition, SDCF ORs are used exclusively for donor organ recovery and staffed by experienced donor coordinators, which streamlines scheduling and increases the efficiency of recovery.[3–5] Indeed, donor recovery at the SDCF has been shown to be more efficient with a reduction in cold ischemia times.[3]

Cost

The regional OPO becomes responsible for the cost of donor management and organ recovery after authorization for organ donation is obtained. In the traditional model, donors are managed by critical care physicians while in the ICU and by anesthesia providers during organ recovery in the OR. Hospital charges for donor evaluation, management, and organ recovery are billed at a premium to the OPO.[4,9] The OPO subsequently bills transplant centers an organ acquisition charge (OAC), which represents an adjusted average annual cost of donor care.[4,9]

The SDCF model requires a significant start-up cost of building a facility capable of providing donor care and performing organ recovery. This cost can be offset by the increased efficiency of the donor care provided. At the SDCF, all donor evaluation and management can be provided by donor coordinators, limiting the need for on-site physician support and reducing cost.[4,8,9] In addition, coordinators manage donors in the OR during organ recovery, eliminating the need for anesthesia provider support and further reducing cost.[4,8,9] Indeed, prior evaluation of the SDCF model has shown a greater than 50% reduction in the cost of organ recovery over a 5-year period compared with the OPOs utilizing the traditional model.[4] In this evaluation, OPOs utilizing the traditional model displayed increasing OACs while the SDCF was able to sustain a stable OAC over the 5-year period.[4] Furthermore, economic modeling has shown that universal adoption of the SDCF model in the United States could increase organ transplants while significantly reducing cost.[9] This finding was particularly impactful for thoracic organ transplantations, estimating an additional 156 transplants and nearly $25 million reduction in cost.[9]

IMPACT ON SURGEON BURNOUT

High-stress procedures, long and unpredictable working hours, significant call responsibilities, and a requirement for frequent travel contribute to feelings of emotional exhaustion, inefficacy, and cynicism associated with burnout among transplant surgeons.[28–31] The SDCF model addresses some of the major components that drive transplant surgeon burnout.[32]

In the traditional model, multiple recovery teams coordinate to schedule an OR time and travel to the donor hospital for organ procurement. Travel to acute care hospitals for donor organ recovery can be scheduled at odd hours, to remote locations, and in a wide range of weather conditions.[7,33–35] Such organ recovery exposes procurement teams to significant risk with over 30 travel-related deaths since the first kidney transplant in 1954.[3,7,34,35] The risks associated with travel for organ procurement can be reduced in the SDCF model. Over a 10-year period, one center reduced travel for nonlocal donors within

the OPO's donation service area by 93%.[3] In addition, some centers are utilizing local surgical teams for organ recovery, though most procurements continue to be performed by the accepting center's recovery team.

In the SDCF model, scheduling donor organ procurement operations is more efficient allowing both organ recovery and subsequent transplant to be performed during daytime hours.[4,32] Indeed, nighttime operations, both procurements and transplants, have been associated with an increased risk of postoperative complications and recipient mortality.[36–41] Prior studies evaluating the effect of nighttime procedures on lung transplant outcomes have shown an increased risk of airway dehiscence and increased 90-day mortality.[41] A different analysis showed an increased risk of postoperative complications along with decreased 5-year bronchiolitis obliterans syndrome-free and overall survival associated with nighttime operations.[42] By limiting nighttime operations, the SDCF model can not only contribute to improved outcomes but also improve quality of life and reduce burnout among transplant surgeons.[32]

EX VIVO LUNG PERFUSION RESUSCITATION FACILITIES

One other model currently in use is a centralized *ex vivo* lung assessment and repair center. The advent of the normothermic *ex vivo* lung perfusion (EVLP) platform has revolutionized the field of clinical lung transplantation by allowing for an increased utilization of extended criteria donor lungs, which would have otherwise been rejected for the purposes of transplantation.[43] Recognizing the value of this system to increase lung transplant volumes through the broadening of a viable donor pool, usage of EVLP has increasingly become a part of clinical practices in several continents around the world.[44–53] Clinical EVLP can be performed either through the establishment of a single-center program, or by outsourcing the procedure through dedicated EVLP facilities. Single-center EVLP is typically favored based on geographic criteria (small number of transplant centers in a large area), health care system models (in Canada and the United States, EVLP is a reimbursable procedure), and by centers who have established lung transplant research programs. The development of a single-center EVLP program requires technical expertise, initial large capital funding, and infrastructure, and thus, is mostly confined to high-volume transplant centers.

Given that a majority of centers today still perform fewer than 40 lung transplants per year and share a small geographic region, centralization of EVLP through dedicated organ resuscitation facilities is actively being explored to overcome the barrier to entry for these programs.[54] The model for this concept begins with donor lungs being retrieved and transported to a nearby dedicated EVLP facility. Once the lungs arrive at the EVLP center, they are perfused by organ perfusion specialists who follow strict standard operative procedures, and if the organ is deemed suitable for transplantation, it is offered to surrounding centers. The receiving transplant team has excellent access to the lung assessment information via a high-quality video and Web platform. Consultation with EVLP experts is available to transplant teams upon request. Once a recipient hospital has accepted these lungs, they are transported and prepared for transplantation (**Fig. 1**). A proof-of-concept clinical trial (identifier: NCT03641677) evaluating the feasibility of this approach is currently underway in the United States, with dedicated facilities built in Jacksonville, FL, and Baltimore, MD. To date, more than 280 lung assessments have been performed at these facilities with nearly 200 patients being transplanted (data based on personal communication with United Therapeutics Corporation). The emergence of these centralized facilities within appropriate geographic areas rests mainly upon the validation of this model alongside the overcoming of associated regulatory issues. A case report demonstrating the feasibility of "remote EVLP" has been published. In this report, extended criteria donor lungs were procured at a tertiary medical center in Chicago and subsequently flown to Toronto for EVLP evaluation.[55] After evaluation, the lungs were deemed suitable for transplantation and transported back to Chicago for transplantation. Although total ischemic times exceeded 15 hours, no primary graft dysfunction was observed. This is consistent with recent retrospective data which show that greater than 12 hours of preservation can be achieved with the interjection of EVLP during long periods of ischemia.[56]

Establishing these facilities poses several advantages. First, through continuous encounters with higher-risk lungs offered from these facilities, smaller transplant centers will likely be encouraged to transplant extended criteria lungs, which are generally transplanted by large centers at the

present time. Moreover, as noted previously, dedicated EVLP facilities will allow for centralization of expertise in performing these procedures and allow for certain programs to overcome barriers to entry. Together, this may allow for increased transplant volume and utilization rates within these geographic regions. Furthermore, clinical trials examining interventions toward better preparation of donor lungs such as anti-inflammatory, anticell death, and antiviral therapies before transplantation can be conducted at these EVLP facilities.

Cost structures and logistics for these dedicated facilities are still being explored and refined. Different cost models have been proposed, but in general, the cost of performing EVLP at individual centers or at a centralized facility has been compared on a case-by-case basis. However, the latter is not associated with initial capital costs of purchasing EVLP equipment and training of personnel. Furthermore, higher lung utilization rates following EVLP at these facilities increase the ratio of perfusion/transplant optimizing the financial model.

DISCUSSION

Although the SDCF model confers many advantages over the traditional model, barriers to more widespread implementation include a considerable start-up cost, utilization of resources to train donor coordinators, and a minimum donor volume (estimated at 100 donors/y) to maintain cost-effectiveness.[9,10] Some approaches to overcome these barriers include close association with local centers, outsourcing of testing to diminish start-up cost, and gradual growth to establish satisfactory outcomes and rapport with transplant centers.[10] In 2001, only stable, local, brain-dead donors were transferred to the MTS SDCF and only abdominal organs were procured.[8] Donor coordinators were trained over the course of 2 years after which physician oversight was relaxed.[10] Over time, the MTS SDCF demonstrated satisfactory outcomes and built trust with the transplant centers it serviced, allowing it to expand gradually into the comprehensive donor care facility that exists today.

MTS is fortunate to have all the transplant centers it services in one city. Although certain geographic and financial constraints such as large or noncontiguous DSAs, transplant centers

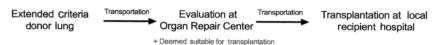

Extended Criteria donor lung → *Transportation* → Evaluation at Organ Repair Center → *Transportation* → Transplantation at local recipient hospital

+ Deemed suitable for transplantation

Fig. 1. Flowchart of EVLP performed at an Organ Repair Center.

separated by hundreds of miles, and locations with expensive real estate have posed challenges, other OPOs have been able to adapt the SDCF model to fit their particular geographic and medical situation. Some OPOs have established free-standing facilities like MTS, whereas others use facilities within a local transplant center or a surgical center. In addition, many OPOs with an SDCF manage donors at the hospital where brain death is declared for the first 24 hours to complete certain evaluations that the SDCF may not be equipped to perform, such as right and left cardiac catheterizations. A recent evaluation suggests that 38 OPOs have sufficient donor volume to support an SDCF from a cost-effectiveness perspective.[9] To date, 12 of 57 OPOs have adopted the SDCF model in some form.[9,10] However, data from SDCFs other than MTS remain limited to date.

OPOs are regulated by the Centers for Medicare and Medicaid Services (CMS) and the Organ Procurement and Transplantation Network (OPTN). As an example, CMS and OPTN prohibit SDCFs from managing living donors, and thus donation after cardiac death is not possible in the SDCF model at the present time. Although these organizations regulate OPOs, and therefore the SDCFs they operate, no consensus guidelines currently exist that specifically address the establishment or management of SDCFs.

Alternative strategies for reducing OAC have been proposed, including models of reducing travel, standardization of organ retrieval teams, and streamlining the donor evaluation process.[4,5,7] Unfortunately, implementation of these strategies has been largely unsuccessful to date because of challenges with organization and financial deterrents.[4,5,7,34,57,58]

For lungs that do not meet standard criteria for immediate transplantation, or lungs that require increased preservation time due to logistics of organ allocation, centralized EVLP centers can add a major value to transplant centers aiming at safely increasing lung transplant activities. This model is currently experiencing growth in the United States and is likely to expand to other countries in the future.

SUMMARY

The development of centralized organ recovery and reconditioning centers has been driven by an increased focus on improving efficiency and decreasing costs associated with donor management and organ recovery. The SDCF model uses a free-standing facility to provide highly efficient and cost-effective donor care. This model has been associated with improved organ yield and

shorter ischemic times. In addition, the SDCF model is associated with decreased travel and fewer nighttime operations, which can not only improve outcomes but also enhance the surgeons' quality of life and reduce burnout. EVLP has been shown to improve utilization of extended criteria donor lungs and ongoing clinical trials are evaluating the role of dedicated EVLP facilities. Indeed, dedicated EVLP facilities have the potential to centralize expertise associated with this modality and improve utilization rates and volumes for smaller-volume centers. These models are increasingly being used in the United States to combat the ongoing donor organ shortage and decrease waitlist mortality.

DISCLOSURE

M. Cypel is a founder of XOR Labs Toronto and a consultant for Lung Bioengineering Inc. D. Kreisel has a pending patent entitled "Compositions and methods for detecting CCR2 receptors" (application number 15/611,577). DK is supported by National Institutes of Health grants 1P01AI116501, R01HL094601, R01HL151078, The Cystic Fibrosis Foundation, and The Foundation for Barnes-Jewish Hospital. AB is supported by National Institutes of Health grant 5T32HL007317-44.

REFERENCES

1. Valapour M, Lehr CJ, Skeans MA, et al. OPTN/SRTR 2019 annual data report: lung. Am J Transplant 2021;21(Suppl 2):441–520. https://doi.org/10.1111/ajt.16495.

2. United Network for Organ Sharing - Transplant Trends. United network for organ sharing. https://unos.org/data/transplant-trends/. Accessed June 10, 2021.

3. Doyle MBM, Vachharajani N, Wellen JR, et al. A novel organ donor facility: a decade of experience with liver donors. Am J Transplant 2014;14(3):615–20. https://doi.org/10.1111/ajt.12607.

4. Doyle M, Subramanian V, Vachharajani N, et al. Organ donor recovery performed at an organ procurement organization-based facility is an effective way to minimize organ recovery costs and increase organ yield. J Am Coll Surg 2016;222(4):591–600. https://doi.org/10.1016/j.jamcollsurg.2015.12.032.

5. Chang SH, Kreisel D, Marklin GF, et al. Lung focused resuscitation at a specialized donor care facility improves lung procurement rates. Ann Thorac Surg 2018;105(5):1531–6. https://doi.org/10.1016/j.athoracsur.2017.12.009.

6. Bollinger RR, Heinrichs DR, Seem DL, et al. UNOS Council for Organ Availability. United Network for Organ Sharing. Organ procurement organization

(OPO), best practices. Clin Transplant 2001; 15(Suppl 6):16–21. https://doi.org/10.1034/j.1399-0012.2001.00003.x.

7. Lynch RJ, Mathur AK, Hundley JC, et al. Improving organ procurement practices in Michigan. Am J Transplant 2009;9(10):2416–23. https://doi.org/10.1111/j.1600-6143.2009.02784.x.

8. Jendrisak MD, Hruska K, Wagner J, et al. Cadaveric-donor organ recovery at a hospital-independent facility. Transplantation 2002;74(7):978–82. https://doi.org/10.1097/00007890-200210150-00014.

9. Gauthier JM, Doyle MBM, Chapman WC, et al. Economic evaluation of the specialized donor care facility for thoracic organ donor management. J Thorac Dis 2020;12(10):5709–17. https://doi.org/10.21037/jtd-20-1575.

10. Bery A, Marklin G, Itoh A, et al. The Specialized Donor Care Facility (SDCF) model and advances in management of thoracic organ donors. Ann Thorac Surg 2021. https://doi.org/10.1016/j.athoracsur.2020.12.026.

11. Marklin GF, Klinkenberg WD, Helmers B, et al. A stroke volume-based fluid resuscitation protocol decreases vasopressor support and may increase organ yield in brain-dead donors. Clin Transplant 2020; 34(2):e13784. https://doi.org/10.1111/ctr.13784.

12. Dhar R, Cotton C, Coleman J, et al. Comparison of high- and low-dose corticosteroid regimens for organ donor management. J Crit Care 2013;28(1):111.e1–7. https://doi.org/10.1016/j.jcrc.2012.04.015.

13. Gauthier JM, Bierhals AJ, Liu J, et al. Chest computed tomography imaging improves potential lung donor assessment. J Thorac Cardiovasc Surg 2019;157(4): 1711–8.e1. https://doi.org/10.1016/j.jtcvs.2018.11.038.

14. Marklin GF, O'Sullivan C, Dhar R. Ventilation in the prone position improves oxygenation and results in more lungs being transplanted from organ donors with hypoxemia and atelectasis. J Heart Lung Transplant 2021;40(2):120–7. https://doi.org/10.1016/j.healun.2020.11.014.

15. Kotloff RM, Blosser S, Fulda GJ, et al. Management of the potential organ donor in the ICU: Society of Critical Care Medicine/American College of Chest Physicians/Association of Organ Procurement Organizations Consensus Statement. Crit Care Med 2015;43(6):1291–325. https://doi.org/10.1097/CCM.0000000000000958.

16. Anwar ASMT, Lee J-M. Medical management of brain-dead organ donors. Acute Crit Care 2019;34(1): 14–29. https://doi.org/10.4266/acc.2019.00430.

17. Avlonitis VS, Fisher AJ, Kirby JA, et al. Pulmonary transplantation: the role of brain death in donor lung injury. Transplantation 2003;75(12):1928–33. https://doi.org/10.1097/01.TP.0000066351.87480.9E.

18. Mascia L, Mastromauro I, Viberti S, et al. Management to optimize organ procurement in brain dead donors. Minerva Anestesiol 2009;75(3):125–33.

19. Venkateswaran RV, Patchell VB, Wilson IC, et al. Early donor management increases the retrieval rate of lungs for transplantation. Ann Thorac Surg 2008;85(1):278–86. https://doi.org/10.1016/j.athoracsur.2007.07.092 [discussion 286].

20. Amado JA, López-Espadas F, Vázquez-Barquero A, et al. Blood levels of cytokines in brain-dead patients: relationship with circulating hormones and acute-phase reactants. Metab Clin Exp 1995;44(6):812–6. https://doi.org/10.1016/0026-0495(95)90198-1.

21. Mascia L, Pasero D, Slutsky AS, et al. Effect of a lung protective strategy for organ donors on eligibility and availability of lungs for transplantation: a randomized controlled trial. JAMA 2010;304(23): 2620–7. https://doi.org/10.1001/jama.2010.1796.

22. Angel LF, Levine DJ, Restrepo MI, et al. Impact of a lung transplantation donor-management protocol on lung donation and recipient outcomes. Am J Respir Crit Care Med 2006;174(6):710–6. https://doi.org/10.1164/rccm.200603-432OC.

23. Gabbay E, Williams TJ, Griffiths AP, et al. Maximizing the utilization of donor organs offered for lung transplantation. Am J Respir Crit Care Med 1999;160(1):265–71. https://doi.org/10.1164/ajrccm.160.1.9811017.

24. Dhar R, Stahlschmidt E, Yan Y, et al. A randomized trial comparing triiodothyronine (T3) with thyroxine (T4) for hemodynamically unstable brain-dead organ donors. Clin Transplant 2019;33(3):e13486. https://doi.org/10.1111/ctr.13486.

25. Dhar R, Stahlschmidt E, Marklin G. A randomized trial of intravenous thyroxine for brain-dead organ donors with impaired cardiac function. Prog Transplant 2020;30(1):48–55. https://doi.org/10.1177/1526924819893295.

26. Dhar R, Stahlschmidt E, Paramesh A, et al. A randomized controlled trial of naloxone for optimization of hypoxemia in lung donors after brain death. Transplantation 2019;103(7):1433–8. https://doi.org/10.1097/TP.0000000000002511.

27. Frye CC, Gauthier JM, Bery A, et al. Donor management using a specialized donor care facility is associated with higher organ utilization from drug overdose donors. Clin Transplant 2021;35(3): e14178. https://doi.org/10.1111/ctr.14178.

28. Karasek R, Brisson C, Kawakami N, et al. The Job Content Questionnaire (JCQ): an instrument for internationally comparative assessments of psychosocial job characteristics. J Occup Health Psychol 1998;3(4): 322–55. https://doi.org/10.1037//1076-8998.3.4.322.

29. Jesse MT, Abouljoud M, Eshelman A. Determinants of burnout among transplant surgeons: a national survey in the United States. Am J Transplant 2015; 15(3):772–8. https://doi.org/10.1111/ajt.13056.

30. Bertges Yost W, Eshelman A, Raoufi M, et al. A national study of burnout among American transplant surgeons. Transplant Proc 2005;37(2):1399–401. https://doi.org/10.1016/j.transproceed.2005.01.055.

31. Pondrom S. Has transplantation lost its luster? Am J Transplant 2011;11(6):1109–10. https://doi.org/10.1111/j.1600-6143.2011.03629.x.

32. Lindemann J, Dageforde LA, Brockmeier D, et al. Organ procurement center allows for daytime liver transplantation with less resource utilization: may address burnout, pipeline, and safety for field of transplantation. Am J Transplant 2019;19(5):1296–304. https://doi.org/10.1111/ajt.15129.

33. Englesbe MJ, Merion RM. The riskiest job in medicine: transplant surgeons and organ procurement travel. Am J Transplant 2009;9(10):2406–15. https://doi.org/10.1111/j.1600-6143.2009.02774.x.

34. Englesbe MJ, Shah S, Cutler JA, et al. Improving organ procurement travel practices in the United States: proceedings from the Michigan Donor Travel Forum. Am J Transplant 2010;10(3):458–63. https://doi.org/10.1111/j.1600-6143.2009.02964.x.

35. Schenk AD, Washburn WK, Adams AB, et al. A survey of current procurement travel practices, accident frequency, and perceptions of safety. Transpl Direct 2019;5(10):e494. https://doi.org/10.1097/TXD.0000000000000942.

36. Sugünes N, Bichmann A, Biernath N, et al. Analysis of the effects of day-time vs. night-time surgery on renal transplant patient outcomes. J Clin Med 2019;8(7). https://doi.org/10.3390/jcm8071051.

37. Ren S-S, Xu L-L, Wang P, et al. Circadian rhythms have effects on surgical outcomes of liver transplantation for patients with hepatocellular carcinoma: a retrospective analysis of 147 cases in a single center. Transplant Proc 2019;51(6):1913–9. https://doi.org/10.1016/j.transproceed.2019.03.033.

38. Hendrikx J, Van Raemdonck D, Pirenne J, et al. Outcome of transplantation performed outside the regular working hours: a systematic review and meta-analysis of the literature. Transpl Rev (Orlando) 2018;32(3):168–77. https://doi.org/10.1016/j.trre.2018.05.001.

39. de Boer J, Van der Bogt K, Putter H, et al. Surgical quality in organ procurement during day and night: an analysis of quality forms. BMJ Open 2018;8(11):e022182. https://doi.org/10.1136/bmjopen-2018-022182.

40. Lonze BE, Parsikia A, Feyssa EL, et al. Operative start times and complications after liver transplantation. Am J Transplant 2010;10(8):1842–9. https://doi.org/10.1111/j.1600-6143.2010.03177.x.

41. George TJ, Arnaoutakis GJ, Merlo CA, et al. Association of operative time of day with outcomes after thoracic organ transplant. JAMA 2011;305(21):2193–9. https://doi.org/10.1001/jama.2011.726.

42. Yang Z, Takahashi T, Gerull WD, et al. Impact of nighttime lung transplantation on outcomes and costs. Ann Thorac Surg 2021;112(1):206–13. https://doi.org/10.1016/j.athoracsur.2020.07.060.

43. Cypel M, Yeung JC, Liu M, et al. Normothermic ex vivo lung perfusion in clinical lung transplantation. N Engl J Med 2011;364(15):1431–40. https://doi.org/10.1056/NEJMoa1014597.

44. Aigner C, Slama A, Hötzenecker K, et al. Clinical ex vivo lung perfusion-pushing the limits: clinical ex vivo lung perfusion. Am J Transplant 2012;12(7):1839–47. https://doi.org/10.1111/j.1600-6143.2012.04027.x.

45. Slama A, Schillab L, Barta M, et al. Standard donor lung procurement with normothermic ex vivo lung perfusion: A prospective randomized clinical trial. J Heart Lung Transplant 2017;36(7):744–53. https://doi.org/10.1016/j.healun.2017.02.011.

46. Sage E, Mussot S, Trebbia G, et al. Lung transplantation from initially rejected donors after ex vivo lung reconditioning: the French experience. Eur J Cardiothorac Surg 2014;46(5):794–9. https://doi.org/10.1093/ejcts/ezu245.

47. Valenza F, Citerio G, Palleschi A, et al. Successful transplantation of lungs from an uncontrolled donor after circulatory death preserved in situ by alveolar recruitment maneuvers and assessed by ex vivo lung perfusion. Am J Transplant 2016;16(4):1312–8. https://doi.org/10.1111/ajt.13612.

48. Wallinder A, Riise GC, Ricksten S-E, et al. Transplantation after ex vivo lung perfusion: a midterm follow-up. J Heart Lung Transplant 2016;35(11):1303–10. https://doi.org/10.1016/j.healun.2016.05.021.

49. Warnecke G, Moradiellos J, Tudorache I, et al. Normothermic perfusion of donor lungs for preservation and assessment with the Organ Care System Lung before bilateral transplantation: a pilot study of 12 patients. Lancet 2012;380(9856):1851–8. https://doi.org/10.1016/S0140-6736(12)61344-0.

50. Boffini M, Ricci D, Bonato R, et al. Incidence and severity of primary graft dysfunction after lung transplantation using rejected grafts reconditioned with ex vivo lung perfusion. Eur J Cardiothorac Surg 2014;46(5):789–93. https://doi.org/10.1093/ejcts/ezu239.

51. Zych B, Popov AF, Stavri G, et al. Early outcomes of bilateral sequential single lung transplantation after ex-vivo lung evaluation and reconditioning. J Heart Lung Transplant 2012;31(3):274–81. https://doi.org/10.1016/j.healun.2011.10.008.

52. Henriksen ISI, Møller-Sørensen H, Møller CH, et al. First Danish experience with ex vivo lung perfusion of donor lungs before transplantation. Dan Med J 2014;61(3):A4809.

53. Zhang ZL, van Suylen V, van Zanden JE, et al. First experience with ex vivo lung perfusion for initially discarded donor lungs in the Netherlands: a single-centre study. Eur J Cardiothorac Surg 2019;55(5):920–6. https://doi.org/10.1093/ejcts/ezy373.

54. Khush KK, Cherikh WS, Chambers DC, et al. The international thoracic organ transplant registry of the international society for heart and lung transplantation: thirty-fifth adult heart transplantation report-2018; focus theme: Multiorgan transplantation.

J Heart Lung Transplant 2018;37(10):1155–68. https://doi.org/10.1016/j.healun.2018.07.022.

55. Wigfield CH, Cypel M, Yeung J, et al. Successful emergent lung transplantation after remote *ex vivo* perfusion optimization and transportation of donor lungs: *ex vivo* lung perfusion transplantation after ECMO. Am J Transplant 2012;12(10):2838–44. https://doi.org/10.1111/j.1600-6143.2012.04175.x.

56. Yeung JC, Krueger T, Yasufuku K, et al. Outcomes after transplantation of lungs preserved for more than 12 h: a retrospective study. Lancet Respir Med 2017;5(2):119–24. https://doi.org/10.1016/S2213-2600(16)30323-X.

57. Abecassis M. Organ acquisition cost centers part I: medicare regulations–truth or consequence. Am J Transplant 2006;6(12):2830–5. https://doi.org/10.1111/j.1600-6143.2006.01582.x.

58. Abecassis M. Organ acquisition cost centers part II: reducing the burden of cost and inventory. Am J Transplant 2006;6(12):2836–40. https://doi.org/10.1111/j.1600-6143.2006.01583.x.

Anesthetic Management During Lung Transplantation – What's New in 2021?

Marek Brzezinski, MD, PhD[a],*, Domagoj Mladinov, MD, PhD[b],
Arne Neyrinck, MD[c]

KEYWORDS

- Lung transplantation • Anesthesiology • Intraoperative management

KEY POINTS

- The risk profile of patients scheduled for LTx has steadily increased driven by survival improvements in high-risk patients.
- There is growing appreciation that many of the postoperative complications, such as primary graft dysfunction (PGD) or extrapulmonary organ failure, have medical rather than surgical origin.
- Lung transplantation (LTx) even in high-risk patients requiring perioperative ECMO support can offer excellent results.

INTRODUCTION

Currently, the intraoperative management of patients requiring lung transplantation (LTx) is defined by 2 trends:

- A steady increase in the risk profile of lung transplant candidates driven by survival improvements in high-risk patients.[1–4] The consequence has been a substantial increase in the acuity of clinical presentations and utilization of advanced bridge-to-transplant (BTT) support.[2] In parallel and equally important, there has been an increase in patients without prior evaluation for LTx presenting with acutely deteriorating respiratory failure requiring BTT support with extracorporeal membrane oxygenation (ECMO) followed by LTx (de novo waitlisting).[2,5] Overall, the growing number of patients on ECMO-BTT may increase the need to use marginal organs,[6,7] and the risk of PGD.
- Growing appreciation that many of the postoperative complications, such as primary graft dysfunction (PGD) or end-organ failures, have medical rather than surgical origin.[8–13] Consequently, the intraoperative management of potential risk factors has received increasing attention.

The goal of this article is to provide a summary of the key concepts of state-of-the-art intraoperative anesthesia management for LTx, with emphasis on hemodynamic stability, prevention of extrapulmonary complications, and preservation of allograft function. The article concludes with a review of the most recent literature on outcomes in the high-risk patient population requiring BTT, a group growing in size and relevance.

[a] Department of Anesthesia and Perioperative Care, University of California, VA Medical Center, Anesthesiology Service (129), 4150 Clement Street, San Francisco, CA 94121, USA; [b] Anesthesia Department of Anesthesiology and Perioperative Medicine University of Alabama at Birmingham JT 923, 619 19th Street South, Birmingham, AL 35249-6810, USA; [c] Department of Anaesthesiology Associate Professor, Department of Cardiovascular Sciences, KU Leuven University Hospitals Leuven Herestraat 49B-3000, Leuven, Belgium
* Corresponding author.
E-mail address: marek.brzezinski@ucsf.edu

Thoracic Surg Clin 32 (2022) 175–184
https://doi.org/10.1016/j.thorsurg.2022.01.001
1547-4127/22/

KEY CONCEPTS OF INTRAOPERATIVE ALLOGRAFT AND EXTRAPULMONAY END-ORGAN PROTECTION

Primary graft dysfunction remains the main allograft complication in the early postoperative period.[14–17] Currently, perioperative risk factors for PGD include the volume of administrated fluids as well as the transfused volume of red blood cells, hypotension, elevated pulmonary pressure and vascular resistance, use of cardiopulmonary bypass (CPB), fraction of inspired oxygen (Fio_2) ≥ 0.4 during reperfusion, donor factors, prolonged ischemia time and anastomotic complications.[10,15,18–23] These risk factors are also shared by many of the perioperative extrapulmonary end-organ complications.[11,24,25] Therefore, the anesthesiologist can actively protect the allograft function and prevent extrapulmonary complications by.

a) Maintaining hemodynamic stability, optimal perfusion, and oxygenation, as well as reducing pulmonary pressure and vascular resistance,
b) Using lung-protective ventilation strategies
c) Avoiding CPB, and
d) Reducing surgical complications and ischemia time (eg, transesophageal echocardiography (TEE) evaluation of pulmonary artery (PA) and venous anastomosis).

MAINTENANCE OF HEMODYNAMIC STABILITY DURING KEY INTRAOPERATIVE PERIODS

Patients undergoing LTx should be considered, *a priori*, at high risk for hypotension, acute right ventricular (RV) failure, hypoxia, and hypercarbia.[11,23–25] This risk is highest during induction, PA clamping, and after allograft implantation.

Management during the induction of general anesthesia and intubation. The overarching goal of induction should be maintaining hemodynamic stability with the surgeon and perfusionist immediately available to provide emergent cardio-circulatory-pulmonary support (eg, sternotomy, cannulation, ECMO). In patients at high risk for hemodynamic collapse, (eg, suprasystemic pulmonary hypertension with reduced RV function $\pm$ hemodynamic instability) preinduction ECMO cannulation should be strongly considered.[11,24,25] Given the lack of clinical evidence to support the use of a particular anesthesia induction agent, the anesthesia technique should be selected based on the cardiovascular and pulmonary risk profile. The induction agents should be administered slowly and incrementally with high clinical vigilance.[11,24,25] Of note, a recent survey of LTx anesthesiologists, identified propofol as the most commonly used anesthesia induction agent.[26] Anesthesia may be maintained using inhalational agents or total intravenous anesthesia (TIVA) alone or in combination, tailored to the patient's underlying pulmonary disease. For example, in patients at risk of inadequate pulmonary blood flow or ventilation that is, unpredictable uptake of inhaled anesthetic, TIVA should be strongly considered. Similarly, TIVA may be also the preferred technique in patients requiring ECMO.[11,24,25] Notably, there is currently no evidence that the method of maintaining anesthesia during one-lung ventilation affects patient outcomes (eg, by affecting pulmonary vascular tone, intrapulmonary shunt, or hypoxemia).[27,28] Although there is a growing number of lung isolation techniques, double-lumen tubes (DLT) remain the most common choice in LTx as they offer ease of use, reliable positioning, superior lung isolation, as well as the ability to perform bronchoscopy and mucus suctioning in both lungs. The left-sided DLT is more commonly used for double-lung transplants given the length of the left mainstem bronchus as opposed to the right-sided DLT. The tube is placed as proximally as possible to allow room for the bronchial anastomosis.[11,13,24,25]

Management During Pulmonary Artery Clamping, Pneumonectomy of the Native Lung, and Allograft Implantation. The process of native lung pneumonectomy (ie, PA clamping) results in increased PA pressure potentially leading to hemodynamic instability in patients with pre-existing pulmonary hypertension and impaired RV function.[11,13,24,25] Anticipation of those events, continuous monitoring including TEE, and timely commencement of hemodynamic optimization with inotropic and vasoactive medications is key to successful management.[11,13,24,25,29] Hemodynamic instability can be also anticipated during the implantation of the donor lung, due to retraction for surgical exposure and access to structures such as the atrium and hilum. After the completion of anastomoses and reperfusion of the graft, hypotension may occur secondary to blood loss through vascular anastomoses, wash-out of ischemic metabolites, and pneumoplegia from the allograft, or entrainment of air in the coronary arteries. High doses of inotropes and vasopressors may be required during those events.

Overall, 20% to 40% of patients require mechanical circulatory support (MCS).[26,30,31] MCS can be provided by CPB or veno-arterial (VA) extracorporeal membrane oxygenation (ECMO); venovenous (VV) ECMO while not providing circulatory support can also provide crucial respiratory support and is discussed later (see later in discussion).[26,30–32] Although MCS provides hemodynamic stability and gas exchange, it involves cannulation and heparinization, and may also incite systemic and local inflammatory response—all leading to potential technical and medical complications. Decision to deploy MCS is frequently based on surgeon and institutional preference.[26,30,31] Patients with severe pulmonary hypertension and significantly reduced RV function are more likely to require MCS.[11,13,24–26,30,31] In such patients establishing elective MCS before starting lung resection should be considered. Patients who require preoperative bridge to transplant with ECMO will also be supported with MCS during transplantation.[2] Finally, MCS may need to be instituted intraoperatively due to inadequate gas exchange with one lung ventilation, inability to maintain blood pressure, and organ perfusion during the surgical manipulation of mediastinal structures, or large blood loss.

Some authors advocate routine use of intraoperative MCS to allow for controlled reperfusion and immediate initiation of lung-protective ventilation following the implantation of the first lung.[33,34] Without MCS the first lung receives the full cardiac output, which increases PA pressure and hydrostatic pressure. This may worsen alveolar edema as well as right heart failure. Mechanical devices enable the diversion of some (or all) of the cardiac output away from the graft. This strategy may reduce ischemia-reperfusion injury and the incidence of PGD. Some studies demonstrated improved survival with VA ECMO used intraoperatively; however, improved outcomes have not been consistently supported by current literature.[35]

Advantages and disadvantages of using CPB versus ECMO have been a topic of growing interest and debate. CPB may provide better hemodynamic control and resuscitative ability in the hemorrhaging patient, which is facilitated by the presence of a blood reservoir and cardiotomy suction. However, CPB requires full anticoagulation, which is associated with higher rates of blood transfusion and increased transfusion-related lung injury.[36] Further, its larger priming volume results in more hemodilution and coagulopathy. On the other hand, ECMO has a simpler setup and may cause less inflammatory response due to a smaller blood–air interface and shorter extracorporeal circuit. ECMO also requires less heparin: for ECMO support initiated intraoperatively, anticoagulation is typically established using 5000 units of IV heparin at the time of ECMO initiation with the goal to maintain the activated clotting time (ACT) within a range of 180 to 210 seconds, while in patients with ECMO-BTT the heparin dose may vary according to their risk profile. Additionally, ECMO may provide mechanical cardiac and/or pulmonary support in the postoperative period depending on the system/s needing support. The recent trend toward increased intraoperative ECMO utilization is supported by a growing body of literature showing that compared with CPB, ECMO use is associated with decreased incidence of PGD, reduced postoperative bleeding and blood transfusion, less reoperations, reduced kidney injury as well as shorter intensive care unit (ICU) length of stay.[37–39] While several transplant centers report routine use of ECMO with good outcomes, no significant difference in mortality between the 2 MCS modalities has been demonstrated.[38–40]

When LTx is performed with no MCS ("off-pump"), management during one lung ventilation of the severely diseased lung may be challenging, as hypoxia and hypercapnia resulting in acidosis may increase pulmonary vascular resistance and further worsen the RV function:

- Patients with advanced primary pulmonary hypertension frequently suffer from hemodynamic instability due to RV failure.[11,13,24,25] In those cases, aggressive avoidance or treatment of hypoxemia and hypercarbia, inotropic medications for RV support, and judicious (restrictive) fluid therapy may be required. Addition of inhaled pulmonary vasodilator, such as inhaled nitric oxide, or prostanoid (eg, epoprostenol at 0.01–0.05 mcg/kg/min via jet nebulizer) may be considered.[25,26,41,42]
- Norepinephrine and vasopressin are the most commonly used vasopressor agents to treat hypotension in the setting of pulmonary hypertension and RV dysfunction.[26] Of note, vasopressin is considered to have a small effect on pulmonary vascular resistance (PVR).[43]
- In patients with evidence of heart failure, RV dysfunction, and/or end-organ hypoperfusion the use of inotropes (epinephrine, dobutamine, or milrinone) should be considered.[44] Ideally, sinus rhythm should be maintained.
- Anticoagulation during LTx without *MCS* is commonly established using 5000 units of IV heparin administered before vascular occlusion and subsequently re-dosed before the second lung transplant.

During allograft reperfusion, the risk of PGD should be reduced using controlled reperfusion of the allograft (low PA pressures, use of pulmonary vasodilators) and low Fio_2 (preferably <0.3).[23,25,45]

KEY CONCEPTS OF MECHANICAL CIRCULATORY SUPPORT DURING LUNG TRANSPLANTATION

Despite their differences, the MCS devices typically share several main components: an inflow cannula that diverts patients' blood from their venous system into the device, a blood pump, an oxygenator, a heat exchanger, and an outflow cannula that returns blood back to the patient. MCS devices that are typically used during LTx include, CPB, and VA or VV ECMO:

- *Cardiopulmonary bypass* provides full circulatory and respiratory support. Drainage of venous blood is typically achieved by gravity and aided by suction. Blood is returned to the arterial system via the aorta or a large artery, depending on the cannulation strategy. Unlike other MCS devices, CPB contains suction catheters and a blood reservoir, enabling blood salvage from the surgical field and quick transfusions of large blood volumes. Also, during specific stages of the procedure, a quick temporary decrease in blood flow/pressure can be achieved by decreasing blood return to the patient (while filling the CPB reservoir). In addition to continuously delivering oxygen and removing carbon dioxide from the blood, CPB is also equipped to deliver volatile anesthetics, a particularly important feature in the setting of impaired alveolar gas exchange.
- VA-ECMO, similar to CPB, provides both cardiac and respiratory support.[46] Blood is removed from the venous system typically via one or 2 large veins. Unlike CPB, drainage insufficiency may limit the pump preload and reduce blood flow. Blood is typically returned through a large artery or aorta when centrally cannulated. As a blood reservoir is not part of the standard ECMO device, the extracorporeal circuit cannot be used for volume resuscitation nor can the patient's blood be retained and pooled in the extracorporeal circuit as needed. Lack of a venous reservoir also means that any obstruction or kinking of the venous inflow cannula will result in a significant drop or complete cessation of pump flow. Unlike CPB, the ECMO circuit does not have air traps, which carries a risk of catastrophic air embolism.
- VV-ECMO is used for respiratory support only.[46] Blood is drained from and returned back to the venous system via venous cannulas of various configurations. The device pump maintains blood flow through the extracorporeal circuit, while the patient's native heart delivers blood to the body.

MCS cannulation can be broadly divided into central and peripheral:

- *Central cannulation* requires sternotomy, is almost always conducted in the operating room, and with general anesthesia. It entails the placement of the arterial cannula in the ascending aorta, and the venous cannula in the right atrium and inferior vena cava or the inferior and superior vena cava when 2 cannulas are used. Central cannulation is frequently used for CPB; however, utilization of a particular circulatory support device does not dictate the cannulation site, and central cannulation is also frequently used for VA ECMO.
- *Peripheral cannulation* can be performed with an
  - *Open surgical access (cut-down) or a percutaneous approach* via a femoral or axillary artery. When femoral artery is cannulated, blood supply distal to the cannulation site can be obstructed, resulting in limb ischemia.[47] To decrease the risk of malperfusion, an antegrade distal perfusion cannula may be placed into the ipsilateral superficial femoral artery. Another potential complication associated with femoral artery cannulation is unequal oxygenation between the upper and lower body, a phenomenon known as North-south or Harlequin syndrome.[48] The phenomenon occurs when lung function is severely impaired, and poorly oxygenated blood (ejected from the heart) mixes with well-oxygenated blood (delivered by the femoral cannula) in the distal arch. This may result in myocardial and cerebral hypoxemia and preferential oxygenation of the body that is perfused by the descending aorta.
  - *Peripheral VV-ECMO dual-site cannulation* can be via the left and right femoral veins, or a femoral and internal jugular (IJ) vein. For single-site VV-ECMO cannulation, a double-lumen cannula is typically placed in the internal jugular or subclavian vein. Such configuration is commonly used in awake and ambulating patients as a BTT.[49] If dual-lumen VV ECMO cannula is planned to be placed intraoperatively for LTx, then the placement of a standard central vein catheter in the right IJ should be avoided.

Mechanical ventilation

Following intubation, lung ventilation is commonly initiated using low-tidal volume (4–6 mL/kg), positive end-expiratory pressure (PEEP) < 10 cm H2O, with respiratory rate (RR) and Fio_2 adjusted to maintain oxygen saturation 92%-96% and preoperative baseline P_aCO_2.[23–26,44] Several strategies can be implemented to improve oxygenation and ventilation depending on the native lung pathology:[23,25,26]

- In patients with predominantly obstructive airway pathology at risk for dynamic hyperinflation, barotrauma, and tension pneumothorax (eg, chronic obstructive pulmonary disease or emphysema) pressure control ventilation with small volumes may minimize dynamic hyperinflation. Increasing exhalation time relative to inspiration time (I:E 1:3–1:4) may minimize auto-PEEP, and no extrinsic or low PEEP (3–4 cm H2O), should be used.
- In patients with thick copious secretions or severe hypercapnia, seen with cystic fibrosis or bronchiectasis, one may consider first intubating with a single lumen tube as opposed to a DLT to facilitate bronchoscopy with extensive airway suctioning and utilization of higher airway pressures and higher extrinsic PEEP.
- Restrictive lung disease characteristic of pulmonary fibrosis may require high driving pressures, increased inspiratory time (I:E 1:1–1:2), and higher extrinsic PEEP (8–10 cm H2O).

After allograft implantation is completed and the patient has been weaned off MCS, recommendation for intraoperative mechanical ventilation include a tidal volume of 6 mL/kg ideal body weight (when the allograft is undersized consider using donor's body weight), PEEP 6 to 8 cmH$_2$O, PIP less than 30 cmH$_2$O, lowest Fio_2 to maintain $Pao_2 \geq$ 70 mm Hg.[10,45,50–52] The rationale for frequent utilization of iNO is to provide pulmonary vasodilation in the ventilated parts of the lung, which subsequently results in improved ventilation-perfusion match and oxygenation. Its clinical effects on mitigating lung injury of the transplanted allograft and improving outcomes have not been clearly demonstrated.[53,54] A recent randomized clinical trial in LTx recipients that compared inhaled nitric oxide versus inhaled epoprostenol, found both to be associated with similar risks for severe grade 3 primary graft dysfunction (PGD-3) and other postoperative outcomes.[55]

Fluid management

Administration of excessive fluid volumes has been reported to increase the risk of pulmonary edema, lung injury, prolonged need of postoperative mechanical ventilation, as well as predisposition to PGD.[18–20] Therefore, a restrictive fluid strategy is used, with most institutions using crystalloids for fluid maintenance and colloids such as 5% albumin for volume resuscitation.[23] Obviously, this must be balanced with the goal of maintaining adequate cardiac output and perfusion pressure.

Intraoperative transfusion of red blood cells should be minimized as it represents a risk factor for PGD, and guided primarily by clinical criteria (eg, mixed/central venous oxygen saturation) rather than using a hemoglobin trigger.[10,20,21,56] Although transfusion of fresh frozen plasma (FFP) or platelets has not been reported to increase the risk of PGD, a restrictive approach guided by clinical and laboratory (point-of-care) assessments of prolonged/uncontrolled bleeding and coagulopathy is reasonable.[10,20,21]

In patients at risk for fluid overload and/or right heart failure, the use of prothrombin complex concentrates (PCC) over FFP may be considered. Given the associated increased risk of thrombotic events, it may be prudent to avoid or use cautiously recombinant Factor VII, in small incremental doses.

Transesophageal echocardiography

Surprisingly, despite its utility and diagnostic relevance, TEE still remains only a class IIb indication for intraoperative monitoring in LTx surgery according to the American Society of Echocardiography.[57] Moreover there are no consensus guidelines defining diagnostic criteria for the PA stenosis.[13,29,58] Despite that, TEE is frequently (and at some centers routinely) performed at high-volume institutions, as its clinical utility spans across the entire LTx procedure:[13,23,26,29,58–62]

- In the beginning, a full TEE examination may confirm the preoperative workup findings, and help detect interval changes especially in regard to RVfunction and size, tricuspid valve regurgitation as well as the presence of intracardiac shunts (eg, patent foramen ovale, atrial or ventricular septal defects) that may directly change the course of the procedure (eg, need of ECMO, or surgical closure).
- TEE may assist in continuously monitoring the left and right heart size and function, assessment of volume status, and guidance of hemodynamic interventions, (such as inotropic medications). This is especially relevant at the time of PA clamping, unclamping, and reperfusion of the new lungs as the information may directly affect the decision to initiate CPB or ECMO. TEE examination should also monitor

for the presence of air in the left atrium and ventricle during the reperfusion phase.

- Finally, one crucial role of TEE in LTx surgery is the assessment of pulmonary arterial (PA) and venous (PV) anastomosis.[29,60]

PA anastomosis: While there are no consensus guidelines outlining diagnostic criteria for PA stenosis, few recommendations can be made. The examination should include the measurement of the PA diameter, rule out thrombi in PAs (2-dimensional TEE), followed by spectral and color Doppler. In lieu of official guidelines, a diameter less than 75% of the ipsilateral native PA is commonly used as a cutoff concerning for PA stenosis (mean PA diameter in healthy male volunteers: right PA, 16.6 ± 2.8 mm and left PA, 17.3 ± 2.5 mm).[60,63–65] Turbulent flow or significant gradient across PA anastomosis should also raise concerns for stenosis.

o PV anastomosis: Measurement of the PV diameter, as well as rule out thrombi in PVs (2-dimensional TEE), followed by spectral and color Doppler. PV diameter of less than 0.5 cm and a PV velocity of greater than 1 m/s (normal PV velocity for S and D waves: 30–60 cm/s) should raise concerns for PV stenosis; PV diameter of less than 0.25 cm has been associated with graft failure.[29,60,66–69] A recent systematic review identified PV diameter of 0.48 ± 0.02 cm and a PV velocity of 1.59 ± 0.66 m/s in LTx surgery as predictors of PV dysfunction (stenosis or thrombosis), with a reported mortality rate of 32%.[70] Importantly, the diagnosis of PV stenosis should be based on the presence of multiple features as false positives can be frequently encountered in an uneventful LTx surgery (eg, hyperdynamic circulation, contralateral PA stenosis, vasoconstriction of the donor vein, implantation phase of the second lung, and so forth).[29]

Outcomes of lung transplantation in high-risk patients

With improvement in surgical techniques, intra- and postoperative management, the survival following LTx has improved with a median survival of 6.7 years, though still lagging behind other solid organ transplants.[71] As such, transplant centers are pushing the boundaries on several fronts with older, sicker and higher risk profile candidates getting listed and transplanted. Age more than 65 years used to be considered a relative contraindication[72] and still is in Belgium, for instance. However, ISHLT consensus document for the selection of lung transplant candidates published earlier this year did not acknowledge an upper age limit as an absolute contraindication.

Currently, in the US, 30% of waitlisted candidates are more than 65 years of age and this cohort is being transplanted at the highest rate.[73] Between 2004 and 2016 there has been a 430% increase in the number of lung transplant recipients more than 65 years of age in the US. Globally, similar trends have been seen though to a lesser degree.[74] Data on survival outcomes for those greater than 60 years of age remain conflicting, however.[75–77] Mosher and colleagues retrospectively examined close to 6000 recipients in the Scientific Registry of Transplant Recipients to identify risk factors for mortality in patients more than 65 years of age.[78] They found a median survival of 4.41 years with a worsening survival with increasing age. In addition, in the multivariable analysis, they identified several other risk factors associated with poorer outcomes in the elderly: creatinine level, bilirubin level, hospital admission for exacerbation before transplant, single lung transplant, CMV mismatch, and donor diabetes. Of note, those hospitalized before transplant, especially those in the ICU, had much worse short-term survival compared with outpatients $\geq$ 65 of years age.[78] Therefore, despite advances in perioperative care, certain risk factors may still preclude successful outcomes in the elderly.

Historically, patients requiring pre-LTx invasive mechanical ventilation (IMV) displayed higher postoperative mortality than those not requiring IMV,[79–82] hence, IMV was classified as a relative contraindication to LTx.[83,84] However, a recently published study by Hamilton and colleagues suggests that advances in perioperative management have led to significant improvements in survival.[1] In this retrospective study, the authors examined the safety and outcomes of pre-LTx IMV between 2005 and 2018 in 21,375 patient undergoing LTx using data from the Organ Procurement and transplantation Network registry from the United Network for Organ Sharing.[1] Using propensity score-matching and multivariable modeling, the authors compared outcomes between the period 2005–2011 vs 2011–2018 and reported 2 main findings: (1) The survival for IMV recipients significantly improved over time, despite increase in severity and acuity of patients requiring IMV: Compared with 2005–2011 period, the IMV recipients transplanted between 2011 and 2018, had a 25-fold lower hazard of death at 30 days, 2-fold at 14 months, and 1.4-fold lower hazard of death at 3 years.[1] (2) When compared with non-IMV, IMV recipients transplanted in the 2011 to 2018 period displayed significantly increased mortality *only* at 30-day time point (9.53; CI, 4.57–19.86; adjusted analysis), with no significant differences at subsequent time points.[1] The authors attributed the improved outcomes to advancements in organ preservation as well as in ICU management.

Similarly, pre-LTx use of ECMO had historically poor survival.[79] With advances in ECMO technology and perioperative management, the outcomes of ECMO-BTT in the current era have improved.[2,5,85,86] The success rate of ECMO-BTT has been reported to be as high as 89%.[5,86,87] Even in older populations with high ILD prevalence, the 1-year survival ranged between 86%[2] and 93%[5] (with 1-year survival conditional on discharge range of 88%[86] and 97%[2]). As such, over the last decade the use of ECMO-BTT has increased 271%, while IMV-BTT has decreased 38%.[88] With this success, the acuity and age of patients requiring ECMO-BTT has also increased over time.[86,87,89]

Additonally, authors have witnessed an increase in de novo waitlisting for patients *without* prior evaluation for LTx presenting with acute on chronic respiratory failure, also requiring mechanical support (MV and/or ECMO) as BTT.[2,5] This presents the care team with ethical and moral concerns regarding the optimal treatment. Kukreja and colleagues, recently compared the outcomes of emergently waitlisted (EWL) *after* ECMO deployment to patients actively waitlisted (AWL) before ECMO initiation in a retrospective, single-center study of 62 patients (EWL: 20, AWL: 42) between 2010 and 2018. The authors reported 2 main findings: (1) There was no statistical difference in BTT success between AWL and EWL and (2) similarly, there was no significant difference in survival (survival to hospital discharge: 100% and 87% in the EWL and AWL group, respectively).[2] The 1-year survival conditional on discharge was 91% in the EWL and 100% in the AWL group, while the unconditional survival was 91% (EWL) and 83% (AWL).

SUMMARY

There has been a steady increase in the medical complexity of lung transplant candidates as well as a steady rise in the number of candidates requiring ECMO-BTT support. This has led to a growing appreciation of the importance of intraoperative management of potentially modifiable risk factors on postoperative outcomes. Multiple interventions within the domain of the intraoperative (anesthetic) management that may mitigate those factors have been identified and discussed.

REFERENCES

1. Hamilton BCS, Dincheva GR, Matthay MA, et al. Improved survival after lung transplantation for adults requiring preoperative invasive mechanical ventilation: A national cohort study. J Thorac Cardiovasc Surg 2020;160(5):1385–1395 e1386.

2. Kukreja J, Tsou S, Chen J, et al. Risk Factors and Outcomes of Extracorporeal Membrane Oxygenation as a Bridge to Lung Transplantation. Semin Thorac Cardiovasc Surg 2020;32(4):772–85.

3. Stehlik J, Chambers DC, Zuckermann A, et al. Increasing complexity of thoracic transplantation and the rise of multiorgan transplantation around the world: Insights from the International Society for Heart and Lung Transplantation Registry. J Heart Lung Transplant 2018;37(10):1145–54.

4. Chambers DC, Cherikh WS, Goldfarb SB, et al. The International Thoracic Organ Transplant Registry of the International Society for Heart and Lung Transplantation: Thirty-fifth adult lung and heart-lung transplant report-2018; Focus theme: Multiorgan Transplantation. J Heart Lung Transplant 2018; 37(10):1169–83.

5. Banga A, Batchelor E, Mohanka M, et al. Predictors of outcome among patients on extracorporeal membrane oxygenation as a bridge to lung transplantation. Clin Transpl 2017;31(7).

6. Kukreja J, Chen J, Brzezinski M. Redefining marginality: donor lung criteria. Curr Opin Organ Transpl 2020;25(3):280–4.

7. Tsou S, Chen J, Brzezinski M, et al. Lung transplantation from swimming pool drowning victims: A case series. Am J Transplant 2021;21(6):2273–8.

8. Kinaschuk K, Nagendran J. Improving long-term survival by preventing early complications after lung transplantation: Can we prevent ripples by keeping pebbles out of the water? J Thorac Cardiovasc Surg 2016;151(4):1181–2.

9. Chan EG, Bianco V 3rd, Richards T, et al. The ripple effect of a complication in lung transplantation: Evidence for increased long-term survival risk. J Thorac Cardiovasc Surg 2016;151(4):1171–9.

10. Diamond JM, Lee JC, Kawut SM, et al. Clinical risk factors for primary graft dysfunction after lung transplantation. Am J Respir Crit Care Med 2013;187(5):527–34.

11. Kachulis B, Mitrev L, Jordan D. Intraoperative anesthetic management of lung transplantation patients. Best Pract Res Clin Anaesthesiol 2017;31(2):261–72.

12. Marczin NKL, Wright IG, Simon AR. Anaesthesia for lung transplantation. In: R Peter Alston PSM, Ranucci Marco, editors. Oxford textbook of cardiac anaesthesia. Oxford University Press; 2015.

13. Sellers D, Cassar-Demajo W, Keshavjee S, et al. The Evolution of Anesthesia for Lung Transplantation. J Cardiothorac Vasc Anesth 2017;31(3):1071–9.

14. Yusen RD, Edwards LB, Kucheryavaya AY, et al. The Registry of the International Society for Heart and Lung Transplantation: Thirty-second Official Adult

Lung and Heart-Lung Transplantation Report–2015; Focus Theme: Early Graft Failure. J Heart Lung Transplant 2015;34(10):1264–77.

15. Snell GI, Yusen RD, Weill D, et al. Report of the ISHLT Working Group on Primary Lung Graft Dysfunction, part I: Definition and grading-A 2016 Consensus Group statement of the International Society for Heart and Lung Transplantation. J Heart Lung Transplant 2017;36(10):1097–103.

16. Gelman AE, Fisher AJ, Huang HJ, et al. Report of the ISHLT Working Group on Primary Lung Graft Dysfunction Part III: Mechanisms: A 2016 Consensus Group Statement of the International Society for Heart and Lung Transplantation. J Heart Lung Transplant 2017;36(10):1114–20.

17. Van Raemdonck D, Hartwig MG, Hertz MI, et al. Report of the ISHLT Working Group on primary lung graft dysfunction Part IV: Prevention and treatment: A 2016 Consensus Group statement of the International Society for Heart and Lung Transplantation. J Heart Lung Transplant 2017; 36(10):1121–36.

18. McIlroy DR, Pilcher DV, Snell GI. Does anaesthetic management affect early outcomes after lung transplant? An exploratory analysis. Br J Anaesth 2009; 102(4):506–14.

19. Assaad S, Kratzert WB, Perrino AC Jr. Extravascular lung water monitoring for thoracic and lung transplant surgeries. Curr Opin Anaesthesiol 2019; 32(1):29–38.

20. Geube MA, Perez-Protto SE, McGrath TL, et al. Increased Intraoperative Fluid Administration Is Associated with Severe Primary Graft Dysfunction After Lung Transplantation. Anesth Analg 2016; 122(4):1081–8.

21. Cernak V, Oude Lansink-Hartgring A, van den Heuvel ER, et al. Incidence of Massive Transfusion and Overall Transfusion Requirements During Lung Transplantation Over a 25-Year Period. J Cardiothorac Vasc Anesth 2019;33(9):2478–86.

22. Hamilton BCS, Dincheva GR, Zhuo H, et al. Elevated donor plasminogen activator inhibitor-1 levels and the risk of primary graft dysfunction. Clin Transpl 2018;32(4):e13210.

23. Gerlach RM. Lung transplantation: Anesthetic management. In: O'Connor MF, Marks JB, eds. UpToDate. Waltham, MA.2021.

24. Buckwell E, Vickery B, Sidebotham D. Anaesthesia for lung transplantation. BJA Educ 2020;20(11):368–76.

25. Nicoara A, Anderson-Dam J. Anesthesia for Lung Transplantation. Anesthesiol Clin 2017;35(3): 473–89.

26. Tomasi R, Betz D, Schlager S, et al. Intraoperative Anesthetic Management of Lung Transplantation: Center-Specific Practices and Geographic and Centers Size Differences. J Cardiothorac Vasc Anesth 2018;32(1):62–9.

27. Pruszkowski O, Dalibon N, Moutafis M, et al. Effects of propofol vs sevoflurane on arterial oxygenation during one-lung ventilation. Br J Anaesth 2007; 98(4):539–44.

28. Modolo NS, Modolo MP, Marton MA, et al. Intravenous versus inhalation anaesthesia for one-lung ventilation. Cochrane Database Syst Rev 2013;(7): CD006313.

29. Abrams BA, Melnyk V, Allen WL, et al. TEE for Lung Transplantation: A Case Series and Discussion of Vascular Complications. J Cardiothorac Vasc Anesth 2020;34(3):733–40.

30. Moreno Garijo J, Cypel M, McRae K, et al. The Evolving Role of Extracorporeal Membrane Oxygenation in Lung Transplantation: Implications for Anesthetic Management. J Cardiothorac Vasc Anesth 2019;33(7):1995–2006.

31. Martin AK, Jayaraman AL, Nabzdyk CG, et al. Extracorporeal Membrane Oxygenation in Lung Transplantation: Analysis of Techniques and Outcomes. J Cardiothorac Vasc Anesth 2021;35(2):644–61.

32. Kiziltug H, Falter F. Circulatory support during lung transplantation. Curr Opin Anaesthesiol 2020;33(1): 37–42.

33. Marczin N, Royston D, Yacoub M. Pro: lung transplantation should be routinely performed with cardiopulmonary bypass. J Cardiothorac Vasc Anesth 2000;14(6):739–45.

34. Nazarnia S, Subramaniam K. Pro: Veno-arterial Extracorporeal Membrane Oxygenation (ECMO) Should Be Used Routinely for Bilateral Lung Transplantation. J Cardiothorac Vasc Anesth 2017;31(4):1505–8.

35. Hoetzenecker K, Schwarz S, Muckenhuber M, et al. Intraoperative extracorporeal membrane oxygenation and the possibility of postoperative prolongation improve survival in bilateral lung transplantation. J Thorac Cardiovasc Surg 2018;155(5):2193–2206 e2193.

36. Bennett SCBE, Dumond CA, Preston T, et al. Mechanical circulatory support in lung transplantation: Cardiopulmonary bypass, extracorporeal life support, and ex-vivo lung perfusion. World J Respirol 2015;5(2):78–93.

37. Biscotti M, Yang J, Sonett J, et al. Comparison of extracorporeal membrane oxygenation versus cardiopulmonary bypass for lung transplantation. J Thorac Cardiovasc Surg 2014;148(5):2410–5.

38. Machuca TN, Collaud S, Mercier O, et al. Outcomes of intraoperative extracorporeal membrane oxygenation versus cardiopulmonary bypass for lung transplantation. J Thorac Cardiovasc Surg 2015;149(4): 1152–7.

39. Bermudez CA, Shiose A, Esper SA, et al. Outcomes of intraoperative venoarterial extracorporeal membrane oxygenation versus cardiopulmonary bypass during lung transplantation. Ann Thorac Surg 2014; 98(6):1936–42.

40. Aigner C, Wisser W, Taghavi S, et al. Institutional experience with extracorporeal membrane oxygenation in lung transplantation. Eur J Cardiothorac Surg 2007;31(3):468–73.

41. Khan TA, Schnickel G, Ross D, et al. A prospective, randomized, crossover pilot study of inhaled nitric oxide versus inhaled prostacyclin in heart transplant and lung transplant recipients. J Thorac Cardiovasc Surg 2009;138(6):1417–24.

42. Kim N, Lee SH, Joe Y, et al. Effects of Inhaled Iloprost on Lung Mechanics and Myocardial Function During One-Lung Ventilation in Chronic Obstructive Pulmonary Disease Patients Combined With Poor Lung Oxygenation. Anesth Analg 2020;130(5): 1407–14.

43. Siehr SL, Feinstein JA, Yang W, et al. Hemodynamic Effects of Phenylephrine, Vasopressin, and Epinephrine in Children With Pulmonary Hypertension: A Pilot Study. Pediatr Crit Care Med 2016;17(5):428–37.

44. Rana M, Yusuff H, Zochios V. The Right Ventricle During Selective Lung Ventilation for Thoracic Surgery. J Cardiothorac Vasc Anesth 2019;33(7): 2007–16.

45. Barnes L, Reed RM, Parekh KR, et al. Mechanical Ventilation for the Lung Transplant Recipient. Curr Pulmonol Rep 2015;4(2):88–96.

46. Barry A, Brzezinski M. Adult Extracorporeal Membrane Oxygenation: An Update for Intensivists. ICU Director 2013;4(3):107–14.

47. Lamb KM, DiMuzio PJ, Johnson A, et al. Arterial protocol including prophylactic distal perfusion catheter decreases limb ischemia complications in patients undergoing extracorporeal membrane oxygenation. J Vasc Surg 2017;65(4):1074–9.

48. St-Arnaud C, Theriault MM, Mayette M. North-south syndrome in veno-arterial extra-corporeal membrane oxygenator: the other Harlequin syndrome. Can J Anaesth 2020;67(2):262–3.

49. Biscotti M, Gannon WD, Agerstrand C, et al. Awake Extracorporeal Membrane Oxygenation as Bridge to Lung Transplantation: A 9-Year Experience. Ann Thorac Surg 2017;104(2):412–9.

50. Martin AK, Yalamuri SM, Wilkey BJ, et al. The Impact of Anesthetic Management on Perioperative Outcomes in Lung Transplantation. J Cardiothorac Vasc Anesth 2020;34(6):1669–80.

51. Verbeek GL, Myles PS. Intraoperative protective ventilation strategies in lung transplantation. Transpl Rev (Orlando) 2013;27(1):30–5.

52. Diamond JM, Arcasoy S, Kennedy CC, et al. Report of the International Society for Heart and Lung Transplantation Working Group on Primary Lung Graft Dysfunction, part II: Epidemiology, risk factors, and outcomes-A 2016 Consensus Group statement of the International Society for Heart and Lung Transplantation. J Heart Lung Transplant 2017; 36(10):1104–13.

53. Bhandary S, Stoicea N, Joseph N, et al. Pro: Inhaled Pulmonary Vasodilators Should Be Used Routinely in the Management of Patients Undergoing Lung Transplantation. J Cardiothorac Vasc Anesth 2017; 31(3):1123–6.

54. Ramadan ME, Shabsigh M, Awad H. Con: Inhaled Pulmonary Vasodilators Are Not Indicated in Patients Undergoing Lung Transplantation. J Cardiothorac Vasc Anesth 2017;31(3):1127–31.

55. Ghadimi K, Cappiello J, Cooter-Wright M, et al. Inhaled Pulmonary Vasodilator Therapy in Adult Lung Transplant: A Randomized Clinical Trial. JAMA Surg 2021;157(1):e215856.

56. Huddleston SJ, Jackson S, Kane K, et al. Separate Effect of Perioperative Recombinant Human Factor VIIa Administration and Packed Red Blood Cell Transfusions on Midterm Survival in Lung Transplantation Recipients. J Cardiothorac Vasc Anesth 2020; 34(11):3013–20.

57. Ramadan ME, Shabsigh M, Awad H. Con: Inhaled Pulmonary Vasodilators Are Not Indicated in Patients Undergoing Lung Transplantation. J Cardiothorac Vasc Anesth. 2017 Jun;31(3):1127–31. https://doi.org/10.1053/j.jvca.2016.08.035. Epub 2016 Aug 31. PMID: 27856154.

58. Iyer MH, Bhatt A, Kumar N, et al. Transesophageal Echocardiography for Lung Transplantation: A New Standard of Care? J Cardiothorac Vasc Anesth 2020;34(3):741–3.

59. American Society of A, Society of Cardiovascular Anesthesiologists Task Force on Transesophageal E. Practice guidelines for perioperative transesophageal echocardiography. An updated report by the American Society of Anesthesiologists and the Society of Cardiovascular Anesthesiologists Task Force on Transesophageal Echocardiography. Anesthesiology 2010;112(5):1084–96.

60. Evans A, Dwarakanath S, Hogue C, et al. Intraoperative echocardiography for patients undergoing lung transplantation. Anesth Analg 2014;118(4):725–30.

61. Tan Z, Roscoe A, Rubino A. Transesophageal Echocardiography in Heart and Lung Transplantation. J Cardiothorac Vasc Anesth 2019;33(6):1548–58.

62. Serra E, Feltracco P, Barbieri S, et al. Transesophageal echocardiography during lung transplantation. Transpl Proc 2007;39(6):1981–2.

63. Hausmann D, Daniel WG, Mugge A, et al. Imaging of pulmonary artery and vein anastomoses by transesophageal echocardiography after lung transplantation. Circulation 1992;86(5 Suppl):II251–8.

64. Michel-Cherqui M, Brusset A, Liu N, et al. Intraoperative transesophageal echocardiographic assessment of vascular anastomoses in lung transplantation. A report on 18 cases. Chest 1997; 111(5):1229–35.

65. Burman ED, Keegan J, Kilner PJ. Pulmonary artery diameters, cross sectional areas and area changes

measured by cine cardiovascular magnetic resonance in healthy volunteers. J Cardiovasc Magn Reson 2016;18:12.

66. Huang YC, Cheng YJ, Lin YH, et al. Graft failure caused by pulmonary venous obstruction diagnosed by intraoperative transesophageal echocardiography during lung transplantation. Anesth Analg 2000;91(3):558–60.

67. Gentile F, Mantero A, Lippolis A, et al. Pulmonary venous flow velocity patterns in 143 normal subjects aged 20 to 80 years old. An echo 2D colour Doppler cooperative study. Eur Heart J 1997;18(1):148–64.

68. Gonzalez-Fernandez C, Gonzalez-Castro A, Rodriguez-Borregan JC, et al. Pulmonary venous obstruction after lung transplantation. Diagnostic advantages of transesophageal echocardiography. Clin Transpl 2009;23(6):975–80.

69. Cartwright BL, Jackson A, Cooper J. Intraoperative pulmonary vein examination by transesophageal echocardiography: an anatomic update and review of utility. J Cardiothorac Vasc Anesth 2013;27(1):111–20.

70. Kumar N, Essandoh M, Bhatt A, et al. Pulmonary cuff dysfunction after lung transplant surgery: A systematic review of the evidence and analysis of its clinical implications. J Heart Lung Transplant 2019;38(5):530–44.

71. Valapour M, Skeans MA, Heubner BM, et al. OPTN/SRTR 2012 Annual Data Report: lung. Am J Transplant 2014;14(Suppl 1):139–65.

72. Orens JB, Estenne M, Arcasoy S, et al. International guidelines for the selection of lung transplant candidates: 2006 update–a consensus report from the Pulmonary Scientific Council of the International Society for Heart and Lung Transplantation. J Heart Lung Transplant 2006;25(7):745–55.

73. Leard LE, Holm AM, Valapour M, et al. Consensus document for the selection of lung transplant candidates: An update from the International Society for Heart and Lung Transplantation. J Heart Lung Transpl 2021;40(11):1349–79.

74. Courtwright A, Cantu E. Lung transplantation in elderly patients. J Thorac Dis 2017;9(9):3346–51.

75. Ehrsam JP, Benden C, Seifert B, et al. Lung transplantation in the elderly: Influence of age, comorbidities, underlying disease, and extended criteria donor lungs. J Thorac Cardiovasc Surg 2017;154(6):2135–41.

76. Hayanga AJ, Aboagye JK, Hayanga HE, et al. Contemporary analysis of early outcomes after lung transplantation in the elderly using a national registry. J Heart Lung Transplant 2015;34(2):182–8.

77. McCarthy F, Savino D, Graves D, et al. Cost and Readmission of Single and Double Lung Transplantation in the U.S. Medicare Population. J Heart Lung Transplant 2017;36:S115.

78. Mosher CL, Weber JM, Frankel CW, et al. Risk factors for mortality in lung transplant recipients aged >/=65 years: A retrospective cohort study of 5,815 patients in the scientific registry of transplant recipients. J Heart Lung Transplant 2021;40(1):42–55.

79. Mason DP, Thuita L, Nowicki ER, et al. Should lung transplantation be performed for patients on mechanical respiratory support? The US experience. J Thorac Cardiovasc Surg 2010;139(3):765–73.e761.

80. Elizur A, Sweet SC, Huddleston CB, et al. Pre-transplant mechanical ventilation increases short-term morbidity and mortality in pediatric patients with cystic fibrosis. J Heart Lung Transplant 2007;26(2):127–31.

81. O'Brien G, Criner GJ. Mechanical ventilation as a bridge to lung transplantation. J Heart Lung Transplant 1999;18(3):255–65.

82. Singer JP, Blanc PD, Hoopes C, et al. The impact of pretransplant mechanical ventilation on short- and long-term survival after lung transplantation. Am J Transplant 2011;11(10):2197–204.

83. Maxwell BG, Mooney JJ, Lee PH, et al. Increased resource use in lung transplant admissions in the lung allocation score era. Am J Respir Crit Care Med 2015;191(3):302–8.

84. Weill D, Benden C, Corris PA, et al. A consensus document for the selection of lung transplant candidates: 2014–an update from the Pulmonary Transplantation Council of the International Society for Heart and Lung Transplantation. J Heart Lung Transplant 2015;34(1):1–15.

85. Hoopes CW, Kukreja J, Golden J, et al. Extracorporeal membrane oxygenation as a bridge to pulmonary transplantation. J Thorac Cardiovasc Surg 2013;145(3):862–7.

86. Tipograf Y, Salna M, Minko E, et al. Outcomes of Extracorporeal Membrane Oxygenation as a Bridge to Lung Transplantation. Ann Thorac Surg 2019;107(5):1456–63.

87. Hoetzenecker K, Donahoe L, Yeung JC, et al. Extracorporeal life support as a bridge to lung transplantation-experience of a high-volume transplant center. J Thorac Cardiovasc Surg 2018;155(3):1316–1328 e1311.

88. Hayanga JWA, Hayanga HK, Holmes SD, et al. Mechanical ventilation and extracorporeal membrane oxygenation as a bridge to lung transplantation: Closing the gap. J Heart Lung Transplant 2019;38(10):1104–11.

89. Benazzo A, Schwarz S, Frommlet F, et al. Twenty-year experience with extracorporeal life support as bridge to lung transplantation. J Thorac Cardiovasc Surg 2019;157(6):2515–2525 e2510.

Early Postoperative Management of Lung Transplant Recipients

Binh N. Trinh, MD, PhD[a], Marek Brzezinski, MD, PhD[b],
Jasleen Kukreja, MD, MPH[a],*

KEYWORDS

- Critical care management • Immunosuppression • Infection prophylaxis
- Lung transplant complication • Primary graft dysfunction • Extracorporeal membrane oxygenation

KEY POINTS

- The focus of postoperative management is preservation of allograft function while maintaining adequate end organ perfusion.
- Good pain management facilitates early ambulation and pulmonary toilet, which reduces risk of allograft pneumonia.
- Early recognition of primary graft dysfunction and selected use of extracorporeal membrane oxygenation are key to a successful outcome.
- Arrhythmias are common, and rate control is the primary goal.
- Other common complications include infections, acute kidney injury, and pleural effusions.

INTRODUCTION

As lung transplantation has become standard therapy for end-stage lung disease, the annual case volume as reported by the International Thoracic Organ Transplant Registry has increased to more than 4000 cases per year.[1] Although long-term survival remains poor with a median survival of 6.7 years, short-term survival has improved over the past 4 decades owing to improved surgical techniques and perioperative management.[1,2]

The leading causes of morbidity and mortality in the early postoperative period are graft failure and infection not related to cytomegalovirus (CMV). To a lesser extent, survival is adversely affected by cardiovascular event, multisystem organ failure, and technical reasons.[1] A multidisciplinary team approach is critical to ensure a successful outcome.[3,4] Herein, the authors review management strategies in the postoperative period.

PATIENT SELECTION

Postoperative management begins with recipient selection and is greatly affected by medical and physical optimization before transplant.[5] As experience is growing, transplant centers are considering candidates with conditions that were previously contraindicated. For example, lung transplantation is now being performed in older patients with comorbidities,[6,7] those with prior chest operations,[6,8,9] or patients requiring multiorgan transplants.[10] Moreover, an increasing number of patients are being bridged to transplantation with mechanical ventilation and/or extracorporeal membrane oxygenation (ECMO) support.[2,11,12] These patients are less mobile, are more frail, and are at higher risk for morbidity and mortality.[13] Growing evidence suggests, however, that even in these high-risk candidates, good outcomes can be achieved with careful patient selection, preoperative optimization, operative planning, and postoperative management.[2,7,9,11,12]

[a] Division of Cardiothoracic Surgery, University of California, San Francisco, 500 Parnassus Avenue, Suite MUW-405, San Francisco, CA 94143-0118, USA; [b] Department of Anesthesia, University of California, San Francisco, 500 Parnassus Avenue, Suite MUW-405, San Francisco, CA 94143-0118, USA
* Corresponding author.
E-mail address: jasleen.kukreja@ucsf.edu

Thorac Surg Clin 32 (2022) 185–195
https://doi.org/10.1016/j.thorsurg.2021.11.006
1547-4127/22/© 2022 Elsevier Inc. All rights reserved.

Respiratory failure from the recent emergence of SARS-CoV-2 (severe acute respiratory syndrome coronavirus 2) has produced an unprecedented, high-risk recipient cohort that is often ventilator and ECMO dependent for weeks, or months in the authors' center experience, before transplantation.[14,15] Although short-term outcomes are relatively satisfactory, their long-term survival remains to be seen. It is important to highlight that successful outcomes depend on nutritional optimization,[5,16] pulmonary rehabilitation,[17,18] and recognition of biological factors that can pose a challenge, such as short stature, rare blood groups, and pulmonary hypertension.[12] Management of pulmonary hypertension and close surveillance of right ventricular function with transthoracic echocardiography (TTE) can help to optimize the conduct of surgery.[19]

INTRAOPERATIVE MANAGEMENT

Preoperative planning and intraoperative conduct help set the stage for success in the postoperative period.[5,16] The authors briefly discuss their surgical philosophy. Regarding donor selection, an analysis of height and weight matching found that donor undersizing leads to inferior survival, except for the group transplanted for fibrotic lung disease.[1] It has been hypothesized that undersized donor lungs are at risk of being overventilated and therefore more prone to primary graft dysfunction (PGD) development.[20] Because bilateral lung transplant has superior survival,[10] the authors' practice is to perform double-lung transplantation for those less than 70 years of age barring major comorbidities. The transplant can be carried out with ECMO or cardiopulmonary bypass (CPB) or without extracorporeal support.[21] Because the use of CPB is associated with increased transfusion requirement and risk for PGD, ECMO support with its superior coagulation profile and outcomes has essentially replaced CPB for double-lung transplants at the authors' center and others.[22–25] There is ongoing debate on whether all lung transplants should be performed with ECMO support regardless of the underlying cause or pathophysiology. The authors selectively use CPB for high-risk cases, such as patients with adhesive lung disease on ECMO bridge-to-transplant, where massive blood loss (>10 units of packed red blood cells) at explant is expected. Despite the "hostile" pleural cavities of the COVID adult respiratory distress syndrome (ARDS), the authors have managed them successfully with ECMO intraoperatively.[12,25] Chronic obstructive pulmonary disease (COPD) and single-lung transplants without severe pulmonary hypertension at the authors' center are generally performed without extracorporeal support.

Prolonged ischemic time is associated with increased risk of PGD,[8,26] although good outcomes with ischemia in excess of 6 hours have been described.[27] The authors' center has successfully performed lung transplants with ischemia time in excess of 11 hours, without ex vivo lung perfusion. Close monitoring for significant reperfusion injury is advised before closing the chest. A Pao_2/Fio_2 (PF ratio) less than 150 should prompt a search for reversible causes and consideration for ECMO support. In severe cases, leaving the chest partially open, with or without ECMO, minimizes airway pressure and potential for pulmonary tamponade, allowing time for the allograft to improve.[28–30] A temporary open chest strategy helps to address issues of ongoing coagulopathy and initial graft dysfunction before a later-staged chest washout and definitive closure.

POSTOPERATIVE MANAGEMENT OF HEMODYNAMICS

On arrival to the intensive care unit, low-dose vasopressor and inotropic support with judicious use of fluids (crystalloid or colloid) is advisable, aiming to keep the allograft dry while preserving end-organ perfusion.[21] The presence of major pulmonary edema portends significant reperfusion injury, and opacities with anemia may indicate hemothoraces. Bedside TTE can be a helpful adjunct to assess biventricular function and volume status and to rule out tamponade.

Hemodynamic goals include the maintenance of adequate preload and optimization of cardiac output by controlling heart rate and stroke volume. Reduced myocardial contractility can occur after transplant because of metabolic acidosis, hypoxemia, hypotension, and electrolyte disturbances. TTE evaluation can help guide the delivery of inotropic supportive drugs, such as dobutamine, epinephrine, dopamine, and milrinone. Although milrinone improves cardiac contractility, significant systemic vasodilation remains a concern. Therefore, the authors seldom use milrinone in the perioperative period. Given that many patients with interstitial lung disease have preexisting pulmonary hypertension and right ventricular dysfunction, special attention is needed to avoid PGD.[12,19] Use of inhaled nitric oxide and prostacyclin can improve oxygenation but has not been shown to improve survival or length of stay.[21,31,32]

Arrhythmias also contribute to a low-cardiac output state. Mason and colleagues[33] reported a 20% incidence of atrial fibrillation after lung transplant, which was associated with increased length of stay and higher mortality.[34] Up to 70% of cases occurred in the first 4 days.[33] Rate control strategies with ß-blockade and replacement of serum magnesium are effective. Use of ß-blocker, calcium channel blockers, or amiodarone is supported by class II evidence per the 2014 American Association for Thoracic Surgery guidelines.[35] Current best practices aim at rate control with rhythm control as a secondary goal.[35] Intravenous amiodarone can be useful for pharmacologic cardioversion. Hemodynamically unstable patients are urgently cardioverted by R-wave direct current synchronization. Class I recommendations include weaning or withdrawing catecholaminergic inotropic agents, optimizing electrolytes, and treating trigger events, such as pain, bleeding, and infection.[35] A recent multicenter randomized trial in patients undergoing cardiac surgery found that performing left atrial appendage occlusion with anticoagulation was associated with reduction of stroke from 7% to 4.8%[36]; however, this has not been studied in lung transplantation.

The transplanted lung benefits from avoidance of volume overload. However, the early postoperative period is commonly marked by a low-cardiac output state owing to hypovolemia caused by intraoperative bleeding, lung explantation, and vasoplegia. The combination of low central venous pressure (CVP), stroke volume, and pulmonary capillary wedge pressures (PCWP) further supports hypovolemia. Laboratory results can reveal marked metabolic acidosis and elevated serum lactate levels that are responsive to volume replacement with colloids and crystalloids.[37,38]

The syndrome of anemia, hypotension, declining urine output, low CVP, low PCWP, and low mixed venous oxygen saturation (SVO$_2$) is suggestive of ongoing blood loss. These patients often require blood product resuscitation. Significant bleeding has been reported in 9% to 18% of cases.[25,39,40] Extrapleural dissection for severe pleural symphysis and use of ECMO or CPB, which require anticoagulation, exacerbate bleeding, leading to a vicious cycle of coagulopathy, hypofibrinogenemia, and thrombocytopenia.[25] Hypocalcemia secondary to blood transfusion should be corrected, as calcium has a central role in cardiac contractility. Prompt recognition and treatment of ongoing blood loss are important to prevent excessive transfusion, potential transfusion-related acute lung injury, pulmonary edema, and alloimmunization.[41–43] If ongoing coagulopathy ensues, hypotension with increasing vasopressor requirement, reduced lung compliance, and hypoxemia could lead to thoracic compartment syndrome.[28,29] This is caused by pulmonary edema, oversized lungs, and a restricted chest cavity compounded by ongoing intrathoracic bleeding. Prompt recognition is necessary to allow surgical decompression. Refractory cases may require the use of ECMO support as a bridge to recovery.[44]

SEDATION AND PAIN MANAGEMENT

The authors' program uses conventional short-acting propofol for sedation.[45] Low-dose dexmedetomidine is a useful adjunct with both sedative and analgesic properties.[45,46] Adequate postoperative analgesia is an important component of perioperative management.[47] Pain control with a multimodal approach allows the patient to mobilize, ambulate, and participate in pulmonary toiletry, which in turn prevents atelectasis and pneumonia. Opioids, such as fentanyl and hydromorphone, can be given intravenously or via a patient-controlled analgesia pump. Alternatively, thoracic epidural anesthesia (TEA) can offer excellent pain relief using local anesthetics (eg, bupivacaine) and opioid combinations. Its use has been associated with less pulmonary complications.[47] TEA can be placed before extubation, although perioperative coagulopathy can delay epidural catheter placement. Useful nonopioid alternatives include intravenous acetaminophen, gabapentin, and lidocaine patches. Typically, the authors add stool softeners to prevent opioid-induced constipation and use oral naloxone or methylnaltrexone if needed. Nonsteroidal anti-inflammatory drugs are usually avoided to reduce the risk of renal injury. Finally, pain control studies in repair of pectus excavatum suggest that intercostal cryoanalgesia is effective at reducing opioid requirement and need for TEA.[48,49] In the authors' experience, this approach has essentially replaced TEA, providing effective analgesia in lung transplant recipients without significant morbidity.[50,51]

MANAGEMENT OF GRAFT FUNCTION

The goals of mechanical ventilation are to minimize plateau airway pressure, avoid high tidal volumes, and prevent hypoxia.[52] Choice of tidal volumes is generally based on donor body weight.[20,52–54] Inhaled nitric oxide may alleviate perfusion-ventilation mismatching in severely hypoxic patients with pulmonary hypertension but has not been shown to prevent PGD.[55,56] Most patients without significant PGD can be extubated safely in the first 72 hours.[25] Practice patterns show that 32% of centers extubate within 24 hours and another 32% extubate within 48 hours.[52] Noninvasive ventilation can help to reduce the work of breathing and support existing respiratory weakness. Preventive strategies against atelectasis and pneumonia include incentive spirometry, chest physiotherapy, and early ambulation. Bronchoscopy performed as needed is an important tool to survey airway health and helps to mobilize thick secretions.[57] Patients with prolonged duration of intubation are at risk for associated complications, such as atrial arrhythmias and need for tracheostomy.[52]

Transplanted lungs in the early period exhibit decreased compliance owing to a combination of cardiac, pulmonary, and chest cavity factors. A major management goal is to increase lung compliance while reducing airway resistance and avoid fluid overload when possible. High CVP and PCWP suggest volume overload and warrant diuresis.[21] Mucus plugging contributes to airway resistance, increased ventilation perfusion mismatch, and low oxygen saturation. As the allograft airway is relatively ischemic from the loss of bronchial artery supply, mucosal sloughing occurs, which needs to be cleared routinely. Cases of airway necrosis, stenosis, and dehiscence can occur in up to 20% of cases in some series.[58] Thus, bronchoscopy is an important part of the diagnostic and therapeutic armamentarium.[57] With impaired surfactant function, poor pain control, and airway secretions, the transplanted lungs often exhibit early atelectasis and noncompliance.[59] Pleural space complications and diaphragmatic dysfunction can restrict the chest cavity and contribute to pulmonary derecruitment. Bleeding, infection, and loss of lymphatic drainage can all lead to pleural space complications.[60] Some patients with preexisting chest restriction based on severely reduced total lung capacity and forced vital capacity or diaphragmatic dysfunction can exhibit significant compressive atelectasis.

PGD is an important cause of early and late mortality and is linked to the development of chronic lung allograft dysfunction (CLAD).[8,26,61,62] It typically occurs in the first 72 hours and is characterized by hypoxemia, pulmonary edema, reduced compliance, and bilateral radiographic infiltrates not explained by other causes. It can range from mild to severe. The International Society for Heart and Lung Transplantation grading scheme based on PF ratio, ranging from grade 1 to 3 with increasing severity, has been adopted to standardize classification.[63] The overall incidence of PGD is about 30%, with grade 3 PGD occurring in 15% to 20% of recipients at 48 and 72 hours after implantation.[8] Preexisting pulmonary hypertension is an important risk factor, as are prolonged ischemic time, obesity, pretransplant diagnoses of sarcoidosis and idiopathic pulmonary

hypertension, and donor risk factors (eg, smoking, age >65 years).[8,26,55] Early recognition helps to develop management strategies to reduce their risk.[64–66] PGD management is largely supportive with preventive measures geared toward optimal donor selection, proper size matching, and improved perioperative management. An example includes using the lowest Fio_2 to support saturation, as high Fio_2 has been associated with allograft reperfusion injury.[26] Similarly, keeping CVP low helps to minimize graft edema. Delayed chest closure has been used as a strategy to manage grade 3 PGD.[28,29] Selected use of ECMO can protect the allograft from diffuse alveolar damage and improve survival.[67] Prophylactic early institution of ECMO may lead to improved outcomes.[68] Venovenous (VV) ECMO can be deployed in patients with good hemodynamics, normal right ventricular function, and no significant pulmonary hypertension.[67] In unstable patients with right ventricular dysfunction, venoarterial (VA) ECMO can protect the right heart and reduce ongoing pulmonary edema.[25,44] ECMO allows the transplanted lung to rest with ultraprotective ventilation strategies, with tidal volume less than 3 mL/kg, and addresses any ongoing respiratory acidosis. In a hemodynamically stable patient, the choice between VV and VA ECMO is controversial.[66]

As a special case, single orthotropic lung transplant has been reported as an independent risk factor for PGD,[26] and it is associated with inferior survival.[10] Although the choice of single versus double remains debatable,[69–71] bilateral lung transplant is the procedure of choice for cystic fibrosis and bronchiectasis, where preexisting infection may contaminate the new lung.[69] Furthermore, single-transplant cases can exhibit severe ventilation perfusion mismatch.[72] In patients with COPD, acute native lung hyperinflation[71] can occur during positive pressure ventilation, resulting in contralateral mediastinal shift, extrinsic compression of the single-lung allograft, hypoxemia, and hemodynamic instability. In patients transplanted for interstitial lung disease, acute exacerbation in the native lung can still occur.[73]

IMMUNOSUPPRESSION

Approximately 25% of lung recipients experience at least one episode of rejection in the first year.[1] The topic of lung allograft rejection is discussed elsewhere in this issue. Although individual programs will differ in their practice, a 2017 survey indicates that 80% of transplant programs incorporated an induction strategy.[1] Although there is no strong evidence favoring a particular strategy, the use of lymphocyte-depleting thymoglobulin and monoclonal anti-CD52 alemtuzumab has declined, whereas that of interleukin-2 receptor alpha-chain antagonist (ie, basiliximab) has increased in 75% of transplant programs.[1] This trend is possibly due to favorable patient tolerance and side-effect profiles.[74] Induction therapy increases the risk of opportunistic infections and lymphoproliferative disorders. Thymoglobulin and alemtuzumab are associated with severe myelosuppression and can cause cytokine-release reactions.[74] In the authors' practice, they intraoperatively administer intravenous mycophenolate and basiliximab with a bolus of methylprednisolone before each allograft perfusion. Conventional maintenance therapy uses corticosteroid, a calcineurin inhibitor (CNI) (tacrolimus or cyclosporine), and an antiproliferative agent (mycophenolate or azathioprine). The authors' preference is tacrolimus with mycophenolate, a combination that is used in more than 80% of transplant cases internationally.[74] Tacrolimus has supplanted cyclosporine as first-line therapy because of lower incidence of acute rejection and CLAD.[74,75] Among CNI adverse effects, which include hyperkalemia, hypertension, hyperlipidemia, and neurotoxicity, nephrotoxicity is one of the most detrimental. The mTOR inhibitors, sirolimus and everolimus, are alternative immunosuppressants that help reduce CNI dose and lower nephrotoxicity, but their use is limited because of concerns for poor wound healing, proteinuria, and edema.[76,77] As for mycophenolate versus azathioprine, studies have not supported a particular choice, but mycophenolate is often favored possibly because of better patient tolerance and decreased risk for skin cancers,[74,78] although it is notably associated with myelosuppression and gastrointestinal disturbances.[79–81] In patients with severe gastrointestinal symptoms, the authors have found better tolerance to mycophenolic acid than mycophenolate. Tolerance to mycophenolate can be variable because of leukopenia.[80]

MANAGEMENT OF INFECTION

Infectious complications are a major cause of mortality after lung transplantation and contribute to lower survival rates relative to other solid organ transplants.[82] This is especially prevalent in the first 3 to 6 months after transplant.[83] Bacterial infections are frequently encountered in the form of pneumonia, pleural space, and wound infections, but also occur in the urinary tract and biliary tree. Timing of the infection and culture data can help direct appropriate therapy. Early administration of broad-spectrum antibiotics is desirable to cover nosocomial infections, including multidrug-resistant organisms.[84] Donor culture results and surveillance bronchoalveolar lavage cultures with susceptibility data can help providers formulate a targeted antimicrobial regimen to reduce donor-to-host transmission with the narrowest effective antibiotic spectrum.[85] Prompt removal of indwelling central-line and urinary catheter together with aggressive pulmonary toiletry are well-known preventive measures against hospital-acquired infections.[86] The emergence of multidrug-resistant microbes can affect decision making, and as such, choices of vancomycin and carbapenem are popular initial therapy for methicillin-resistant Staphylococcus aureus and extended spectrum ß-lactamases, respectively.[87] Vancomycin-resistant Enterococcus can be treated with linezolid. Except for ertapenem, carbapenems generally have good empiric coverage against pseudomonal species. Acinetobacter can be challenging but can be covered by colistin and imipenem/cilastatin.[87] More unusual infections with Nocardia, Listeria, and Rhodococcus are less frequently encountered, and Stenotrophomonas maltophilia can be pesky.[88] In patients with cystic fibrosis and bronchiectasis, native colonizers with multidrug resistance in the upper and lower airways are especially problematic, as lung explantation alone does not remove all potential sources of infection.[89–91]

Invasive fungal infection is another important source of morbidity. Mortality from invasive pulmonary Aspergillus can reach 60%. A survey of about 1700 cases showed an infection prevalence of almost 9% in the first year of transplant,[92] with Aspergillus accounting for more than 70% of all cases.[93] Severe immunosuppression with exposure to Aspergillus colonization at ischemic anastomotic sites and tracheobronchitis are major risk factors for serious infection.[94] Thus, fungal prophylaxis has become standard across many programs in the form of voriconazole with or without inhaled liposomal amphotericin B.[95,96] Despite widespread use, fungal prophylaxis is weakly supported by available data.[97] Other fungal sources come from yeast species, such as Candida, Cryptococcus, Pneumocystis jiroveci, and nonaspergillus, such as Scedosporium and Fusarium. At the authors' program, the authors initiate prophylaxis using intravenous voriconazole with isavuconazole as an alternative. With resumption of enteral alimentation, oral posaconazole is then used to reduce known side effects of voriconazole.[98,99] Posaconazole and isavuconazole have more favorable hepatotoxicity profiles. Voriconazole can cause unique hallucinations in 30% of patients, photosensitivity, and periostitis. It also inhibits CNI metabolism, and prolonged use is associated with increased risk of cutaneous squamous cell carcinoma.[100] Azole use is also known to contribute to QTc prolongation and risk for torsade de pointes.[99]

Finally, viral infections have been associated with acute respiratory failure and bronchiolitis obliterans syndrome (BOS) development. The group of community-acquired respiratory virus (influenza A and B, metapneumovirus, rhinovirus, adenovirus, and respiratory syncytial virus) can cause significant morbidity on a seasonal basis.[101] Severe PGD also can result from both recipient and donor-derived viral infection. For example, the authors retransplanted a recipient 30 days following the first transplant for allograft loss owing to donor-derived metapneumovirus causing ARDS. Preventive actions include hand hygiene, avoidance of sick contacts, and thorough surveillance. Treatment is geared toward the specific organism and available antivirals. Ribavirin in combination with steroids has been used for metapneumovirus and respiratory syncytial virus.[102] Adenovirus, which can cause pneumonia and disseminated disease, can be particularly challenging. Cidofovir has been used with some success.[103] CMV infection is an important cause of mortality and is associated with the development of CLAD. Active CMV infection is identified by DNA replication in serum and biopsy of affected organs. Its incidence is higher in patients with lung transplant than those with other organ transplants, potentiated by donor-recipient CMV mismatch and profound immunosuppression. CMV prophylaxis consists of an antiviral drug, usually valganciclovir, given for 12 months or more and serum viral load monitoring by polymerase chain reaction.[104]

MANAGEMENT OF OTHER MEDICAL COMPLICATIONS

Although preservation of the lung function is the primary focus, several medical complications place patients with lung transplant at risk during their index hospitalization. Immunosuppressive drugs will compound preexisting conditions, including osteoporosis, diabetes, hypertension, coronary artery disease, and gastroesophageal reflux disease (GERD).[3,74] Indeed, hyperkalemia, hyperglycemia, and hyperlipidemia are frequent metabolic disturbances. Tremors, leukopenia, anemia, and diarrhea are common adverse effects of tacrolimus, mycophenolate, and valganciclovir.[74,80]

A high GERD prevalence has been observed in pretransplant recipients.[105–107] Pretransplant manometry and pH studies often show associated hiatal hernia, esophageal dysmotility, and elevated DeMeester scores. Acid reflux exposure can worsen after transplantation.[107,108] Indeed, BOS has been linked to GERD.[109] To this end, proton-pump inhibitor therapy is used to counteract acid reflux but may not address microaspiration from nonacid reflux.[106] Early postoperative antireflux surgery is thought to be protective and associated with improved survival and freedom from BOS.[108,110]

Acute kidney injury (AKI) is common after lung transplantation and is a prognostic marker for long-term outcome. Wehbe and colleagues[111] reported that AKI developed in 65% of the patients within 2 weeks of transplant. Those who were discharged without renal recovery had higher incidence of chronic kidney disease and lower survival at 12 months. Interestingly, even those with renal recovery had relatively poorer long-term outcome as compared with those without AKI. Risk factors are multifactorial, including older age, diabetes, poorly controlled hypertension, sepsis, perioperative hypotension, and importantly, the use of CNI.[111,112] This highlights the importance of early awareness of risk factors and aggressive management directed toward more renoprotective strategies, including hypertension control,[113] early referral to a nephrology specialist, minimization of CNI, while balancing the need to prevent rejection.[112,114]

Pleural complications are frequent and negatively impact allograft function.[115,116] Pleural fluid characteristics change with time, and excess drainage is thought to be secondary to increase alveolar capillary permeability and disruption of pulmonary lymphatics.[60] Indeed, the authors' own observation is consistent with the published literature reporting that significant drainage can last for 9 to 19 days,[39,60] and thus, the need for chest tube leads to an increase length of stay. In their cohort, Ferrer and colleagues[39] observed that 12 of their patients had chest tubes in for more than 30 days, and the investigators hypothesized that this may be due to the time needed to reestablish lymphatic drainage. Tang and colleagues[116] reported that, out of 1039 patients, almost 200 patients required more than 300 thoracenteses and 200 thoracostomies. Unfortunately, 140 patients needed an open operation for washouts, and another 88 patients required decortication. In a retrospective study by Marom and colleagues,[117] 31 patients with pleural effusions were treated with percutaneous small-bore catheters, with 16/31 cases categorized as infectious. A median time of 6 days was necessary for drainage, and residual collections were treated with streptokinase as thrombolytic therapy. Furthermore, 9/31 patients required multiple catheter insertions. At the 3-month follow-up, 79% of the patients had a complete response. However, of the 16 patients with empyema, 9 patients died within 6 months of drainage intervention.

Finally, multiple reports have documented the high prevalence of deep vein thrombosis (DVT) in the transplant population.[118] A single-center study showed that routine lower-extremity screening identified a 17% DVT rate in the first 90 days. Another report by Jorge and colleagues[119] suggested that universal DVT screening might be associated with improved 1-year survival. As DVT can negatively impact survival,[120] the authors' program routinely uses prophylaxis with subcutaneous unfractionated heparin in hospitalized patients.

SUMMARY

The early postoperative period after lung transplantation is a critical time. Prompt recognition and treatment of PGD can alter long-term allograft function. Cardiovascular, gastrointestinal, renal, hematologic derangements and infectious complications are common and require close management to limit their negative sequelae.

DISCLOSURE

B.N. Trinh: nothing to disclose. J. Kukreja: TransMedics (research); Lung Bioengineering (data monitoring committee). M. Brzezinski: Trevena and Grifols (research).

REFERENCES

1. Chambers, et al. The International Thoracic Organ Transplant Registry of the International Society for Heart and Lung Transplantation: thirty-sixth adult lung and heart-lung transplantation report-2019; focus theme: donor and recipient size match. J Heart Lung Transplant 2019;38(10):1042–55.
2. Hamilton, et al. Improved survival after lung transplantation for adults requiring preoperative invasive mechanical ventilation: a national cohort study. J Thorac Cardiovasc Surg 2020;160(5):1385–95.e6.
3. Sam, et al. Roles and impacts of the transplant pharmacist: a systematic review. Can J Hosp Pharm 2018;71(5):324–37.
4. Gordon, et al. Reducing length of stay after lung transplant through Implementation of multidisciplinary care coordination rounds. J Heart Lung Transplantation 2020;39(4):S209.
5. Allen, et al. The impact of recipient body mass index on survival after lung transplantation. J Heart Lung Transplant 2010;29(9):1026–33.
6. Weill, et al. A consensus document for the selection of lung transplant candidates: 2014–an update from the Pulmonary Transplantation Council of the International Society for Heart and Lung Transplantation. J Heart Lung Transplant 2015;34(1):1–15.
7. McKellar, et al. Lung transplantation following coronary artery bypass surgery-improved outcomes following single-lung transplant. J Heart Lung Transplant 2016;35(11):1289–94.
8. Diamond, et al. Report of the International Society for Heart and Lung Transplantation Working Group on Primary Lung Graft Dysfunction, part II: epidemiology, risk factors, and outcomes-a 2016 consensus group statement of the International Society for Heart and Lung Transplantation. J Heart Lung Transplant 2017;36(10):1104–13.
9. Wallinder, et al. Outcomes and long-term survival after pulmonary retransplantation: a single-center experience. Ann Thorac Surg 2019;108(4):1037–44.
10. Chambers, et al. The International Thoracic Organ Transplant Registry of the International Society for Heart and Lung Transplantation: thirty-fifth adult lung and heart-lung transplant report-2018; focus theme: multiorgan transplantation. J Heart Lung Transplant 2018;37(10):1169–83.
11. Hoopes, et al. Extracorporeal membrane oxygenation as a bridge to pulmonary transplantation. J Thorac Cardiovasc Surg 2013;145(3):862–7 [discussion: 867–8].
12. Kukreja, et al. Risk factors and outcomes of extracorporeal membrane oxygenation as a bridge to lung transplantation. Semin Thorac Cardiovasc Surg 2020;32(4):772–85.
13. Singer, et al. Frailty phenotypes and mortality after lung transplantation: a prospective cohort study. Am J Transplant 2018;18(8):1995–2004.
14. Bharat, et al. Early outcomes after lung transplantation for severe COVID-19: a series of the first consecutive cases from four countries. Lancet Respir Med 2021;9(5):487–97.
15. Cypel, et al. When to consider lung transplantation for COVID-19. Lancet Respir Med 2020;8(10):944–6.
16. Lederer, et al. Obesity and underweight are associated with an increased risk of death after lung transplantation. Am J Respir Crit Care Med 2009;180(9):887–95.
17. Martinu, et al. Baseline 6-min walk distance predicts survival in lung transplant candidates. Am J Transplant 2008;8(7):1498–505.
18. Rochester pulmonary rehabilitation for patients who undergo lung-volume-reduction surgery or lung transplantation. Respir Care 2008;53(9):1196–202.
19. Chicotka, et al. Increasing opportunity for lung transplant in interstitial lung disease with pulmonary hypertension. Ann Thorac Surg 2018;106(6):1812–9.

20. Eberlein, et al. Lung size mismatch and primary graft dysfunction after bilateral lung transplantation. J Heart Lung Transplant 2015;34(2):233–40.

21. Subramaniam, et al. Anesthetic management of lung transplantation: results from a multicenter, cross-sectional survey by the society for advancement of transplant anesthesia. Clin Transplant 2020;34(8):e13996.

22. Bermudez, et al. Outcomes of intraoperative venoarterial extracorporeal membrane oxygenation versus cardiopulmonary bypass during lung transplantation. Ann Thorac Surg 2014;98(6):1936–42 [discussion: 1942–3].

23. Machuca, et al. Outcomes of intraoperative extracorporeal membrane oxygenation versus cardiopulmonary bypass for lung transplantation. J Thorac Cardiovasc Surg 2015;149(4):1152–7.

24. Nagendran, et al. Should double lung transplant be performed with or without cardiopulmonary bypass? Interact Cardiovasc Thorac Surg 2011; 12(5):799–804.

25. Hoetzenecker, et al. Bilateral lung transplantation on intraoperative extracorporeal membrane oxygenator: an observational study. J Thorac Cardiovasc Surg 2020;160(1):320–327 e1.

26. Diamond, et al. Clinical risk factors for primary graft dysfunction after lung transplantation. Am J Respir Crit Care Med 2013;187(5):527–34.

27. Grimm, et al. Association between prolonged graft ischemia and primary graft failure or survival following lung transplantation. JAMA Surg 2015; 150(6):547–53.

28. Force, et al. Outcomes of delayed chest closure after bilateral lung transplantation. Ann Thorac Surg 2006;81(6):2020–4 [discussion: 2024–5].

29. Shigemura, et al. Delayed chest closure after lung transplantation: techniques, outcomes, and strategies. J Heart Lung Transplant 2014;33(7):741–8.

30. Tsou et al. Delayed chest closure following bilateral lung transplantation: risk factors and outcomes. Mar 2020 - Present. . Mini-oral presentation at the 41st Annual Meeting & Scientific Sessions of the International Society for Heart and Lung Transplantation (ISHLT) April 24-28, 2021,

31. Yerebakan, et al. Effects of inhaled nitric oxide following lung transplantation. J Card Surg 2009; 24(3):269–74.

32. Khan, et al. A prospective, randomized, crossover pilot study of inhaled nitric oxide versus inhaled prostacyclin in heart transplant and lung transplant recipients. J Thorac Cardiovasc Surg 2009;138(6): 1417–24.

33. Mason, et al. Atrial fibrillation after lung transplantation: timing, risk factors, and treatment. Ann Thorac Surg 2007;84(6):1878–84.

34. Waldron, et al. Adverse outcomes associated with postoperative atrial arrhythmias after lung transplantation: a meta-analysis and systematic review of the literature. Clin Transplant 2017;31(4). https://doi.org/10.1111/ctr.12926.

35. Frendl, et al. 2014 AATS guidelines for the prevention and management of perioperative atrial fibrillation and flutter for thoracic surgical procedures. J Thorac Cardiovasc Surg 2014;148(3): e153–93.

36. Whitlock, et al. Left atrial appendage occlusion during cardiac surgery to prevent stroke. N Engl J Med 2021;384(22):2081–91.

37. Worrell, et al. Is lactic acidosis after lung transplantation associated with worse outcomes? Ann Thorac Surg 2020;110(2):434–40.

38. Xu, et al. The prognostic value of peak arterial lactate levels within 72 h of lung transplantation in identifying patient outcome. J Thorac Dis 2020; 12(12):7365–73.

39. Ferrer, et al. Acute and chronic pleural complications in lung transplantation. J Heart Lung Transplant 2003;22(11):1217–25.

40. Navarro C, et al. [Complications after lung transplantation in chronic obstructive pulmonary disease]. Med Clin (Barc) 2013;140(9):385–9.

41. Zimring, et al. Current problems and future directions of transfusion-induced alloimmunization: summary of an NHLBI working group. Transfusion 2011;51(2):435–41.

42. Brand immunological complications of blood transfusions. Presse Med 2016;45(7–8 Pt 2):e313–24.

43. Bux, et al. The pathogenesis of transfusion-related acute lung injury (TRALI). Br J Haematol 2007; 136(6):788–99.

44. Fischer, et al. Extracorporeal membrane oxygenation for primary graft dysfunction after lung transplantation: analysis of the Extracorporeal Life Support Organization (ELSO) registry. J Heart Lung Transplant 2007;26(5):472–7.

45. King, et al. Early postoperative management after lung transplantation: results of an international survey. Clin Transplant 2017;31(7). https://doi.org/10. 1111/ctr.12985.

46. Schlichter Dexmedetomidine is an excellent agent for sedation status-post lung transplant. J Clin Anesth 2010;22(1):1–2.

47. Feltracco, et al. Thoracic epidural analgesia in lung transplantation. Transplant Proc 2010;42(4): 1265–9.

48. Clemence, et al. Cryoablation of intercostal nerves decreased narcotic usage after thoracic or thoracoabdominal aortic aneurysm repair. Semin Thorac Cardiovasc Surg 2020;32(3):404–12.

49. Graves, et al. Intraoperative intercostal nerve cryoablation during the Nuss procedure reduces length of stay and opioid requirement: a randomized clinical trial. J Pediatr Surg 2019;54(11): 2250–6.

50. Haro et al. Intercostal nerve cryoanalgesia versus thoracic epidural analgesia in lung transplantation. The Western Thoracic Surgical Association 2019 Abstract. 2019,

51. Parrado, et al. The use of cryoanalgesia in minimally invasive repair of pectus excavatum: lessons learned. J Laparoendosc Adv Surg Tech A 2019; 29(10):1244–51.

52. Beer, et al. Mechanical ventilation after lung transplantation. An international survey of practices and preferences. Ann Am Thorac Soc 2014;11(4): 546–53.

53. Dezube, et al. The effect of lung-size mismatch on mechanical ventilation tidal volumes after bilateral lung transplantation. Interact Cardiovasc Thorac Surg 2013;16(3):275–81.

54. Mascia, et al. Effect of a lung protective strategy for organ donors on eligibility and availability of lungs for transplantation: a randomized controlled trial. JAMA 2010;304(23):2620–7.

55. Liu, et al. Recipient-related clinical risk factors for primary graft dysfunction after lung transplantation: a systematic review and meta-analysis. PLoS One 2014;9(3):e92773.

56. Meade, et al. A randomized trial of inhaled nitric oxide to prevent ischemia-reperfusion injury after lung transplantation. Am J Respir Crit Care Med 2003;167(11):1483–9.

57. Trulock. Flexible bronchoscopy in lung transplantation. Clin Chest Med 1999;20(1):77–87.

58. Machuzak, et al. Airway complications after lung transplantation. Thorac Surg Clin 2015;25(1): 55–75.

59. Amital, et al. Surfactant as salvage therapy in life threatening primary graft dysfunction in lung transplantation. Eur J Cardiothorac Surg 2009;35(2): 299–303.

60. Judson, et al. Pleural effusions following lung transplantation. Time course, characteristics, and clinical implications. Chest 1996;109(5):1190–4.

61. Christie, et al. Primary graft failure following lung transplantation. Chest 1998;114(1):51–60.

62. Huang, et al. Late primary graft dysfunction after lung transplantation and bronchiolitis obliterans syndrome. Am J Transplant 2008;8(11):2454–62.

63. Snell, et al. Report of the ISHLT Working Group on Primary Lung Graft Dysfunction, part I: definition and grading-a 2016 consensus group statement of the International Society for Heart and Lung Transplantation. J Heart Lung Transplant 2017; 36(10):1097–103.

64. de Perrot, et al. Report of the ISHLT Working Group on Primary Lung Graft Dysfunction part III: donor-related risk factors and markers. J Heart Lung Transplant 2005;24(10):1460–7.

65. Barr, et al. Report of the ISHLT Working Group on Primary Lung Graft Dysfunction part IV: recipient-related risk factors and markers. J Heart Lung Transplant 2005;24(10):1468–82.

66. Van Raemdonck, et al. Report of the ISHLT Working Group on primary lung graft dysfunction part IV: prevention and treatment: a 2016 consensus group statement of the International Society for Heart and Lung Transplantation. J Heart Lung Transplant 2017;36(10):1121–36.

67. Hartwig, et al. Improved survival but marginal allograft function in patients treated with extracorporeal membrane oxygenation after lung transplantation. Ann Thorac Surg 2012;93(2): 366–71.

68. Wigfield, et al. Early institution of extracorporeal membrane oxygenation for primary graft dysfunction after lung transplantation improves outcome. J Heart Lung Transplant 2007;26(4):331–8.

69. Puri, et al. Single versus bilateral lung transplantation: do guidelines exist? Thorac Surg Clin 2015; 25(1):47–54.

70. Brown, et al. Outcomes after single lung transplantation in older patients with secondary pulmonary arterial hypertension. J Heart Lung Transplant 2013;32(1):134–6.

71. Siddiqui, et al. Lung transplantation for chronic obstructive pulmonary disease: past, present, and future directions. Curr Opin Pulm Med 2018; 24(2):199–204.

72. Stevens, et al. Regional ventilation and perfusion after lung transplantation in patients with emphysema. N Engl J Med 1970;282(5):245–9.

73. Marron, et al. Acute hypoxemic respiratory failure and native lung idiopathic pulmonary fibrosis exacerbation in single-lung transplant patients with cytomegalovirus disease: a case series. Transplant Proc 2019;51(10):3391–4.

74. Chung, et al. Immunosuppressive strategies in lung transplantation. Ann Transl Med 2020;8(6): 409.

75. Treede, et al. Tacrolimus versus cyclosporine after lung transplantation: a prospective, open, randomized two-center trial comparing two different immunosuppressive protocols. J Heart Lung Transplant 2001;20(5):511–7.

76. Gottlieb, et al. A randomized trial of everolimus-based quadruple therapy vs standard triple therapy early after lung transplantation. Am J Transplant 2019;19(6):1759–69.

77. Groetzner, et al. Airway anastomosis complications in de novo lung transplantation with sirolimus-based immunosuppression. J Heart Lung Transplant 2004;23(5):632–8.

78. Palmer, et al. Results of a randomized, prospective, multicenter trial of mycophenolate mofetil versus azathioprine in the prevention of acute lung allograft rejection. Transplantation 2001;71(12): 1772–6.

79. Ceschi, et al. Acute mycophenolate overdose: case series and systematic literature analysis. Expert Opin Drug Saf 2014;13(5):525–34.

80. Tokman, et al. Clinical outcomes of lung transplant recipients with telomerase mutations. J Heart Lung Transplant 2015;34(10):1318–24.

81. A blinded, randomized clinical trial of mycophenolate mofetil for the prevention of acute rejection in cadaveric renal transplantation. The Tricontinental Mycophenolate Mofetil Renal Transplantation Study Group. Transplantation 1996;61(7):1029–37.

82. Parada, et al. Early and late infections in lung transplantation patients. Transplant Proc 2010;42(1): 333–5.

83. Christie, et al. The registry of the International Society for Heart and Lung Transplantation: 29th adult lung and heart-lung transplant report-2012. J Heart Lung Transplant 2012;31(10):1073–86.

84. Remund, et al. Infections relevant to lung transplantation. Proc Am Thorac Soc 2009;6(1):94–100.

85. Ruiz, et al. Donor-to-host transmission of bacterial and fungal infections in lung transplantation. Am J Transplant 2006;6(1):178–82.

86. Septimus, et al. Prevention of device-related healthcare-associated infections. F1000Res 2016; 5. F1000 Faculty Rev-65.

87. Patel, et al. Carbapenem-resistant Enterobacteriaceae and Acinetobacter baumannii: assessing their impact on organ transplantation. Curr Opin Organ Transplant 2010;15(6):676–82.

88. Khan, et al. Nocardia infection in lung transplant recipients. Clin Transplant 2008;22(5):562–6.

89. Shteinberg, et al. The impact of fluoroquinolone resistance of Gram-negative bacteria in respiratory secretions on the outcome of lung transplant (noncystic fibrosis) recipients. Clin Transplant 2012; 26(6):884–90.

90. Hadjiliadis, et al. Survival of lung transplant patients with cystic fibrosis harboring panresistant bacteria other than Burkholderia cepacia, compared with patients harboring sensitive bacteria. J Heart Lung Transplant 2007;26(8):834–8.

91. Vital, et al. Impact of sinus surgery on pseudomonal airway colonization, bronchiolitis obliterans syndrome and survival in cystic fibrosis lung transplant recipients. Respiration 2013;86(1):25–31.

92. Pappas, et al. Invasive fungal infections among organ transplant recipients: results of the Transplant-Associated Infection Surveillance Network (TRANSNET). Clin Infect Dis 2010;50(8):1101–11.

93. Doligalski, et al. Epidemiology of invasive mold infections in lung transplant recipients. Am J Transplant 2014;14(6):1328–33.

94. Luong, et al. Pretransplant Aspergillus colonization of cystic fibrosis patients and the incidence of post-lung transplant invasive aspergillosis. Transplantation 2014;97(3):351–7.

95. Marino, et al. Prophylactic antifungal agents used after lung transplantation. Ann Pharmacother 2010;44(3):546–56.

96. Neoh, et al. Antifungal prophylaxis in lung transplantation–a world-wide survey. Am J Transplant 2011;11(2):361–6.

97. Pennington, et al. Antifungal prophylaxis in lung transplant recipients: a systematic review and meta-analysis. Transpl Infect Dis 2020;22(4): e13333.

98. Walsh, et al. Treatment of invasive aspergillosis with posaconazole in patients who are refractory to or intolerant of conventional therapy: an externally controlled trial. Clin Infect Dis 2007;44(1): 2–12.

99. Klatt, et al. Review of pharmacologic considerations in the use of azole antifungals in lung transplant recipients. J Fungi (Basel) 2021;7(2):76.

100. Singer, et al. High cumulative dose exposure to voriconazole is associated with cutaneous squamous cell carcinoma in lung transplant recipients. J Heart Lung Transplant 2012;31(7):694–9.

101. Bailey, et al. A mini-review of adverse lung transplant outcomes associated with respiratory viruses. Front Immunol 2019;10:2861.

102. Li, et al. Oral versus inhaled ribavirin therapy for respiratory syncytial virus infection after lung transplantation. J Heart Lung Transplant 2012;31(8): 839–44.

103. Sandkovsky, et al. Adenovirus: current epidemiology and emerging approaches to prevention and treatment. Curr Infect Dis Rep 2014;16(8):416.

104. Zuk, et al. An international survey of cytomegalovirus management practices in lung transplantation. Transplantation 2010;90(6):672–6.

105. Sweet, et al. The prevalence of distal and proximal gastroesophageal reflux in patients awaiting lung transplantation. Ann Surg 2006;244(4):491–7.

106. Blondeau, et al. Gastro-oesophageal reflux and gastric aspiration in lung transplant patients with or without chronic rejection. Eur Respir J 2008; 31(4):707–13.

107. Young, et al. Lung transplantation exacerbates gastroesophageal reflux disease. Chest 2003; 124(5):1689–93.

108. Hartwig, et al. Fundoplication after lung transplantation prevents the allograft dysfunction associated with reflux. Ann Thorac Surg 2011;92(2):462–8 [discussion; 468–8].

109. Davis, et al. Improved lung allograft function after fundoplication in patients with gastroesophageal reflux disease undergoing lung transplantation. J Thorac Cardiovasc Surg 2003;125(3):533–42.

110. Linden, et al. Laparoscopic fundoplication in patients with end-stage lung disease awaiting transplantation. J Thorac Cardiovasc Surg 2006; 131(2):438–46.

111. Wehbe, et al. Recovery from AKI and short- and long-term outcomes after lung transplantation. Clin J Am Soc Nephrol 2013;8(1):19–25.

112. Canales, et al. Predictors of chronic kidney disease in long-term survivors of lung and heart-lung transplantation. Am J Transplant 2006;6(9):2157–63.

113. James, et al. 2014 evidence-based guideline for the management of high blood pressure in adults: report from the panel members appointed to the Eighth Joint National Committee (JNC 8). JAMA 2014;311(5):507–20.

114. Snell, et al. Sirolimus allows renal recovery in lung and heart transplant recipients with chronic renal impairment. J Heart Lung Transplant 2002;21(5):540–6.

115. Rappaport, et al. Pleural space management after lung transplant: early and late outcomes of pleural decortication. J Heart Lung Transplant 2021;40(7):623–30.

116. Tang, et al. Natural history of pleural complications after lung transplantation. Ann Thorac Surg 2021;111(2):407–15.

117. Marom, et al. Pleural effusions in lung transplant recipients: image-guided small-bore catheter drainage. Radiology 2003;228(1):241–5.

118. Evans, et al. Venous thromboembolic complications of lung transplantation: a contemporary single-institution review. Ann Thorac Surg 2015;100(6):2033–9 [discussion: 2039–40].

119. Jorge, et al. Routine deep vein thrombosis screening after lung transplantation: incidence and risk factors. J Thorac Cardiovasc Surg 2020;159(3):1142–50.

120. Neto R, et al. Venous thromboembolism after adult lung transplantation: a frequent event associated with lower survival. Transplantation 2018;102(4):681–7.

Surgical Complications of Lung Transplantation

Gabriel Loor, MD[a,b,]*, Aladdein Mattar, MD[a], Lara Schaheen, MD[c,d], Ross M. Bremner, MD, PhD[c,d]

KEYWORDS

- Lung transplant • Wound complications • Primary graft dysfunction • Airway ischemia
- Vascular complications

KEY POINTS

- Lung transplantation is a life-saving intervention for patients with end-stage lung disease.
- Despite the effectiveness of lung transplantation, it is a major operation with several opportunities for complications.
- Knowledge of these complications helps to avoid them, and to detect and mitigate them early should they occur.

INTRODUCTION

Lung transplantation is one of the most challenging surgical specialties, not only because of the technical requirements but also because of the many complications that the surgeon must prevent, detect, and manage. The surgeon's ability to do so has a profound effect on patient outcomes. In this article, we discuss these challenges so that transplant surgeons, medical specialists, and transplant programs can meet their greatest potential.

WOUND COMPLICATIONS

Wound complications affect roughly 15% of patients who undergo lung transplantation. General risk factors for wound complications include diabetes, immunosuppression medications, recipient illness, and obesity.[1–3] However, risk factors that are unique to patients who undergo lung transplantation include high doses of immunosuppression medications, contamination from entry into the airway, and extensive surgical trauma with or without mechanical circulatory support.

Infectious complications are commonly caused by bacterial organisms but can also be caused by fungal species. Characteristic signs are erythema, fever, purulence, and dehiscence, along with positive wound cultures. Initially, the patient is treated with antibiotics against the most likely offending agent. Because lung transplant recipients are immunosuppressed and susceptible to a variety of bacterial organisms, a reasonable approach is to begin with broad antibiotic coverage that addresses gram-positive and gram-negative bacterial organisms until the final cultures return. Treatment of a minor and superficial infectious wound complication may involve opening the incision if a small collection of purulence is present. Iodoform packing or wet-to-dry gauze dressing changes allow for local debridement and healing by secondary intention. However, surgeons should maintain a low threshold to explore the wound in the operating room if there is suspicion that it is deep or contiguous with foreign bodies, such as surgical wires (**Fig. 1**). A computed tomography scan of the chest is helpful for identifying the extent of the infection.

[a] Department of Surgery and Baylor Lung Institute, Baylor College of Medicine, One Baylor Plaza, MS: BCM390, Houston, TX 77030, USA; [b] Division of Cardiothoracic Transplantation and Circulatory Support, Texas Heart Institute, 6720 Bertner Avenue Suite C355K, Houston, TX 77030, USA; [c] Norton Thoracic Institute, St. Joseph's Medical Center, 500 W Thomas Rd Ste 500, Phoenix, AZ 85013, USA; [d] Creighton University School of Medicine–Phoenix Regional Campus, 350 W. Thomas Rd, Phoenix, AZ 85013, USA
* Corresponding author. Department of Surgery, Baylor College of Medicine, One Baylor Plaza, MS: BCM390, Houston, TX 77030.
E-mail address: Gabriel.Loor@bcm.edu

Thorac Surg Clin 32 (2022) 197–209
https://doi.org/10.1016/j.thorsurg.2022.01.003

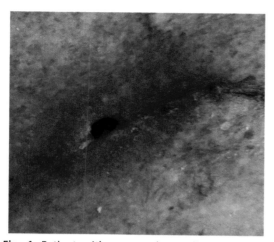

Fig. 1. Patient with a wound complication of the clamshell incision showing erythema and dehiscence initially treated with antibiotics, local incision, and drainage. Surgical exploration, debridement, pulse lavage, removal of sternal hardware, and vacuum-assisted closure followed. A plastic surgeon assisted with delayed closure by using a muscle flap.

If the infectious wound complication is deep with a contained purulent collection or foreign body, operative exploration is required. In such cases, the surgeon debrides and removes all infected material so that only healthy tissue remains. This involves sharp dissection, pulse lavage with antibiotic irrigation, and application of temporary wet-to-dry dressings, or more commonly a vacuum-assisted closure device.[4,5] Typically, such wounds close with vacuum-assisted closure therapy by secondary intention, but another option to expedite healing is primary closure with or without muscle flaps.[6] If, during operative debridement, foreign bodies such as wires or sutures are removed, the stability of the wound should be assessed. If the sternum or thoracotomy is stable, ideally a vacuum-assisted closure device is applied until there is confidence that the wound has been debrided free of the infective inoculum. If the removal of wires or sutures leaves the sternum or thoracotomy unstable, the concern becomes injury to the underlying heart or lung. As soon as most of the infection is gone, fixation with sutures, plates, wires, biologic, or artificial mesh material is necessary.[7] If rigid fixation is not possible, the advancement of biologic tissue, such as muscle or omentum, can provide some protection to the underlying lung or heart, depending on the scenario.

Lung herniation occurs in approximately 2% of thoracic surgery incisions; however, in lung transplantation, its prevalence may be higher secondary to immunosuppression. Meticulous attention to closure technique can prevent lung herniation, but this complication is sometimes unavoidable because of patient mobility, body habitus, or impaired wound healing. Such lung herniation is treated in the operating room by dissecting out the herniated lung segment from the chest wall and either primarily closing the defect or suturing a polypropylene mesh to secure the defect.[8]

Surgeons can reduce surgical site infections by using a variety of techniques including the use of meticulous closure technique; the maintenance of good glycemic control, excellent hemostasis, and normothermia; the treatment of remote infections; and the appropriate use of perioperative antibiotics.[3] Although there is no consensus on the best antibiotic regimens to use, many centers tailor antibiotics depending on history of colonization.[9] Most centers use gram-positive and gram-negative agents for up to 7 days in transplant recipients without evidence of prior colonization and for at least 14 days in recipients with colonization.[9] Considering prior resistant strains is important when choosing perioperative antimicrobials.

The choice of surgical exposure may contribute to wound complications. The bilateral thoracotomy with transverse sternotomy incision (also known as the clamshell incision) is the most common approach for lung transplantation.[10] However, this approach sacrifices the bilateral mammary artery, which in turn compromises blood flow for healing. Elde and colleagues[11] showed that using a median sternotomy approach when feasible for lung transplantations performed with cardiopulmonary bypass (CPB) support was associated with a 0% incidence of major wound complications, whereas the incidence was 20% over 3 years when a clamshell incision was used. Another option for reducing the incidence of wound infections is using an isolated thoracotomy incision without transverse sternotomy. In our opinion, the clamshell approach currently remains the most versatile incision. Its excellent exposure and flexibility allow transplantation to proceed without mechanical circulatory support or with limited support from extracorporeal membrane oxygenation (ECMO), providing ease of central cannulation access.

PRIMARY GRAFT DYSFUNCTION

Primary graft dysfunction (PGD) is the most common cause of early morbidity and mortality after lung transplantation.[12] Operative decisions greatly influence the development of PGD, beginning with the choice and management of the donor organ. A reasonable selection strategy to prevent severe PGD is to avoid combination of donor and recipient risk factors when feasible.[13] The combination of recipient risk factors for PGD (eg, elevated body mass index, pulmonary hypertension, sarcoidosis) and donor risk factors (eg, history of smoking) may increase the chance of severe PGD, especially if adding operative variables that are associated with PGD, such as a large-volume blood transfusion or use of CPB. An area of active investigation is the use of novel preservation methods to reduce the risk of PGD in the donor. In a randomized, controlled study on portable ex vivo lung perfusion, use of the Organ Care System Lung (TransMedics, Inc, Andover, MA) was shown to reduce the incidence of PGD by 50%.[14]

Moreover, extracorporeal life support strategies used during the operation have been shown to affect PGD. Diamond and colleagues[13] showed that the use of CPB during lung transplantation was the most significant operative risk factor for the development of PGD. However, Hoetzenecker and colleagues[15] reported low rates of PGD when the surgeon used intraoperative central venoarterial (VA) ECMO during lung transplantation, regardless of the indication for transplant. Although the transplant community has shown enthusiasm for the use of ECMO over CPB, it remains unclear whether ECMO should be preferred over an off-pump approach as a support strategy for reducing PGD. Finally, the development of PGD may be affected by the use of intraoperative blood products, the fraction of inspired oxygen at reperfusion, and clamp release practices.[13,16,17]

When PGD occurs, it is immediately life threatening and contributes to long-term graft dysfunction.[12,18,19] Once detected, PGD should prompt heightened vigilance by the operating team to ensure adequate oxygen delivery to support end-organ function with the least amount of collateral injury. To avoid collateral damage, surgeons should consider ECMO as a mainstay of management for severe PGD.[20] Typically, venovenous ECMO provides adequate oxygenation, facilitates CO_2 clearance, and normalizes oxygen delivery with a significant reduction in ventilator and vasopressor requirements. However, if marked right- or left-sided ventricular dysfunction is present, VA ECMO should be considered.

AIRWAY ISCHEMIA

Airway ischemia is a potential complication of lung transplantation, with an incidence between 15% and 35%, depending on the definition.[21–23] Airway ischemia occurs because of limited blood supply at the level of the anastomosis, leading to necrosis with or without dehiscence. As the airway heals, it

has a tendency to overgranulate, leading to stenosis. Risk factors inherent to the procedure make some degree of airway ischemia almost unavoidable. Such risk factors include donor ischemia, ischemia-reperfusion injury, immunosuppression, scarce collateral blood supply at the bronchial anastomosis, and bacterial colonization.

Researchers have identified several donor and recipient risk factors for airway ischemia, some of which are potentially modifiable. A study by the Leuven lung transplant group published in 2007[23] showed that donors who were on a ventilator for 50 to 70 hours were at the greatest risk of airway complications, which was attributed to untreated ventilator-associated pneumonia. In a study by Ruttmann and colleagues,[24] graft reperfusion injury and rejection were identified as significant risk factors on multivariate analysis. Thus, strategies that reduce graft dysfunction may conceivably reduce airway ischemia.

Large size mismatches between the donor and recipient airways could result in airway complications. If the recipient has large mainstem bronchi and the donor is very small, the radial tension could impair healing. Similarly, if a smaller recipient airway telescopes into a donor larger airway, the telescoped segment may develop ischemia, presumably because of compromised collateral blood supply.[23] A report by Keshava and colleagues[25] highlights this scenario in pediatric donors.

Investigators have identified donor preservation factors that are potential contributors to airway ischemia. In a study by Necki and colleagues,[22] prolonged cold ischemic time was a strong risk factor for the development of airway complications. Conversely, in a study by Li and colleagues,[21] recipients of extended criteria donor lungs preserved with portable warm perfusion by using the Organ Care System Lung (TransMedics, Inc) developed airway ischemia more commonly than did recipients of lungs preserved with ice in the standard fashion, particularly when the anastomosis was performed with a continuous running rather than an interrupted suture technique.

Several investigators have examined the importance of surgical techniques in the prevention of airway ischemia. A study by Van Berkel and colleagues[26] showed that trimming the donor airway to one ring or less from the secondary carina decreased the incidence of airway complications (dehiscence, obstruction, or malacia) from 13% to 2%. Similarly, a study by FitzSullivan and colleagues[27] showed that trimming the airway back to the secondary carina and incorporating an interrupted figure-of-eight suture technique to the anterior cartilaginous portion of the anastomosis decreased the incidence of airway complications from 18% to 2%.

A potentially important surgical advancement aimed at reducing airway ischemia is bronchial artery revascularization. This technique requires procurement of the donor lungs en bloc with the descending aorta so that a cuff of the main bronchial artery or arteries is fashioned and sewn to the recipient's left mammary artery or aorta.[28,29] The technical challenge of this procedure, along with the increased bleeding risk associated with its use, have limited its widespread adoption. However, we believe this technique deserves additional attention and its outcomes further analysis.

From a perioperative standpoint, some considerations may reduce the risk of airway ischemia. Avoiding hypotension, improving nutrition, and maintaining good cardiac output and mixed venous oxygen levels may help to reduce ischemia. Although these concepts are intuitive, they have not been well evaluated in the literature. Physicians should also be careful to limit aggressive steroid use in patients at risk to prevent airway ischemia.[24]

With the updated International Society for Heart and Lung Transplantation consensus report on airway complications in 2018,[30] the detection and classification of airway complications have improved. These guidelines capture changes in the mucosa affecting variable portions of the anastomosis rather than just capturing dehiscence or stricture, making them more sensitive than prior grading schemes.[21] Surgeons would typically regard any ischemia graded as B2 or greater, or any dehiscence, stricture, or malacia requiring surveillance or intervention, as clinically significant airway ischemia (**Fig. 2**).

The treatment of airway ischemia involves surveillance, recipient optimization, and endobronchial interventions when needed. Rarely is surgical intervention or retransplantation considered. Most of the time, surgeons or pulmonologists monitor airway ischemia without dehiscence by using surveillance bronchoscopies and gentle debridement, as needed. The same is true for limited dehiscence.[31,32] If ischemia turns into stenosis because of excessive healing, balloon dilation or placement of a stent may be required.[30,33] If dehiscence increases in size, placement of a stent may help to bridge the gap and allow healing.[31,32] In severe cases where the stent is not providing adequate coverage, the surgeon may need to consider an open repair. In our experience, such repair is seldom necessary and rarely successful because of the scarcity of adequate tissue to hold sutures. Furthermore, omental or pericardial tissue may be limited as a result of immunosuppression and malnutrition. Surgeons may consider a pneumonectomy as an alternative, depending on the quality of the contralateral lung. In these extreme cases in which operative intervention is required, one should also consider the idea of a salvage single-lung transplant.

VASCULAR COMPLICATIONS

Vascular complications occur in approximately 1% to 3% of cases affecting either the pulmonary artery or the pulmonary veins.[34,35] Any obstruction of the pulmonary blood flow can compromise the allograft, which depends entirely on the pulmonary artery flow, with the rare exception of a heart-lung block or bronchial artery revascularization procedure. Obstruction to pulmonary arterial flow can lead to parenchymal necrosis or airway ischemia. Obstruction to pulmonary venous flow leads to parenchymal edema. Chest radiography findings showing unilateral increase in opacification not explained by mucous plugging or another cause should prompt immediate evaluation for a vascular complication. This is done with a computed tomography scan with contrast (arterial and venous phase), transesophageal echocardiogram, or nuclear perfusion scan (**Fig. 3**).

The most common vascular complication in patients who undergo lung transplantation is pulmonary embolism (**Fig. 4**). Patients may be prothrombotic for several reasons, including recent surgery, manipulation of the pulmonary artery, limited mobility, indwelling venous catheters, and steroid therapy. The incidence of pulmonary embolism after lung transplantation ranges between 6% and 24%, and the mortality rate from this complication is 45%.[36–38] An embolism can be massive in the main pulmonary arteries or subtle and scattered throughout smaller arterial branches. The latter scenario is amenable to conservative therapy with anticoagulation, whereas the former requires endovascular or surgical intervention. Endovascular suction thrombectomy with or without thrombolytics is a minimally invasive option for effectively clearing the thrombus.[39,40] If unstable with severe right heart strain, the patient should be placed immediately on VA ECMO.[41,42] Although surgical pulmonary embolectomy is rarely performed after transplantation, it is used in patients who are good operative candidates to treat a major clot burden that is easily accessible in the main pulmonary arteries. CPB and limited exploration of the pulmonary artery with embolectomy are sufficient to clear most of the clot burden.

	Type	A	Within 1 cm of anastomosis
Ischemia		B	> 1 cm from anastomosis
		C	Extending into distal airways
	Grade	1	< 50% circumferential ischemia
		2	> 50% circumferential ischemia
Stenosis	Severity		< 50%
			> 50%
Dehiscence	Presence of any		

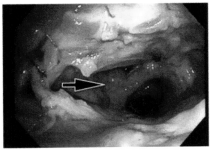

Example
Right Anastomosis
Ischemia: C2
Stenosis: No
Dehiscence: Yes (arrow)

Fig. 2. International Society for Heart and Lung Transplantation 2018 airway ischemia grading system. Image shows a patient with greater than 50% circumferential ischemia with some extension into the distal airways and a dehiscence. The patient underwent stent placement; over time, the anastomosis healed (image not shown).

Anastomotic complications of the pulmonary artery most commonly include narrowing caused by kinking, torsion, purse string effect, intimal hyperplasia, or surrounding tissue (**Fig. 5**). Surgical back walling can also occur. To avoid the possibility of kinking, the surgeon should minimize excessive length on the pulmonary artery anastomosis.

Careful size matching helps achieve the most ideal hemodynamic flow patterns. Moreover, the

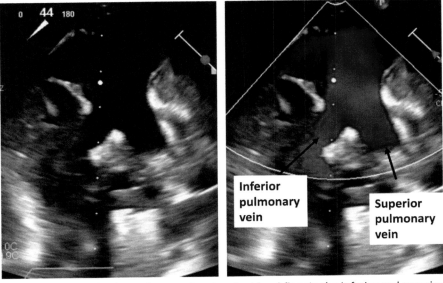

Fig. 3. Normal transesophageal echocardiogram showing the blood flow in the inferior and superior pulmonary veins.

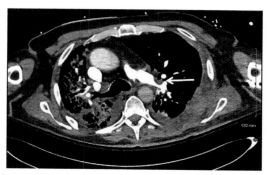

Fig. 4. Large blood clot in the left main pulmonary artery (*arrow*) associated with right ventricular strain on echocardiogram. Given hemodynamic instability, the patient required emergent peripheral venoarterial extracorporeal membrane oxygenation insertion at the bedside and subsequent suction thrombectomy.

pulmonary artery must be sewn while paying careful attention to the orientation of the upper and lower lobar branches to avoid twisting. If significant tension or unusual angulation is present, a patch augmentation of the anterior wall with bovine pericardium or autologous pericardium may be helpful.[43]

If hemodynamic and symptomatic narrowing occur, options include surgical reintervention or balloon angioplasty with or without a stent. Surgery is rarely performed unless it is within a week of the index transplant and there are concerns about the effects of ballooning on the suture line. In that case, the surgeon may choose an operative repair with or without a patch. If the suture line is mature and the narrowing is most likely caused by intimal hyperplasia or fibrosis, balloon and stenting is helpful.[44]

Pulmonary vein obstruction is an uncommon but potentially lethal complication after lung transplantation that can occur because of technical factors, such as twisting or abnormal angulation of the pulmonary veins. Pulmonary vein obstruction can also occur from a purse string effect or back walling of the vessel. The surgeon can easily avoid these issues by using meticulous technique. Pseudo-obstruction can occur as a result of excessive tension on the cuff and flattening of the orifice. This problem may result from size mismatch or inadequate donor cuff length. The pressure from the excessive tension can lead to pulmonary venous hypertension and congestion of the lung. An important preventive solution is to perform a patch augmentation to reduce the pressure in the left atrial cuff (**Fig. 6**). This is done by first suturing the backwall, next estimating the area needed to approximate the front wall, and then trimming a piece of pericardium to fill the gap.

Pulmonary venous stenosis can result from intimal hyperplasia and be successfully managed by using balloon angioplasty with or without stenting.[35] Fortunately, this complication is uncommon because the pulmonary veins are sewn to the recipient by using a large wide-mouthed atrial confluence that is not susceptible to stenosis.

Strokes are another important complication that can occur after lung transplantation because of technical factors affecting the left atrial closure. The left atrial cuff is in direct communication with the central arterial system; thus, it may be an important source of thromboembolic material. A stroke after lung transplantation should raise suspicion for possible emboli from the left atrium (**Fig. 7**). Imbricating the left atrium to exclude the muscular side of the atrium and carefully irrigating to remove debris can help to reduce embolic debris.

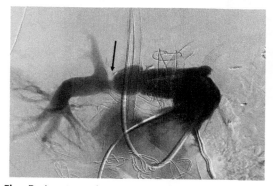

Fig. 5. Anastomotic narrowing (*arrow*) in the right main pulmonary artery noted on a pulmonary angiogram. There was a 50% difference in pressure gradient. This was treated conservatively because the patient's main cause of hypoxia was attributed to a major pulmonary embolism in the contralateral lung.

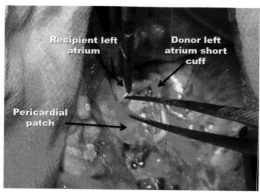

Fig. 6. Pulmonary vein patch augmentation of the anterior surface of a donor atrial cuff cut short.

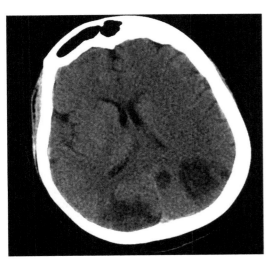

Fig. 7. Stroke in a patient following lung transplantation. Although no clot was identified in the pulmonary veins or the left atrium, this is a potential source for air or embolic debris. This complication is reduced by using an imbricated suture technique with extensive irrigation of the cuff before completing the anastomosis.

Finally, torsion is an important vascular complication of lung transplantation that can affect the veins, arteries, and bronchi.[45–49] Prompt recognition may allow the surgeon to correct the torsion through operative exploration before the onset of necrosis. In questionable cases, a second look may help the surgeon to track improvement of the lung parenchyma. For obvious lung necrosis, the surgeon should be prepared to perform a pneumonectomy or a lobectomy. For complete torsion with lung necrosis requiring a pneumonectomy, retransplant could be considered.

BLEEDING COMPLICATIONS

Lung transplantation is frequently associated with bleeding either at the time of the procedure or during the immediate postoperative period, and occasionally in the later stages of recovery. Despite advancements in surgical techniques and patient blood management and increased awareness of the adverse effects of blood product transfusion, bleeding remains a common complication after lung transplantation.

Intraoperative Bleeding

Blood loss with a chance of significant bleeding should be anticipated for any lung transplantation. Understanding the factors that increase the risk of intraoperative hemorrhage may help transplant surgeons and anesthesiologists anticipate and

prepare for blood product use during the operation. A previous history of thoracic or cardiac surgery, prior pleural interventions, and the presence of suppurative lung disease may be associated with increased vascular adhesions between the native lungs and the chest wall, often resulting in more perioperative hemorrhage. Wang and colleagues[50] demonstrated that blood product use was significantly higher in bilateral than in single-lung transplants, which was attributed to the increased surgical complexity. Eisenmenger syndrome and cystic fibrosis have also been identified as risk factors for blood loss and transfusion requirements during lung transplantation.[51,52]

During surgery, intraoperative blood loss, decreased fibrinogen levels, decreased platelet count, and concomitant fluid replacement may lead to coagulopathy. Adelmann and colleagues[53] identified the presence of coagulopathy as a contributory cause of postoperative bleeding in 69% of reoperations. The same group also found that low postoperative fibrinogen levels and preoperative and postoperative use of ECMO were risk factors for bleeding after lung transplantation.

Recipient factors, such as severe pulmonary hypertension, anatomic variants, and redo transplantation, make many of the major vascular structures prone to injury during dissection. In the case of a challenging hilar dissection, obtaining proximal control of the main pulmonary arteries and ensuring availability of cardiopulmonary support and blood products are of utmost importance.

Although many lung transplantations are performed without the use of cardiopulmonary support, candidates who present with high pulmonary artery pressures, refractory hypoxemia, and other cardiopulmonary instabilities often require support from ECMO or CPB. Although ECMO offers the advantage of less anticoagulation, it has limited ability to decompress the heart and to use cell-saver for blood salvage. However, CPB has the advantage of providing better cardiac decompression and pump cardiotomy suction in the event of massive hemorrhage. Wang and colleagues[50] demonstrated that patients on CPB used significantly more units of blood products than patients without the need for cardiopulmonary support (red blood cells, 8.28 vs 1.45; fresh frozen plasma, 9.70 vs 0.73; platelets, 1.86 vs 0.14; $P < .001$), correlating with time on bypass.

Postoperative Bleeding

Early postoperative hemorrhage is a common complication of lung transplantation. Hong and colleagues[54] found that hemothorax requiring surgical intervention occurred in 13% of cases, often after 48 hours (**Fig. 8**). Sources of bleeding include vascular anastomoses, divided mammary or bronchial arteries, raw surfaces of the pleural spaces, and chest wall incisions. Aggressive correction of postoperative coagulative deficits is often necessary, in cases requiring a large amount of blood products or performed on CPB. Added positive end-expiratory pressure may help tamponade any chest wall bleeding in the case of pleural adhesions. Close attention to drainage from the chest tubes in the early postoperative period may indicate the need to return to the operating room for exploration. The presence of brisk drainage of blood early on arrival to the intensive care unit followed by decreased chest tube drainage despite the patient requiring increased inotropic or vasopressor support warrants an urgent chest radiograph. The presence of significant hemothorax and the inability to obtain adequate chest tube drainage often warrants operative evacuation. Determining the optimal timing to return to the operating room is complex. Stability of the patient, continued or increasing need for support, and coagulation profiles must be considered. In the event of an acute clinical decompensation, such as tamponade and sudden brisk bleeding, bedside exploration may be required. Several studies have demonstrated that blood transfusions contribute to increased hospital stay and mortality after lung transplantation.[55]

Adelmann and colleagues[53] found that severe postoperative hemorrhage was associated with decreased 60-day survival, delayed hemothorax was more commonly associated with the need for anticoagulation, and postoperative hemothorax was associated with decreased 90-day survival. In addition, the economic impact of blood

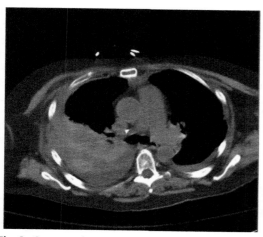

Fig. 8. Computed tomography scan showing right hemothorax after bilateral lung transplant.

transfusion should not be underestimated. In the United States, the cost of one unit of packed red blood cells ranges between $700 and $1200.[56]

PLEURAL SPACE COMPLICATIONS

Pleural space complications, including pleural effusion, pneumothorax, and empyema, are common after lung transplantation. According to Kao and colleagues,[57] pleural complications occur in 22% to 42% of lung transplant recipients. Risk factors for the development of pleural complications include previous thoracic surgery, pleural adhesions, and donor-recipient size mismatch.[58,59] The increased amount of pleural fluid after lung transplantation is related to capillary leak caused by allograft ischemia-reperfusion, recipient fluid overload, bleeding, and surgical interruption of allograft lymphatics at the time of organ recovery.[58,59]

Effusions are troublesome after transplantation, often leading to increased length of stay and additional surgical intervention. Pleural effusions in lung transplant recipients are complicated, such as hemothorax, empyema, and chylothorax, and require careful evaluation. Pleural fluid analysis may include bacterial, fungal, and mycobacterial cultures, polymerase chain reaction assays, cell counts, and measurements of lactate dehydrogenase, protein, glucose, and triglycerides.[58,60]

Late pleural effusions (>2 weeks after transplantation) are often a consequence of infection, rejection, trapped lung from pleural fibrosis, or malignancy.[61,62] Infection of the pleural space or empyema complicate about 3% to 7% of lung transplantations, and approximately one-quarter of pleural effusions that develop within 90 days of lung transplantation are infected.[59,63,64] Lung transplant recipients may have a blunted clinical presentation of empyema as a result of their immunosuppressed status; thus, a high clinical suspicion is required for all patients. Complex pleural effusions have been associated with negative patient outcomes and are treated with a range of medical and surgical procedures depending on the condition and severity. For example, a chylothorax may need surgical ligation of the thoracic duct or a hemothorax may need operative intervention to identify and stop the source of bleeding or to decorticate the lung.

Transplant patients are somewhat unique in that they do not follow "the rules" of pleural space problems. High-dose steroids delay healing and may have an impact on pleural adhesions. Furthermore, the extensive exposure and large incisions that are required for dissection and pneumonectomy frequently contribute to complex adhesions and fusion of the parietal and visceral pleural surfaces. Consequently, managing a loculated effusion (**Fig. 9**) is challenging with a surgical approach and is often not possible with a minimally invasive approach. A decortication that results in a fixed space with multiple air leaks may be difficult to manage long term, especially if this space becomes infected. Careful consideration of the benefits of surgery is important to avoid this situation. A trial of thrombolytic agents with carefully placed image-guided pleural catheters may obviate surgery and decortication.[65]

The Cleveland group[66] has recently published their findings on pleural space problems after lung transplantation. The authors found that 45% of lung transplant recipients in their study experienced a pleural complication: effusion in 26%, pneumothorax in 15%, hemothorax in 12%, empyema in 5%, and chylothorax in 1%. They noted that the presence of a pleural complication was associated with worse long-term survival.[66] Boffa and colleagues[67] looked at the need for and the results of decortication after lung transplantation. The results are illuminating: complete lung expansion was achieved in only 70% of cases, infection was cleared in only 64% of cases, and 30-day operative mortality was 23%. Decortication may be useful in some patients, but a decision to perform this procedure should be tempered by the substantial surgical risk.[67]

CHALLENGES IN MATCHING DONOR AND RECIPIENT SIZE

Although careful attention is paid to sizing the donor organ with the recipient, frequently there is a donor-recipient mismatch (**Fig. 10**). A size mismatch between the donor lung and the recipient's thoracic cage may lead to mechanical complications following lung transplantation. Whereas undersized lungs may contribute to pleural space problems, such as persistent effusions, oversized organs cause different problems, such as areas of persistent atelectatic lung. A size difference of up to 25% between a donor lung and a recipient's thoracic cage has been reported to be acceptable.[68]

Undersized Lung Allograft

A pneumothorax after lung transplantation can result from bronchopleural or parenchymal-pleural fistulas that occur secondary to operative injury. However, bronchial anastomoses dehiscence or a complication of transbronchial biopsies occur more commonly when the donor organ is undersized. A stable or small pneumothorax after lung transplantation can often be managed by watchful waiting, although a larger or symptomatic pneumothorax may require chest tube drainage. Persistent pneumothorax after lung transplantation is uncommon but may occur after chest drain removal when the donor lung is smaller than the recipient's thoracic cavity. This type of donor-recipient size mismatch is most often seen in patients with emphysema and significant hyperinflation of the native lungs before transplantation. Pneumothorax may also occur in the nontransplanted native lung in single-lung transplant recipients with emphysema or pulmonary fibrosis. Additionally, in patients who undergo single-lung transplantation for emphysema, the implantation of a small donor lung within a thoracic cage that is too large may result in allograft compression by the hyperexpanded emphysematous native lung.

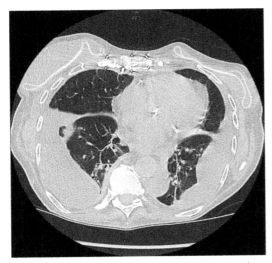

Fig. 9. Computed tomography scan showing loculated effusions after bilateral lung transplant.

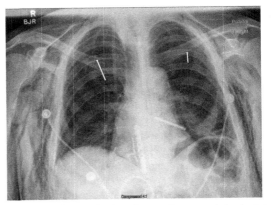

Fig. 10. Radiograph showing a donor-recipient size mismatch (undersized allografts shown by *arrows*).

Oversized Lung Allograft and Volume Reduction

In patients with severe pulmonary fibrosis, the pleural space is often quite restricted and does not necessarily correlate with the patient's height. The diaphragms of these patients are often very elevated, but it is expected that with time and well-sized donor lungs, the donor lungs will expand and the diaphragm will move down, allowing the thoracic cavity volume to increase. There are instances, however, when it is clear that the donor organ is too large for the recipient's chest cavity. Atelectasis and impaired ventilation may result from implanting a large donor lung in a thoracic cage that is too small. These complications are often immediately evident on postoperative radiographs when the patient is still receiving positive pressure ventilation.[68]

In the case of a significantly oversized lung allograft for the recipient's chest cavity, volume reduction may be required to close the chest. Shigemura and colleagues[69] reported that, in cases of oversized lungs, allograft volume reduction was associated with better early and midterm results in terms of allograft function and overall complications. Graft volume is reduced by either lobectomy or serial wedge resections. Removing the right middle lobe and the lingula of the left lobe is often adequate for resizing, but further wedge resections of the lower lobes may be required. Of note, staple lines may leak air or result in a poor fit of the lungs in the chest, which may be troublesome in the postoperative period. For these reasons, an effort to correctly size the donor organ with the recipient's chest cavity is optimal.

RETRANSPLANTATION

Retransplantation poses unique challenges and is covered elsewhere in this issue. A few important points are highlighted here. First, careful patient selection is key. Retransplantation is often reserved for patients with chronic lung allograft dysfunction that is not of the restrictive subcategory and who have survived at least 2 to 3 years after the first transplant.[70–72] In addition, the operation has several aspects that bear discussion. Reentry is complicated by injury to the heart. The dissection is complicated by injury to the phrenic nerves. Extracorporeal life support strategies are often necessary for support. Pulmonary artery dissection in retransplantation is challenging, often necessitating the rapid need for bypass. Therefore, considering more proximal control of the pulmonary artery intrapericardially is recommended. In the authors' practice, preemptive placement of some nearby soft tissue (from either the donor or the recipient) between the bronchial and arterial anastomoses can facilitate dissection in case the patient requires a second transplant at a later date. If significant adhesions are encountered and there are significant raw surfaces after dissection (especially if CPB is required), the surgical team should consider leaving the chest open at the end of the procedure. Outcomes of retransplantation in carefully selected patients approximate those of initial transplantations in some centers.[72,73]

SUMMARY

Lung transplantation is a life-saving intervention for thousands of patients worldwide battling irreversible end-stage lung disease every year. There are many factors that influence outcomes after transplantation. Ensuring a safe and positive surgical outcome is a substantial step toward providing the best possible long-term result.

CLINICS CARE POINTS

- Airway ischemia after lung transplantation may be affected by surgical anastomotic technique.
- Pulmonary embolism is the most common vascular complication affecting lung transplant recipients.
- The incidence of wound complications after lung transplantation may be affected by the choice of operative exposure.
- The occurrence of primary graft dysfunction may be affected by intraoperative factors.

ACKNOWLEDGMENTS

The authors thank Nicole Stancel, PhD, ELS(D), of the Department of Scientific Publications at the Texas Heart Institute, and Kristine Nally, BS, ELS, of Norton Thoracic Institute, for editorial review of the manuscript.

DISCLOSURE

Dr G. Loor is a consultant for Abiomed Breethe, and his institution (Baylor College of Medicine) has received grant support from Maquet and Transmedics, Inc. for involvement in clinical trials related to extracorporeal membrane oxygenation and ex vivo lung perfusion.

REFERENCES

1. Lemaignen A, Birgand G, Ghodhbane W, et al. Sternal wound infection after cardiac surgery: incidence and risk factors according to clinical presentation. Clin Microbiol Infect 2015;21(7):674 e11–8.
2. Ridderstolpe L, Gill H, Granfeldt H, et al. Superficial and deep sternal wound complications: incidence, risk factors and mortality. Eur J Cardiothorac Surg 2001;20(6):1168–75.
3. Young PY, Khadaroo RG. Surgical site infections. Surg Clin North Am 2014;94(6):1245–64.
4. Bakaeen FG, Haddad O, Ibrahim M, et al. Advances in managing the noninfected open chest after cardiac surgery: negative-pressure wound therapy. J Thorac Cardiovasc Surg 2019;157(5): 1891–18903 e9.
5. Seidel D, Diedrich S, Herrle F, et al. Negative pressure wound therapy vs conventional wound treatment in subcutaneous abdominal wound healing impairment: the SAWHI randomized clinical trial. JAMA Surg 2020;155(6):469–78.
6. Nadir A, Kaptanoglu M, Sahin E, et al. Post-thoracotomy wound separation (DEHISCENCE): a disturbing complication. Clinics (Sao Paulo). 2013;68(1):1–4.
7. Pancholy B, Raman J. Chest wall reconstruction using sternal plating in patients with complex sternal dehiscence. Ann Thorac Surg 2015;99(6):2228–30.
8. Athanassiadi K, Bagaev E, Simon A, et al. Lung herniation: a rare complication in minimally invasive cardiothoracic surgery. Eur J Cardiothorac Surg 2008;33(5):774–6.
9. Coiffard B, Prud'Homme E, Hraiech S, et al. Worldwide clinical practices in perioperative antibiotic therapy for lung transplantation. BMC Pulm Med 2020;20(1):109.
10. Ius F, Raemdonck D, Hartwig M, et al. Effect of surgical exposure on outcomes in lung transplantation: insight from the International Multicenter Extracorporeal Life Support (ECLS) in Lung Transplantation registry. J Heart Lung Transplant 2021;40:S164.
11. Elde S, Huddleston S, Jackson S, et al. Tailored approach to surgical exposure reduces surgical site complications after bilateral lung transplantation. Surg Infect (Larchmt) 2017;18(8):929–35.
12. Snell GI, Yusen RD, Weill D, et al. Report of the ISHLT working group on primary lung graft dysfunction, part I: definition and grading. A 2016 Consensus Group statement of the International Society for Heart and Lung Transplantation. J Heart Lung Transpl 2017;36(10):1097–103.
13. Diamond JM, Lee JC, Kawut SM, et al. Clinical risk factors for primary graft dysfunction after lung transplantation. Am J Respir Crit Care Med 2013;187(5): 527–34.
14. Warnecke G, Van Raemdonck D, Smith MA, et al. Normothermic ex-vivo preservation with the portable Organ Care System Lung device for bilateral lung transplantation (INSPIRE): a randomised, open-label, non-inferiority, phase 3 study. Lancet Respir Med 2018;6(5):357–67.
15. Hoetzenecker K, Benazzo A, Stork T, et al. Bilateral lung transplantation on intraoperative extracorporeal membrane oxygenator: an observational study. J Thorac Cardiovasc Surg 2019;160(1):320–7. https://doi.org/10.1016/j.jtcvs.2019.10.155.
16. Subramaniam K, Gabriel L, Bottiger B, et al. Intraoperative red blood cell transfusion is associated with primary graft dysfunction after lung transplantation. Am J Respir Crit Care Med 2021;203.
17. Van Raemdonck D, Hartwig MG, Hertz MI, et al. Report of the ISHLT Working Group on primary lung graft dysfunction Part IV: prevention and treatment. A 2016 Consensus Group statement of the International Society for Heart and Lung Transplantation. J Heart Lung Transpl 2017;36(10):1121–36.
18. DerHovanessian A, Weigt SS, Palchevskiy V, et al. The role of TGF-beta in the association between primary graft dysfunction and bronchiolitis obliterans syndrome. Am J Transplant 2016;16(2):640–9.
19. Whitson BA, Prekker ME, Herrington CS, et al. Primary graft dysfunction and long-term pulmonary function after lung transplantation. J Heart Lung Transpl 2007;26(10):1004–11.
20. Hadaya J, Benharash P. Extracorporeal membrane oxygenation. JAMA 2020;323(24):2536.
21. Li G, Mankidy B, Liu Z, et al. A closer look at risk factors associated with airway complications in lung transplantation. J Heart Lung Transplant 2021;40.
22. Necki M, Antonczyk R, Pandel A, et al. Impact of cold ischemia time on frequency of airway complications among lung transplant recipients. Transpl Proc 2020;52(7):2160–4.
23. Van De Wauwer C, Van Raemdonck D, Verleden GM, et al. Risk factors for airway complications within the first year after lung transplantation. Eur J Cardiothorac Surg 2007;31(4):703–10.
24. Ruttmann E, Ulmer H, Marchese M, et al. Evaluation of factors damaging the bronchial wall in lung transplantation. J Heart Lung Transpl 2005;24(3):275–81.
25. Keshava HB, Mason DP, Murthy SC, et al. Pediatric donor lungs for adult transplant recipients: feasibility and outcomes. Thorac Cardiovasc Surg 2012;60(4): 275–9.
26. van Berkel V, Guthrie TJ, Puri V, et al. Impact of anastomotic techniques on airway complications after lung transplant. Ann Thorac Surg 2011;92(1):316–20.
27. FitzSullivan E, Gries CJ, Phelan P, et al. Reduction in airway complications after lung transplantation with novel anastomotic technique. Ann Thorac Surg 2011;92(1):309–15.
28. Guzman-Pruneda FA, Orr Y, Trost JG, et al. Bronchial artery revascularization and en bloc lung transplant in children. J Heart Lung Transpl 2016;35(1):122–9.

29. Pettersson GB, Karam K, Thuita L, et al. Comparative study of bronchial artery revascularization in lung transplantation. J Thorac Cardiovasc Surg 2013;146(4):894–900 e3.

30. Crespo MM, McCarthy DP, Hopkins PM, et al. ISHLT consensus statement on adult and pediatric airway complications after lung transplantation: definitions, grading system, and therapeutics. J Heart Lung Transpl 2018;37(5):548–63.

31. Machuzak M, Santacruz JF, Gildea T, et al. Airway complications after lung transplantation. Thorac Surg Clin 2015;25(1):55–75.

32. Santacruz JF, Mehta AC. Airway complications and management after lung transplantation: ischemia, dehiscence, and stenosis. Proc Am Thorac Soc 2009;6(1):79–93.

33. Mahajan AK, Folch E, Khandhar SJ, et al. The diagnosis and management of airway complications following lung transplantation. Chest 2017;152(3):627–38.

34. de la Torre M, Fernandez R, Fieira E, et al. Postoperative surgical complications after lung transplantation. Rev Port Pneumol (2006) 2015;21(1):36–40.

35. Loyalka P, Cevik C, Nathan S, et al. Percutaneous stenting to treat pulmonary vein stenosis after single-lung transplantation. Tex Heart Inst J 2012;39(4):560–4.

36. Krivokuca I, van de Graaf EA, van Kessel DA, et al. Pulmonary embolism and pulmonary infarction after lung transplantation. Clin Appl Thromb Hemost 2011;17(4):421–4.

37. Kroshus TJ, Kshettry VR, Hertz MI, et al. Deep venous thrombosis and pulmonary embolism after lung transplantation. J Thorac Cardiovasc Surg 1995;110(2):540–4.

38. Saez-Gimenez B, Berastegui C, Loor K, et al. Deep vein thrombosis and pulmonary embolism after solid organ transplantation: an unresolved problem. Transpl Rev (Orlando) 2015;29(2):85–92.

39. Spratt JR, Shrestha P, Loor G, et al. Pulmonary transplant salvage using ultrasound-assisted thrombolysis of subacute occlusive main pulmonary artery embolus. Innovations (Phila). 2017;12(3):214–6.

40. Tu T, Toma C, Tapson VF, et al. A prospective, single-arm, multicenter trial of catheter-directed mechanical thrombectomy for intermediate-risk acute pulmonary embolism: the FLARE study. JACC Cardiovasc Interv 2019;12(9):859–69.

41. Ghoreishi M, Pasrija C, Kon Z. VA-ECMO for massive pulmonary embolism: when is the time to wean? Ann Thorac Surg 2020. https://doi.org/10.1016/j.athoracsur.2020.09.047.

42. Thomas B, Hassan I, Nobre C. Surgical embolectomy, ECMO, or thrombolytic therapy in massive pulmonary embolism. J Am Coll Cardiol 2020;76(23):2797.

43. Alnajar A, Chen PC, Burt B, et al. Left pulmonary artery patch augmentation for lung transplant in a patient with situs inversus. Tex Heart Inst J 2021;48(1).

44. Sheikh MA, Chowdhury MA, Moukarbel GV. Safety and clinical outcomes of endovascular treatment of adult-onset pulmonary artery stenosis. J Invasive Cardiol 2016;28(5):202–8.

45. Cox CS, Decker SJ, Rolfe M, et al. Middle lobe torsion after unilateral lung transplant. J Radiol Case Rep 2016;10(5):15–21.

46. David A, Liberge R, Corne F, et al. Whole-lung torsion complicating double lung transplantation: CT features. Diagn Interv Imaging 2016;97(9):927–8.

47. Lin MW, Huang SC, Kuo SW, et al. Lobar torsion after lung transplantation. J Formos Med Assoc 2013;112(2):105–8.

48. Nguyen JC, Maloney J, Kanne JP. Bilateral whole-lung torsion after bilateral lung transplantation. J Thorac Imaging 2011;26(1):W17–9.

49. Stephens G, Bhagwat K, Pick A, et al. Lobar torsion following bilateral lung transplantation. J Cardiovasc Surg 2015;30(2):209–14.

50. Wang Y, Kurichi JE, Blumenthal NP, et al. Multiple variables affecting blood usage in lung transplantation. J Heart Lung Transpl 2006;25(5):533–8.

51. Hoechter DJ, von Dossow V, Winter H, et al. The Munich Lung Transplant Group: intraoperative extracorporeal circulation in lung transplantation. Thorac Cardiovasc Surg 2015;63(8):706–14.

52. Triulzi DJ, Griffith BP. Blood usage in lung transplantation. Transfusion 1998;38(1):12–5.

53. Adelmann D, Koch S, Menger J, et al. Risk factors for early bleeding complications after lung transplantation: a retrospective cohort study. Transpl Int 2019;32(12):1313–21.

54. Hong A, King CS, Brown AW, et al. Hemothorax following lung transplantation: incidence, risk factors, and effect on morbidity and mortality. Multidiscip Respir Med 2016;11:40.

55. Weber D, Cottini SR, Locher P, et al. Association of intraoperative transfusion of blood products with mortality in lung transplant recipients. Perioper Med (Lond) 2013;2(1):20.

56. Shander A, Hofmann A, Ozawa S, et al. Activity-based costs of blood transfusions in surgical patients at four hospitals. Transfusion 2010;50(4):753–65.

57. Kao CC, Cuevas JF, Tuthill S, et al. Pleural catheter placement and intrapleural fibrinolysis following lung transplantation. Clin Transpl 2019;33(6):e13592.

58. Arndt A, Boffa DJ. Pleural space complications associated with lung transplantation. Thorac Surg Clin 2015;25(1):87–95.

59. Ferrer J, Roldan J, Roman A, et al. Acute and chronic pleural complications in lung transplantation. J Heart Lung Transpl 2003;22(11):1217–25.

60. Mills NL, Boyd AD, Gheranpong C. The significance of bronchial circulation in lung transplantation. J Thorac Cardiovasc Surg 1970;60(6):866–78.

61. Chhajed PN, Bubendorf L, Hirsch H, et al. Mesothelioma after lung transplantation. Thorax 2006;61(10): 916–7.

62. Judson MA, Handy JR, Sahn SA. Pleural effusion from acute lung rejection. Chest 1997;111(4):1128–30.

63. Shields RK, Clancy CJ, Minces LR, et al. Epidemiology and outcomes of deep surgical site infections following lung transplantation. Am J Transplant 2013;13(8):2137–45.

64. Wahidi MM, Willner DA, Snyder LD, et al. Diagnosis and outcome of early pleural space infection following lung transplantation. Chest 2009;135(2): 484–91.

65. Rahman NM, Maskell NA, West A, et al. Intrapleural use of tissue plasminogen activator and DNase in pleural infection. N Engl J Med 2011;365(6):518–26.

66. Tang A, Siddiqui HU, Thuita L, et al. Natural history of pleural complications after lung transplantation. Ann Thorac Surg 2021;111(2):407–15.

67. Boffa DJ, Mason DP, Su JW, et al. Decortication after lung transplantation. Ann Thorac Surg 2008;85(3): 1039–43.

68. Frost AE. Donor criteria and evaluation. Clin Chest Med 1997;18(2):231–7.

69. Shigemura N, Bermudez C, Hattler BG, et al. Impact of graft volume reduction for oversized grafts after lung transplantation on outcome in recipients with end-stage restrictive pulmonary diseases. J Heart Lung Transpl 2009;28(2):130–4.

70. Halloran K, Aversa M, Tinckam K, et al. Comprehensive outcomes after lung retransplantation: a single-center review. Clin Transpl 2018;32(6):e13281.

71. Schaheen L, D'Cunha J. Re-do lung transplantation: keys to success. J Thorac Dis 2019;11(12):5691–3.

72. Biswas Roy S, Panchanathan R, Walia R, et al. Lung retransplantation for chronic rejection: a single-center experience. Ann Thorac Surg 2018;105(1): 221–7.

73. Clausen ES, Weber JM, Neely ML, et al. Predicting survival for lung retransplantation patients at one and five years. J Heart Lung Transplant 2019; 38(4):S225–6.

Infectious Complications in Lung Transplant Recipients

Erika D. Lease, MD, FCCP[a],*, Marie M. Budev, DO, MPH, FCCP[b]

KEYWORDS

• Lung transplant • Infection • Complications • Prophylaxis

KEY POINTS

• Infection remains a common cause of death following lung transplantation
• Antimicrobial prophylaxis may be used after lung transplantation to target a number of different infections
• Infectious organisms include bacteria, viruses, and fungi; all of which have their own risk factors, clinical presentations, and management in lung transplant recipients

INTRODUCTION

Lung transplantation has evolved into a life-saving therapeutic option for end-stage lung disease. Though the long-term survival lags behind that of other solid organ transplants partially due to the direct and indirect impact of infectious complications themselves and partially due to their impact on the development of chronic lung allograft dysfunction (CLAD). International Society of Heart and Lung Transplant (ISHLT) registry data has noted that median survival after lung transplantation has increased to 6.7 years. However, infection remains a common cause of death, accounting for 35% of deaths in the first year and approximately 21% of deaths during 1 to 3 years posttransplant.[1] Therefore, the management and prevention of infections is of paramount importance in the care of lung transplant recipients throughout their entire lifespan. In this article, we will review certain aspects of donor-derived infections during the early perioperative period and later infectious risks over time. In addition, we will discuss the basic principles of posttransplant antibacterial, antifungal, and antiviral prophylaxis and the management of common bacterial, viral, and fungal infections seen in lung transplant recipients.

ANTIMICROBIAL PROPHYLAXIS

Antimicrobial agents are used frequently following lung transplantation as prophylaxis against several different types of organisms (**Table 1**). Prophylaxis strategies may be targeted (specific to those at increased risk or with known previous infection/colonization) or universal (all lung transplant recipients) depending on the organism, time posttransplant, as well as other clinical factors.

Pneumocystis jirovecii, previously known as *Pneumocystis carinii*, is an opportunistic fungal organism that can lead to *P. jirovecii* pneumonia (PJP) particularly in immunocompromised hosts.[2] Before routine universal prophylaxis, the risk of the development of PJP was 5% to 15% in solid organ transplant recipients with the highest risk in the first 6 months after transplant.[3] In a meta-analysis, the use of sulfamethoxazole-trimethoprim prophylaxis reduced the occurrence of PJP by 91% in hematopoietic stem cell and solid organ transplant recipients.[4] Lung transplant recipients are thought to be at particularly high risk for PJP, thus lifelong prophylaxis is generally recommended.[2] Possible prophylaxis regimens include sulfamethoxazole-trimethoprim, dapsone, atovaquone, and inhaled pentamidine. However, a meta-analysis showed

a Department of Medicine, Division of Pulmonary, Critical Care, and Sleep Medicine, University of Washington, 1959 NE Pacific Street, Box 356175, Seattle, WA 98195, USA; b Lerner College of Medicine, Respiratory Institute, Cleveland Clinic, Desk A 90, 9500 Euclid Avenue, Cleveland, OH 44195, USA
* Corresponding author.
E-mail address: edlease@uw.edu

Thorac Surg Clin 32 (2022) 211–220
https://doi.org/10.1016/j.thorsurg.2021.12.002
1547-4127/22/© 2021 Elsevier Inc. All rights reserved.

Table 1
Postlung transplant prophylaxis

Pneumocystis jirovecii	• Sulfamethoxazole-trimethoprim as first-line prophylaxis • Consider desensitization in those with nonsevere allergy • Life-long prophylaxis is preferred • Sulfamethoxazole-trimethoprim may provide prophylaxis for other organisms as well
Antifungal prophylaxis	• Most lung transplant centers routinely prescribe antifungal prophylaxis • Benefits of antifungal prophylaxis, as well as optimal agent and duration, are unknown • May consider targeted prophylaxis for those with known pretransplant colonization/infection with fungi
Antiviral prophylaxis	• CMV prophylaxis is routinely prescribed by most lung transplant centers • Optimal duration of prophylaxis is unknown • For recipients not prescribed anti-CMV prophylaxis, another antiviral agent should be considered for HSV and/or VZV prophylaxis in the early time posttransplant; optimal duration is unknown
Antibacterial prophylaxis	• Targeted prophylaxis should be considered for recipients with pretransplant colonization/infection with bacteria • Optimal duration of antibacterials is unknown

Abbreviations: CMV, cytomegalovirus; HSV, herpes simplex virus; VZV, varicella-zoster virus.

sulfamethoxazole-trimethoprim to be the superior agent with rare break-through cases while on appropriate and consistent dosing.[2,4] Given the preference for sulfamethoxazole-trimethoprim prophylaxis, desensitization can be considered and successfully performed during the index transplant hospitalization in the majority of solid organ transplant recipients with a nonsevere allergy to sulfa.[5,6] Sulfamethoxazole-trimethoprim may also have the added benefit of prophylaxis against other infections such as *Toxoplasma gondii*, *Nocardia* species, *Listeria monocytogenes*, and other common urinary, respiratory, and gastrointestinal pathogens.[7,8]

Antifungal prophylaxis is a widely accepted practice after lung transplantation, though the optimal regimen is still unclear given the paucity of data. A survey of lung transplant centers in the United States found that 90% of centers used a universal strategy for antifungal prophylaxis.[9] Nearly $^3/_4$ of respondents reported using a combination of inhaled amphotericin with a systemic antifungal agent, about 22% reported using a systemic antifungal agent alone, and about 6% reported using inhaled amphotericin alone. The duration of antifungal prophylaxis varied as well with about 89% of respondents reporting continued antifungal prophylaxis

beyond the index transplant hospitalization but nearly 70% reporting a duration of 6 months posttransplant or less. Subsequently, a systematic review and meta-analysis of available data found no difference in the occurrence of fungal infection in lung transplant recipients with universal prophylaxis as compared with no prophylaxis.[10] In addition, there was no difference in the cumulative incidence of fungal infections within the first year after transplantation when inhaled amphotericin was used as compared with a systemic triazole. The duration of prophylaxis also did not seem to impact the incidence of fungal infections in the short- or long-term following lung transplantation. The authors felt, however, that due to significant heterogeneity, a high risk of bias, and a lack of precision when pooling the existing studies, there was insufficient evidence to support or exclude a benefit of antifungal prophylaxis.

Antiviral prophylaxis is a routine practice after lung transplantation. The primary targets for antiviral prophylaxis are the herpesviruses: cytomegalovirus (CMV), herpes simplex virus (HSV), and varicella-zoster virus (VZV). CMV, in particular, is an important contributor to morbidity and mortality following lung transplantation.[10] In the face of immunosuppression, the herpesviruses may reactivate from the latent form in seropositive recipients (recipient positive, or R+). In the case of CMV, there may also be reactivation either from donor-transmitted CMV in a seropositive recipient (donor positive/recipient positive, or D+/R+) or primary infection via transmission through the transplanted organ in an uninfected recipient (donor positive/recipient negative, or D+/R-). Lung transplant recipients are generally considered at higher risk of CMV infection and disease, particularly in the first 6 months after transplant.[11,12] While oral valganciclovir is generally the prophylactic agent of choice, intravenous (IV) ganciclovir (GCV) may be used early after transplant or in those who are intolerant of or unable to take oral medications. The optimal duration of prophylaxis is unknown although one multi-center randomized study found that 12 months of valganciclovir prophylaxis for D+ and/or R+ recipients resulted in significantly lower rates of CMV disease in the first year after transplant than those who received 3 months of prophylaxis.[13] Both study groups had a low incidence of CMV disease in the 6 months following the 12-month trial. Current guidelines recommend 3 months of prophylaxis for CMV R+ lung transplant recipients and 6 to 12 months of prophylaxis for D+/R- lung transplant recipients. Many centers' protocols extend prophylaxis much longer and some continue prophylaxis indefinitely.[14,15]

Data are limited in regard to HSV and VZV prophylaxis in recipients who are not receiving CMV prophylaxis (CMV D-/R-); however, the general consensus is that recipients who are HSV or VZV seropositive should receive antiviral prophylaxis with acyclovir or valacyclovir for the early posttransplant period.[16,17] The optimal duration is unknown though very early experience in heart–lung recipients found early HSV infections occurred within the first 2 months after transplant.[18,19] The current American Society of Transplantation guidelines suggest at least 1 month of prophylaxis following solid organ transplantation.[16]

Some lung transplant candidates, particularly those with cystic fibrosis (CF), may have chronic respiratory colonization or infection with bacteria, fungi, and mycobacteria. A targeted prophylaxis strategy may be used to prevent the contamination of the pleural space, anastomoses, surgical site, and transplanted lungs. In recipients with CF, the consensus is to administer susceptibility-driven antimicrobials when a susceptible antibiotic choice with acceptable toxicity is available.[20] A worldwide survey regarding lung transplant perioperative antibiotic therapy found all respondents used a susceptibility-driven regimen in recipients with chronic colonization before transplantation.[21] In the setting of a pretransplant multi-drug resistant

colonizing organism, nearly 70% of respondents reported incorporating a combined regimen of 2 susceptible antibiotics. Two-thirds of respondents administered antibiotics for a total of 14 days following transplantation, with a range of 7–21 days. Overall, current data do not suggest worse posttransplant outcomes for recipients with pretransplant multi-drug resistant or pan-resistant organisms, including overall survival, incidence of acute rejection, or incidence of CLAD.[22,23]

DONOR-DERIVED INFECTION

Donor-derived infections may occur and can be considered "expected" vs "unexpected" depending on the predonation evaluation. Expected transmissions may arise from donors who are seropositive for CMV or have active Hepatitis C. Expected transmissions are frequent and allow for posttransplant planning and management such as determining the appropriate CMV prophylaxis strategy in the setting of the recipient's CMV serostatus. Additionally, lung transplant recipients may have expected transmission of bacteria identified on the predonation bronchoscopy and lower respiratory tract sampling. The identification of possible pathogenic bacteria on predonation lower respiratory tract culture seems common, ranging from 48% to 89% in recent studies.[24–26] One study found about 5% were multi-drug resistant organisms and none were identified in posttransplant recipient cultures.[25]

Data are conflicting as to the impact of a positive donor lower respiratory tract culture on posttransplant recipient outcomes. Some studies have reported a longer time of posttransplant mechanical ventilation and presence of posttransplant pneumonia in the recipient but most have not reported a difference in overall outcomes or survival after the immediate posttransplant period.[24–28] Currently, there is no data as to which organisms found on a predonation lower respiratory tract sample should be treated as a true or potential pathogen or as to the optimal duration of treatment in the recipient.

Unexpected donor disease transmission seems to be uncommon, with recent data in the United States over a 10-year period showing disease transmission in 0.18% of recipients and with 0.23% of donors transmitting the proven or probable disease to at least 1 recipient.[29] Of these proven or probable disease transmissions, nearly 73% were infections of which 31% were viral, 30% were bacterial, 22% were fungal, 13% were parasitic, and 4% were mycobacterial. Approximately 67% of proven or probable donor-derived infections presented within 30 days after transplant and 88% within 90 days after transplant.

While unexpected donor-derived infections seem to be rare, they result in mortality in 15% of infected recipients, with parasitic infections having the highest mortality at 35%. The high mortality of unexpected donor-derived infections highlights the need for donor risk stratification via medical and social history, careful clinical assessment of the donor and donor organs, and laboratory screening of the donor with additional testing beyond routine testing in cases whereby there is a concern for possible donor infection.[30]

MANAGEMENT OF BACTERIAL INFECTIONS

Early bacterial infections may result from donor transmission, chronic infection and/or colonization in the recipient, or infections associated with the hospitalization and/or critical illness. Additional risk factors for early postoperative infection in the lung transplant recipient include necrotic tissue at the bronchial anastomosis, denervation of the lung allograft leading to decreased mucociliary clearance and cough reflex, and continuous exposure of the allograft to the environment and microorganisms of the upper respiratory tract. Bacterial infections during the lifetime of a lung transplant recipient can be broad, including infections that predominate in immunosuppressed hosts as well as routine community-acquired infections also seen in normal hosts. As such, this section will focus on early posttransplant bacterial infections.

Surgical site infection in a lung transplant recipient may present as cutaneous or soft tissue infection, extrapulmonary infection such in the pleural space or mediastinum, and airway anastomosis infection. In lung transplant recipients, surgical site infections are relatively common, occurring in 5% to 19% of patients.[31] One study found that surgical site infections after lung transplantation occur at a median of 25 days, with empyema being the most common infection in 42%, followed by surgical wound infections in 29%, mediastinitis in 16%, sternal osteomyelitis in 6%, and pericarditis in 6%.[32] Among these infections, gram-negative and gram-positive bacterial pathogens were found equally in 41% of recipients. One-year mortality from surgical site infections in this study was high at 35%. Given the high risk of mortality and broad microbiology, it is recommended that broad-spectrum antimicrobials be considered if a surgical site infection is suspected and then narrowed once a particular pathogen is identified.[31]

INFECTIOUS RISKS OVER TIME

Although overall short- and long-term survival after lung transplantation has improved according to the most recent ISHLT Registry data, infection remains a significant cause of mortality throughout the life of lung transplant recipients.[1] Transplanted lungs are overall more prone to infectious complications compared with normal lungs for multiple reasons. Unlike native lungs which have a dual blood supply consisting of pulmonary and bronchial arteries, transplanted lungs routinely only have one source of blood supply unless bronchial artery revascularization is performed.[33] This limited blood supply can lead to the disruption of the distal epithelium impacting healing and leading to impaired mucus clearance.[34] Even as time goes on, evidence seems to suggest that mucociliary clearance in transplant patients remains impaired.[35] In addition, as the central lymphatics are not reconnected at the time of surgery, impaired lymphatic drainage occurs early posttransplant. The direct exposure of the lungs to the environment and need for high levels of immunosuppression needed to prevent rejection, all play an important role in the increased risk for infection early and late after transplant.[36] Three periods of infection after solid organ transplant have been described by Fishman and Rubin: (1) the first month following transplant characterized by nosocomial infections and donor-derived infections, (2) a period of intense immunosuppression for up to 6 months associated with opportunistic infections, and (3) a period of reduced immunosuppression with community-acquired and rarer infectious agents.[8,37] Recognition of this timeline has yielded improved prophylactic strategies and approaches to empiric therapy. Several studies have noted the risk of bacterial infection is the highest in the first month (17.3 episodes per 1000 transplant days) during the first-year posttransplant as well as between 6 and 12 months (2.6 infections per 1000 transplant-days).[38,39] Of the bacterial infections, respiratory tract infections with *Pseudomonas aeruginosa* and Enterobacteriaceae are most commonly found.[38]

MANAGEMENT OF VIRAL INFECTIONS
Cytomegalovirus

CMV is the most prevalent opportunistic infection in lung transplant recipients and the second most common infection after bacterial infections in the lung transplant population.[40] The morbidity and mortality associated with CMV infection are due to both its direct tissue injury and its indirect association with the development of acute cellular rejection and CLAD.[41,42] In addition, CMV may play an immunomodulatory role promoting other opportunistic bacterial and fungal infections.[43] CMV disease is defined as the presence of CMV replication in tissue, blood or other bodily fluid with clinical signs and symptoms. CMV disease can manifest clinically in a myriad of ways including a viral syndrome, pneumonitis, colitis, or hepatitis.[41] Before the introduction of GCV, CMV disease was associated with a very high mortality. The approach to the treatment of active disease is based on IV GCV and oral valganciclovir. Both drugs need to be adjusted for renal impairment, but inadequate dosing can lead to reduced efficacy and viral resistance. In addition, careful reduction of the intensity of immunosuppression and possible administration of CMV immune globulin could be considered (limited evidence noted).[44] Treatment should be administered until resolutions of symptoms and viremia with 2 consecutive negative serum CMV loads 1 week apart for a minimum of 2 weeks followed by secondary suppression with oral valganciclovir for at least one to 3 months. The CMV viral load needs to be monitored for possible resistance which should be suspected in cases of rising or elevated viral loads despite ongoing antiviral therapy. If resistance is detected, including UL 97 phosphotransferase which confers resistance to GCV, other alternative agents may include IV foscarnet or cidofovir.[45,46]

Community-Acquired Respiratory Viruses

Community-acquired respiratory viruses (CARV) have an impact on mortality postlung transplant including increasing the risk for acute rejection and CLAD. The CARV cause upper respiratory tract infections including: influenza, parainfluenza (PIV), human rhinovirus (HRV) which most commonly occur in patients with lung transplant, respiratory syncytial virus (RSV), adenovirus (ADV), coronaviruses (COV NOT SARS COV-2), human metapneumovirus (hMPV), and bocavirus (BCV). The reported incidence of CARV infections ranges between 7.7% and 64% with the large variation in range due to diagnostic testing techniques and seasonality for viruses.[47,48] Currently, several PCR assays including multiplex assays allow for the rapid identification of viruses on serum, swabs, and bronchoalveolar lavage (BAL).[49] For most CARV, there are no currently available effective treatments except for supportive care. For those viruses in which treatment options are available, it has been demonstrated that timely intervention can limit complications including ICU admissions and mortality. Different treatment options are available for the treatment of particular CARVs . These include oseltamivir or zanamivir for the treatment of influenza A and B. Oral ribavirin for the treatment of parainfluenza, respiratory syncytial virus or human metapneumonvirus. Cidofovir has been for the treatment of adenovirus as well. For the other common CARVs including rhinovirus , non SARS CoV 2 coronavirus and bocavirus supportive care is recommended .[48] . The role of high-dose corticosteroids in the treatment of CARV infection remains controversial but they are used in conjunction with certain therapies due to the association of CARV infections and acute rejection. However, this association is controversial. A systematic review of 34 studies by Vu and colleagues found the association between CARV infections and acute rejection to be limited and only present in a minority of the published reports included.[50] However, this systematic review is limited in its findings due to the lack of control groups in the pooled studies and variability in the definition of acute rejection. Therefore, no firm conclusions regarding the association of CARVs and acute rejection can be established.[50]

Epstein-Barr Virus

Acute Epstein–Barr virus (EBV) infection causes a polyclonal expansion of B cells that host the virus and express viral antigens leading to a T cell response against the infected B cells. When T cell immunity is limited by immunosuppressive agents, the infected B cells can initiate posttransplant lymphoproliferative disorder (PTLD). The rate of PTLD in lung transplant recipients ranges between 5% and 15%.[51] The routine monitoring of EBV viral load by blood PCR sampling may detect PTLD earlier.[51] Certain transplant centers have advocated the use of antiviral agents including ACV or GCV in high-risk patients for primary EBV infection (EBV + donor, EBV-recipient) to prevent the development of PTLD in this population but evidence to support the use of either of these agents in EBV mismatched recipients is lacking.[51]

Varicella-zoster Virus

Lung transplant recipients are at increased risk for VZV complications from cutaneous involvement in the form of herpes zoster (HZ) to life-threating end-organ involvement including pneumonitis, encephalitis and hepatitis. Treatment of VZV and HZ can be managed with antiviral agents including acyclovir or valacyclovir orally for local HZ involvement for 7 days or intravenously with hospitalization in cases of disseminated HZ or acute varicella.[52,53] Human Herpes 6 infection has been known to cause encephalitis in immunocompromised hosts. In addition, human herpes virus 8 (HHV-8) has been associated with disseminated forms of Kaposi's Sarcoma in organ recipients.[53]

COVID-19

Infection with the SARS COV 2 virus has had a profound impact on morbidity and mortality in lung transplant recipients. Among lung transplant recipients who tested positive for COVID-19, the infection was severe with more than 80% requiring hospitalization and 30% needing intensive care. Mortality due to COVID-19 was significant in this population ranging from 14% to 39%.[54–56] Several therapies have been considered as per recommendations from the Infectious Disease Society of America including neutralizing monoclonal antibody agents bamlanivimab and etesevimab for high-risk ambulatory patients and dexamethasone, tocilizumab, and remdesivir for hospitalized patients.[57] In regards to immunosuppressive management in lung transplant recipients, the International Society of Heart Lung Transplant Guidance Document regarding the SARS COV-2 pandemic recommended holding mycophenolate mofetil, mTOR inhibitors and azathioprine in patients who are admitted with moderate to severe illness.[58]

MANAGEMENT OF FUNGAL INFECTIONS

Lung transplant recipients have the highest risk for fungal infections among solid organ transplant recipients.[52] The 1-year cumulative incidence of fungal infections in lung transplant recipients is approximately 8.6% although the rates can vary depending on several factors. The type of fungal infection and timing of occurrence depends on multiple factors including pretransplant colonization with fungal organisms, antimicrobial prophylaxis, the intensity of immunosuppression, and time from transplant.[59–61] The median time to onset is about 11 months posttransplant but late-onset fungal infections have been noted in several studies, including a study from Toronto demonstrating a 9% incidence of invasive aspergillosis in recipients 2 to 4 years posttransplant.[62] Invasive fungal infections (IFIs) postlung transplant are a major contributor to mortality seen among lung transplant recipients. In a single-center study, IFIs were identified as the strongest predictor for mortality in this patient population.[63] The most common IFIs posttransplant reported were invasive mold diseases (IMDs) including most commonly invasive aspergillosis present in the form of pneumonia or tracheobronchitis, which carry the risk for multi-organ dissemination.[61] In the immediate postoperative period, defined as up to 30 days after surgery, Candida infections predominate.[61,63] These infections can present as mediastinitis, pleuritis, empyema or surgical site infections and candidemia usually due to indwelling lines or catheters. Several nonaspergillus mold infections including mucormycosis, Alternaria, Fusarium, and Scedosporium can occur at later time periods posttransplant and have a lower incidence than that of Aspergillus but are associated with worse prognosis than invasive aspergillosis[59,64] Endemic fungi including Histoplasma capsulatum, Blastomyces dermatitidis, and Coccidioides immitis can also lead to infection in patients living in high-risk areas for these endemic fungi.

The gold standard for the diagnosis of fungal infection includes identifying fungal growth on respiratory culture. A positive fungal culture allows for the susceptibility testing and identification of non-Aspergillus molds. The sensitivity is only 50% limiting is utility in clinical practice.[65,66] Fungal biomarkers including galactomannan is the most widely used and identify carbohydrate residues in the Aspergillus cell wall. False positives can occur as galactomannan also resides in the cell walls of other non-Aspergillus infections including Histoplasma, Blastomyces, Fusarium and Penicillium.[67] Serum galactomannan has a low sensitivity rate and should not be used in lung transplant recipients. Instead BAL galactomannan testing has a higher diagnostic value with sensitivity rates ranging from 60% to 82% in solid organ transplant recipients and should be assessed as part of pneumonia workup.[68,69]

The treatment of fungal infections after lung transplantation is multimodal based on several key principles including the antifungal agent used should target a specific fungal pathogen. Secondly, either surgical or bronchoscopic debridement of the infected tissue along with the removal of infected lines/devices should be performed to reduce the fungal load in the infected tissue. Finally, the immunosuppression intensity should be adjusted to allow for the immune system to resolve the infection and also to prevent rejection.[70] The choice of antifungal therapy is based on the particular pathogen being targeted. The general summary of antifungal treatments for specific fungal infections is provided in **Table 2**.[70] It is important to note that the azoles will increase levels of the calcineurin inhibitors including tacrolimus and cyclosporine. Frequent drug level monitoring of the calcineurin inhibitors and the azoles may be necessary to document absorption and to avoid toxicities.[70]

MYCOPLASMA HOMINIS AND UREAPLASMA UREALYTICUM INFECTIONS

Hyperammonemia is a rare but fatal condition that can occur early in the peri-transplant period in lung transplant recipients. Systemic infection with

Table 2
Treatment choices for common fungal infections postlung transplant

Type of Fungal Infection	Antifungal Treatment Recommendations
Aspergillus species	Voriconazole is the treatment of choice for invasive disease Alternatives agents: • Triazoles: posaconazole, isavuconazole • Echinocandins: caspofungin, anidulafungin, micafungin Combination therapy may be considered for infection Inhaled liposomal amphotericin B for tracheobronchitis + systemic therapy
Candida species	Candidemia and invasive candidiasis Initial empiric therapy: Echinocandins including: caspofungin, anidulafungin, micafungin Target therapies based on susceptibility testing Alternative agents: • Fluconazole if azole resistance not a concern • Liposomal amphotericin B
Mucormycosis	Invasive mucormycosis High-dose liposomal amphotericin B Alternative agents: • Triazoles: posaconazole, isavuconazole
Cryptococcus neoformans	Cryptococcal meningitis Induction therapy includes: • liposomal Amphotericin B+ flucytosine for 2–4 wk Consolidation phase: • Fluconazole 400–800 mg for 8 wk Maintenance phase: • Funconazole 200–400 mg for 12 mo Noncentral nervous system infections • Severe disease – same treatment as meningitis • Nonsevere disease – fluconazole
Fusarium	Invasive fusariosis • Unclear optimal therapeutic options • Choices include amphotericin B, voriconazole, posaconazole, isavuconazole
Scedosporium	Invasive scedosporiosis apiospermum Voriconazole is the treatment of choice for invasive disease
Pneumocystis jirovecii	Trimethoprim-sulfamethoxazole ± high-dose steroids

Adapted from Kennedy CC, Razonable RR. Fungal Infections After Lung Transplantation. *Clin Chest Med*. 2017;38(3):511-520.

either *M. hominis* or *U. urealyticum* can cause hyperammonemia in a lung transplant recipient.[71,72] In a single-center study, hyperammonemia was identified in only 8 patients out of 807 lung transplant recipients but was associated with a high mortality of 75%. Hyperammonemia usually presents with symptoms of lethargy, altered mental status, seizures, or coma. Serum ammonia levels should be checked. If elevated, antibiotic therapies should be initiated including a choice of macrolides, fluoroquinolones, or tetracycline keeping in mind possible resistance patterns. BAL fluid should be sent for polymerase chain reaction (PCR) studies and special cultures for both organisms.

SUMMARY

Lung transplant recipients have an increased susceptibility to various infections throughout their lifespan. This is due to the exposure of the graft to the external environment, impaired mucociliary clearance, and high levels of immunosuppression. Long-term outcomes in lung transplant recipients remain poor compared with other solid organ transplants largely due to deaths from infections and chronic allograft dysfunction. The first month after transplant is characterized by the highest burden of infections but the risk for infections continues throughout the lifetime of this patient cohort. Clinicians should have a high degree of suspicion for infection at all times and have patient-tailored prophylaxis and treatments to help ensure graft and patient survival.

CLINICS CARE POINTS

- Infection remains a common cause of death following lung transplantation
- Long-term outcomes in lung transplant recipients remain poor compared with other solid organ transplants due to deaths from infections and chronic allograft dysfunction.
- Antimicrobial, antifungal, and antiviral prophylaxis may be used after lung transplantation to target a number of different opportunistic infections.
- The first month posttransplant is characterized by nosocomial infections and donor-derived infections. Following the first month after transplant and up to 6-months posttransplant, during a period of intense, is associated with opportunistic infections. After the first year posttransplant, immunosuppression is reduced but the infectious risk still with community-acquired and rarer infectious agents implicated most commonly.
- Infectious organisms whether they are bacterial, fungal, or viral have their own individual risk factors and particular presentations and treatment options.
- Clinicians should remain vigilant for infections at all periods posttransplant.

DISCLOSURE

The authors have no pertinent disclosures.

REFERENCES

1. Chambers DC, Cherikh WS, Harhay MO, et al. The International Thoracic Organ Transplant Registry of the International Society for Heart Lung Transplantation: Thirty –Fifth adult lung and heart lung report -2019; Focus theme donor and recipient size match. J Heart Lung Transplant 2019;38:1042–55.
2. Fishman JA, Gans H. *Pneumocystis jirovecii* in solid organ transplantation: guidelines from the American Society of Transplantation Infectious Diseases Community of Practice. Clin Transplant 2019;33(9): e13587.
3. Iriart X, Challan Belval T, Fillaux J, et al. Risk factors of *Pneumocystis* Pneumonia in solid organ recipients in the era of the common use of posttransplant prophylaxis. Am J Transplant 2015;15:190–9.
4. Green H, Paul M, Vidal L, et al. Prophylaxis of *Pneumocystis* pneumonia in immunocompromised non-HIV-infected patients: Systematic review and meta-analysis of randomized controlled trials. Mayo Clin Proc 2007;82(9):1052–9.
5. Ionnidis JP, Cappelleri JC, Sklnik PR, et al. A meta-analysis of the relative efficacy and toxicity of pneumocystis carinii prophylactic regimens. Arch Intern Med 1996;156(2):177–88.
6. Pryor JB, Olyaei AJ, Kirsch D, et al. Sulfonamide desensitization in solid organ transplant recipients: a protocol-driven approach during the index transplant hospitalization. Transpl Infect Dis 2019;21(6): e13191.
7. Fishman JA, Issa NC. Infection in organ transplantation: risk factors and evolving patterns of infection. Infect Dis Clin North Am 2010;24(2):273–83.
8. Fishman JA. Infection in solid-organ transplant recipients. N Engl J Med 2007;357(25):2601–14.
9. Pennington KM, Yost K, Escalante P, et al. Antifungal prophylaxis in lung transplant: a survey of United States' transplant centers. Clin Transpl 2019;33(7): e13630.
10. Pennington KM, Baqir M, Erwin PJ, et al. Antifungal prophylaxis in lung transplant recipients: a systematic review and meta-analysis. Transpl Infect Dis 2020;22(4):e13333.
11. Razonable RR, Humar A. Cytomegalovirus in solid organ transplant recipients – guidelines of the American Society of Transplantation Infectious Diseases Community of Practice. Clin Transpl 2019;33: e13512.
12. Humar A, Kumar D, Preiksaitis J, et al. A trial of valganciclovir prophylaxis for cytomegalovirus prevention in lung transplant recipients. Am J Transt 2005; 5(6):1462–8.
13. Palmer SM, Limaye AP, Banks M, et al. Extended valganciclovir prophylaxis to prevent cytomegalovirus after lung transplantation: a randomized, controlled trial. Ann Intern Med 2010;152(12):761–9.
14. Kotton CN, Kumar D, Caliendo AM, et al. The third international consensus guidelines on the management of cytomegalovirus in solid-organ transplantation. Transplantation 2018;102(6):900–31.
15. Zuk DM, Humar A, Weinkauf JG, et al. An international survey of cytomegalovirus management practices in lung transplantation. Transplant 2010;90(6): 612–76.
16. Lee DH, Zuckerman RA. Herpes simplex virus infections in solid organ transplant transplantation: guidelines from the American Society of Transplantation Infectious Diseases Community of Practice. Clin Transpl 2019;33:e13526.
17. Pergam SA, Limaye AP. Varicella zoster virus in solid organ transplantation: guidelines from the American Society of Transplantation Infectious Diseases Community of Practice. Clin Transpl 2019;33:e13622.

18. Brooks RG, Hofflin JM, Jamieson SW, et al. Infectious Complications in Heart-Lung Transplant Recipients. Am J Med 1985;79(4):412–22.

19. Smyth RL, Higenbottam TW, Scott JP, et al. Herpes simplex virus infection in heart-lung transplant recipients. Transplantation 1990;49(4):735–9.

20. Shah P, Lowery E, Chapparro C, et al. Cystic fibrosis foundation consensus statements for the care of cystic fibrosis lung transplant recipients. J Heart Lung Transpl 2021;40(7):539–56.

21. Coiffard B, Prud'Homme E, Hraich S, et al. Worldwide clinical practices in perioperative antibiotic therapy for lung transplantation. BMC Pulm Med 2020;20(1):109–17.

22. Winstead RJ, Waldman G, Autry EB, et al. Outcome of lung transplantation for cystic fibrosis in the setting of extensively drug-resistant organisms. Prog Transplant 2019;29(3):220–4.

23. Lay C, Law N, Holm AM, et al. Outcomes in cystic fibrosis lung transplant recipients infected with organisms labeled as pan-resistant: An ISHLT Registry-based analysis. J Heart Lung Transpl 2019;38(5):545–52.

24. Ahmad O, Shafii AE, Mannino DM, et al. Impact of donor lung pathogenic bacteria on patient outcomes in the immediate post-transplant period. Transplantation 2018;20(6):e12986.

25. Bunsow E, Los-Arcos I, Martin-Gomez MT, et al. Donor-derived bacterial infections in lung transplant recipients in the era of multidrug resistance. J Infect 2020;80:190–6.

26. Bonde PN, Patel ND, Borja MC, et al. Impact of donor lung organisms on post-transplant pneumonia. J Heart Lung Transpl 2006;25(1):99–105.

27. Weill D, Dey GC, Hicks RA, et al. A positive donor gram stain does not predict outcome following lung transplantation. J Heart Lung Transpl 2002;21(5):555–8.

28. Avlonitis VS, Krause A, Luzzi L, et al. Bacterial colonization of the donor lower airways is a predictor of poor outcome in lung transplantation. Eur J Cardiothorac Surg 2003;24(4):601–7.

29. Kaul DR, Vece G, Blumberg E, et al. Ten years of donor-derived disease: a report of the disease transmission advisory committee. Am J Transpl 2021;21(2):689–702.

30. Wolfe CR, Ison MG. Donor-derived infections: Guidelines from the American Society of Transplantation Infectious Diseases Community of Practice. Clin Transpl 2019;33:e13547.

31. Abb LM, Grossi PA. Surgical site infections: Guidelines from the American Society of Transplantation Infectious Diseases Community of Practice. Clin Transpl 2019;33(9):e13589.

32. Shields RK, Clancy CJ, Minces LR, et al. Epidemiology and outcomes of deep surgical site infections following lung transplantation. Am J Transpl 2013;13(8):2137–45.

33. Yun JJ, Unai S, Pettersson G. Lung transplant with bronchial arterial revascularization: review of surgical technique and clinical outcomes. J Thorac Dis 2019;11:S1821–8.

34. Nørgaard MAB, Andersen CB, Pettersson G. Airway epithelium of transplanted lungs with and without direct bronchial artery revascularization. Eur J Cardiothorac Surg 1999;15(01):37–44.

35. Duarte AG, Myers AC. Cough reflex in lung transplant recipients. Lung 2012;190(01):23–7.

36. Rubin RH, Schaffner A, Speich R, et al. Introduction to the Immunocompromised Host Society Consensus Conference on epidemiology, prevention, diagnosis, and management of infections in solid organ transplant patients. Clin Infect Dis 2001;33:S1–4.

37. Fishman JA, Rubin RH. Infection in organ transplant recipients. N Engl J Med 1998;338:1741–51.

38. Van Delden C, Stampf S, Hirsch HH, et al. Burden and timeline of infectious diseases in the first year after solid organ transplantation in the Swiss Transplant Cohort Study. Clin Infect Dis 2020;71:e159–69.

39. Gagliotti C, Morsillo F, Moro M, et al. Infections in liver and lung transplant recipients. A Natl Prospective Cohort 2018;37:399–407.

40. Fisher RA. Cytomegalovirus infection and disease in the new era of immunosuppression following solid organ transplantation. Transpl Infect Dis 2009;11:195–202.

41. Zamora MR. Cytomegalovirus and lung transplantation. Am J Transpl 2004;4:1219–26.

42. Ducan SR, Paradis IL, Yousem SA, et al. Sequelae of cytomeglovirus pulmonary infections in lung allograft recipients. Am Rev Respir Dis 1992;146:1419–25.

43. Razonable RR, Limaye RR. Cytomegalovirus infection after solid organ transplantation. In: Bowden RA, Ljungman P, Snydman DR, editors. Transplant infections. 3rd edition. Philadelphia (PA): Lippincott Williams and Wilkins; 2010. p. 328.

44. Kotton CN, Kumar D, Caliendo AM, et al. Updated international consensus guidelines on the management of cytomegalovirus in solid-organ transplantation. Transplantation 2013;96:333.

45. Piiparinen H, Hockerstedt K, Gronhagen-Riska C, et al. Comparison of two quantitative CMV PCR tests, Cobas Amplicor CMV Monitor and TaqMan assay, and pp65- antigenemia Assay in the Determination of Viral Loads from Peripheral Blood of Organ Transplant Patients. J Clin Virol 2004;30:258.

46. Hakki M, Chou S. The biology of cytomegalovirus drug resistance. Curr Opin Infect Dis 2011;24:605–11.

47. Shalhoub S, Husain S. Community-acquired respiratory viral infections in lung transplant recipients. Curr Opin Infect Dis 2013;26:302–8.

48. Gottlieb J, Schulz TF, Welte T, et al. Communityacquired respiratory viral infections in lung transplant

recipients: a single season cohort study. Transplantation 2009;87:1530–7.

49. Mahony J, Chong S, Merante F, et al. Development of a respiratory virus panel test for detection of twenty human respiratory viruses by use of multiplex PCR and a fluid microbead-based assay. J Clin Microbiol 2007;45:2965–70.

50. Vu DL, Bridevaux PO, Aubert JD, et al. Respiratory viruses in lung transplant recipients: a critical review and pooled analysis of clinical studies. Am J Transpl 2011;11:1071–8.

51. Neuringer IP. Posttransplant lymphoproliferative disease after lung transplantation. Clin Dev Immunol 2013;2013:430209.

52. Nosotti M, Tarsia P, Morlacchi L. Infections after lung transplant. J Thorac Dis 2018;10:3849–68.

53. Miller GG, Dummer JS. Herpes simplex and varicella zoster viruses: forgotten but not gone. Am J Transpl 2007;7:741–7.

54. Pereira MR, Mohan S, Cohen DJ, et al. COVID-19 in solid organ transplant recipients: initial report from the US epicenter. Am J Transpl 2020;20(07):1800–8.

55. Saez-Giménez B, Berastegui C, Barrecheguren M, et al. COVID-19 in lung transplant recipients: a multi-center study. Am J Transpl 2020. https://doi.org/10.1111/ajt.16364.

56. Messika J, Eloy P, Roux A, et al, French Group of Lung Transplantation. COVID-19 in lung transplant recipients. Transplantation 2021;105(01):177–86.

57. Infectious Diseases Society of America Guidelines on the Treatment and Management of Patients with COVID-19. Available at: https://www.idsociety.org/practice-guideline/%20covid-19-guideline-treatment-and-management/. Accessed September 4, 2021.

58. Guidance from the International Society of Heart and Lung Transplantation regarding the SARS CoV-2 pandemic. Available at: https://ishlt.org/ishlt/media/documents/SARS-CoV-2_Guidance-for-Cardiothoracic-Transplant-and-VAD-center.pdf. Accessed September 4, 2021.

59. Doligalski CT, Benedict K, Cleveland AA, et al. Epidemiology of invasive mold infections in lung transplant recipients. Am J Transpl 2014;14:1328–33.

60. Vazquez R, Vazquez-Guillamet MC, Suarez J, et al. Invasive mold infections in lung and heart-lung transplant recipients: Stanford University experience. Transpl Infect Dis 2015;17:259–66.

61. Pappas PG, Alexander BD, Andres DR, et al. Invasive fungal infections among organ transplant recipients: results of the transplant –associated infection surveillance network (Transnet). Clin Infect Dis 2010;50:1101–11.

62. Herrera S, Davoudi S, Farooq A, et al. Late onset invasive pulmonary aspergillosis in lung transplant recipients in the setting of targeted prophylaxis. Am J Transpl 2014;14:1328–33.

63. Arthurs SK, Eid AJ, Deziel PJ, et al. The impact of invasive fungal disease on survival after lung transplantation. Clin Transpl 2010;24:341–8.

64. Koo S, Kubiak DW, Issa NC, et al. A targeted peri-transplant antifungal strategy for the prevention of invasive fungal disease after lung transplantation: a sequential cohort analysis. Transplantation 2012;94:281–6.

65. Hoenigl M, Prattes J, Spiess B, et al. Performance of glactomannan, beta d-glucan , aspergillus lateral –flow device, conventional culture , pcr tests with bronchoalveolar lavage fluid for diagnosis of invasive pulmonary aspergillosis. J Clin Microbiol 2014;52:2039–45.

66. Geltner C, Lass-Florl C. Invasive pulmonary aspergillosis in organ transplants- focus on lung transplants. Respir Investig 2016;54:76–84.

67. Patterson TF, Thompson GR, Denning DW, et al. Practice guidelines for the diagnosis and management of Aspergillosis:2016 Update by the Infectious Disease Society of America. Clin Infect Dis 2016;63:e1–60.

68. Pfeiffer CD, Fine JP, Safdar N. Diagnosis of invasive aspergillosis using a galactomannan assay: meta-analysis. Clin Infect Dis 2006;42:1417–27.

69. Husain S, Paterson DL, Studer SM, et al. Aspergillus galactomannan antigen in the bronchoalveolar lavage fluid for the diagnosis of invasive aspergillosis in lung transplant recipients. Transplantation 2007;83:1330–6.

70. Kennedy CC, Pennington KM, Bean E, et al. Fungal infection in lung transplantation. Sem Respir Crit Care Med 2021;42:471–82.

71. Lichtenstein GR, Yang YX, Nunes FA, et al. Fatal hyperammonemia after orthotopic lung transplantation. Ann Intern Med 2000;132:283–7.

72. Chen C, Bain KB, Iuppa JA, et al. Hyperammonemia syndrome after lung transplantation: a single center experience. Transplantation 2016;100:678–84.

Lung Allograft Rejection

Deborah J. Levine, MD[a], Ramsey R. Hachem, MD[b],*

KEYWORDS

- Lung transplantation • Acute cellular rejection • Antibody-mediated rejection
- Donor-specific antibodies

KEY POINTS

- Lung allograft rejection is common despite advances in therapeutic immunosuppression.
- Acute cellular rejection and antibody-mediated rejection are common forms of lung rejection.
- Lung allograft rejection is the primary cause for poor long-term outcomes after lung transplantation.

INTRODUCTION

Lung transplantation is the best therapeutic option for many patients with end-stage lung diseases for which there are no other available therapies. The 2019 International Society for Heart and Lung Transplantation (ISHLT) registry revealed that the median survival is 6.7 years,[1] which lags behind other organ transplants. Rejection, the main determinant of allograft failure, is the barrier to successful long-term survival. Because the lung allograft has constant exposure to the environment and an increased susceptibility to injury and infection, it has a greater risk of rejection compared with other organ transplants.[2]

Chronic lung allograft dysfunction (CLAD) is the leading cause of mortality after the first year posttransplantation. Risk factors that influence long-term graft function and the development of CLAD occur early posttransplant and include both immune-mediated and non–immune-mediated processes. Graft injury from acute rejection is the predominant immunologic factor responsible for the development of CLAD.[3] Acute rejection can be mediated either through a T-cell (acute cellular rejection [ACR]) or a B-cell (antibody-mediated rejection [AMR]) process. The risk of CLAD increases with both the severity and frequency of episodes of acute rejection; however, even one episode of minimal ACR has been associated with CLAD.[4,5]

Early identification of acute rejection is important for prompt treatment to protect graft function and recipient survival. A combination of pulmonary function tests (PFTs), antibody assessment, imaging, and histologic assessments are tools currently used to detect acute rejection.[2]

ACUTE CELLULAR REJECTION
Mechanism

ACR is the most frequently identified type of acute rejection after transplantation. It affects the vasculature and small airways, which can lead to irreversible damage to the graft. ACR is mediated predominantly by T-cell recognition of foreign major histocompatibility complex proteins (human leukocyte antigens [HLAs]) and other donor antigens.[6] Recognition of donor antigens activates the innate immune system, triggering the adaptive immune response, which creates a proinflammatory effect. The common pathway of ACR involves recruitment and activation of recipient T cells to the allograft, resulting in allograft injury and loss of function.[7]

Diagnosis

Transplant recipients with ACR may be asymptomatic or may present with nonspecific symptoms, such as dyspnea, fever, cough, or sputum production.[8,9] The nonspecific presentation of ACR makes the diagnosis challenging, and can potentially result in delayed therapy. Monitoring with PFTs, imaging, and laboratory tests should

a Division of Pulmonary and Critical Care Medicine, University of Texas Health San Antonio, 7703 Floyd Curl Drive, San Antonio, TX 78229, USA; b Division of Pulmonary and Critical Care Medicine, Washington University in St. Louis, 4523 Clayton Avenue, Mailstop 8052-0043-14, St Louis, MO 63110, USA
* Corresponding author.
E-mail address: Rhachem@wustl.edu

Thorac Surg Clin 32 (2022) 221–229
https://doi.org/10.1016/j.thorsurg.2021.12.003
1547-4127/22/© 2021 Elsevier Inc. All rights reserved.

be performed routinely to improve diagnostic accuracy.[9]

Serial PFTs are currently the best screening tool for identifying patients at risk for ACR. Spirometry can be the initial assessment that can identify early allograft dysfunction and prompt further investigations.[10] Of note, however, recipients may be asymptomatic with stable PFTs, and still have ACR found on biopsy.[11]

Imaging may be helpful in providing clues to ACR; however, the discriminatory accuracy is limited,[12,13] with only 50% of biopsy-proven ACR having abnormal findings on imaging. Given the poor specificity of clinical findings, PFTs, and imaging, histopathologic analysis of transbronchial biopsies (TBBs) has become most reliable monitoring tool to diagnose ACR.

There is no standardization on the utility, protocol, or implication of surveillance biopsies; however, monitoring with surveillance bronchoscopy with TBB is the most frequent approach used, although it remains highly controversial as TBB is not without risk (ie, pneumothorax, bleeding, respiratory failure, and pneumonia) and protocols vary among centers. An international survey in 2020 reported 87% of centers performed surveillance TBB at variable times.[14] Other centers perform TBB only in the presence of suspected clinical issues.

In 2007, the ISHLT Pathology Council Working Group revised the lung transplant pathology nomenclature for the diagnosis of ACR and established a standardized set of criteria.[15] The findings are well characterized and based on perivascular and interstitial mononuclear infiltrates. They include patchy lymphohistiocytic inflammatory infiltrates centered on small blood vessels (arterioles/venules) or in bronchioles. Grading of ACR is based on the severity of the inflammatory process and the structures involved. The vascular component ranges from grade A0 (no rejection) to grade A4 (severe), with most cases being A1 or A2. The airway component lymphocytic bronchiolitis (LB), is characterized by airway inflammation without identifiable cause and ranges in severity from B0 (no rejection) to B2R (high grade). An ungradable category (BX) exists for biopsies without enough airway tissue to grade.[15] Acute vascular and airway rejection can be found independently or may coexist in the same patient (**Tables 1** and **2**).

There is significant interobserver variability in the diagnosis and interpretation of pathologic specimens for ACR, particularly in lower grade rejection, making it challenging for both individual patient management as well as standardization in multicenter trials. The ISHLT recommends obtaining at least 5 "adequate" samples of alveolated parenchyma for the best interpretation.[15]

Symptoms are more common in patients with grade A2 or higher rejection compared with those with grade A0 or A1.[10] It is quite often that patients with a grade <A2 are asymptomatic and often have stable or increasing PFTs. On the other hand, one study showed that a drop in forced expiratory volume in 1 second (FEV1) by a mean of 10.4% from prerejection values has a sensitivity of greater than 60% for detecting grade A2 ACR or infection; however, it cannot differentiate between the two.[11]

Epidemiology

ACR is most commonly diagnosed within the first 1 to 2 years posttransplantation, with the highest risk being within the first 3 to 6 months.[11] It results in approximately 3.5% of deaths within the first 30 days after transplantation.[5] Thirty percent of adult recipients have at least one episode of ACR within the first year after transplantation.[1] The reported incidence of ACR, however, is inconsistent primarily due to differences in monitoring protocols and interreader variability of histology.[11] Glanville and colleagues[16] reported the incidence of ACR to be 46% in the first year after transplantation, whereas Hachem and colleagues[17] found that 49% of recipients had at least 1 episode of A2 rejection. In 2018, in a multicenter study, Hachem and colleagues[18] reported 64% of patients had at least one episode of ACR. Todd and colleagues[19] reported that in 400 recipients, more than 50% experienced at least 1 episode of ACR, with most episodes occurring within 3 months after transplantation.

Risk Factors

It is important to recognize early risk factors for ACR in order to risk stratify patients and consider additional monitoring if found. Several pretransplantation and posttransplantation recipient and donor factors have been evaluated as potential risk factors, but more evidence is needed for many of these.[20,21] There *are* however, characteristics that *have* been found to be associated with ACR. Recipient age has been associated with ACR events. Patients in different age groups may respond differently to therapy based on immune function related to age. Patients may adhere more or less to their therapy based on their stage of life. Very young recipients (younger than 1 year) have been reported to have low rates of rejection, whereas those in their teenage and young adulthood have some of the highest rates of rejection.[22] Multiple reports in the literature reflect that both anti-HLA antibodies and the

Table 1
Pathologic grading of acute cellular rejection

Grade	Severity	Description
A0	None	Normal parenchyma
A1	Minimal	Scattered, infrequent perivascular mononuclear infiltrates that are 2–3 cells thick
A2	Mild	More frequent perivascular mononuclear infiltrates that are readily recognizable at low magnification; infiltrates may include lymphocytes, macrophages, and eosinophils
A3	Moderate	Dense perivascular mononuclear infiltrates commonly associated with endothelialitis; extension of inflammatory cell infiltrate into alveolar septa and airspaces; eosinophils and occasional neutrophils are common
A4	Severe	Diffuse perivascular, interstitial, and air-space infiltrates of mononuclear cells; alveolar pneumocyte damage and endothelialitis

Data from Stewart S, Fishbein MC, Snell GI, Berry GJ, Boehler A, Burke MM, Glanville A, Gould FK, Magro C, Marboe CC, McNeil KD, Reed EF, Reinsmoen NL, Scott JP, Studer SM, Tazelaar HD, Wallwork JL, Westall G, Zamora MR, Zeevi A, Yousem SA. Revision of the 1996 working formulation for the standardization of nomenclature in the diagnosis of lung rejection. J Heart Lung Transplant. 2007 Dec;26(12):1229-42.

numbers of HLA mismatches are associated with an increased propensity toward ACR events.[23–26] The type of transplant performed has been linked to ACR in that single lung transplantation has been shown to have a higher incidence of ACR than bilateral lung transplantation.[22] The risk of ACR is highest within the first year after transplantation. The risk for recurrent ACR is increased after a previous severe episode.[23] Insufficient immunosuppression has been shown to be a strong risk factor for ACR, so maintaining adequate levels and monitoring are imperative.[27] Cytomegalovirus infection has a strong association with ACR post lung transplantation. Most programs use a prophylactic antiviral regimen, which has decreased the risk in these patients.[28,29] Although the association between gastrointestinal reflux and CLAD is the most well studied, there is an increased risk of ACR in patients with reflux as well.[30,31] The presence of donor-specific antibodies (DSAs) is most often linked to patients with AMR; however, it is also a strong risk factor for ACR.[32]

Management

The therapeutic regimen of ACR varies between transplant centers and grades of ACR. There is general consensus among centers that recipients with Grade A2 and above require therapy. The specific regimen usually depends on the specific patient, and presence or absence of symptoms.[8] Gordon and colleagues[8] revealed that few centers (50% of centers) would treat LB and even fewer (35%) would treat asymptomatic A1 ACR. All regimens require increased immunosuppression, usually with a course of pulse-dosed intravenous corticosteroids as first-line therapy. Most centers use intravenous methylprednisolone of 10 to 15 mg/kg daily or 500 to 1000 mg daily for 3 days with an oral prednisone taper following the pulse. In cases of severe (A3 or A4), or persistent or refractory ACR, additional therapy is given. The calcineurin inhibitor is often changed from cyclosporine to tacrolimus[33] and/or azathioprine is changed to mycophenolate. Antithymocyte globulin (ATG), alemtuzumab,[34] total lymphoid radiation,[35] extracorporeal photopheresis,[36] and inhaled cyclosporine[37] have all been used as well in severe cases. Our knowledge of the pathogenesis, identification, monitoring, and management of ACR has improved over the past decade. However, the low sensitivity and specificity of our existing tools reflect our need for continued collaboration between centers to improve our current protocols and to assess newer diagnostic platforms so that we may more easily identify these entities earlier to delay or prevent chronic graft injury.

ANTIBODY-MEDIATED REJECTION
Historical Perspectives and Hyperacute Rejection

Although AMR has long been established in other solid organ transplants, our understanding of pulmonary AMR is still evolving. Until approximately 15 years ago, the recognition of AMR after lung transplantation was limited to hyperacute rejection.[38–40] This is a fulminant form of lung rejection that is caused by preformed DSAs to mismatched HLAs typically resulting in allograft failure.[38–40]

Table 2
Pathologic grading of lymphocytic bronchiolitis

Grade	Severity	Description
B0	None	No evidence of bronchiolar inflammation
B1R	Low grade	Mononuclear cells within the submucosa of the bronchioles with occasional submucosal eosinophils
B2R	High grade	Large and activated mononuclear cells, eosinophils, and plasmacytoid cells in the submucosa; evidence of epithelial damage with necrosis, metaplasia, and intra-epithelial lymphocytic infiltration
BX	Ungradable	No bronchiolar tissue available

Data from Stewart S, Fishbein MC, Snell GI, Berry GJ, Boehler A, Burke MM, Glanville A, Gould FK, Magro C, Marboe CC, McNeil KD, Reed EF, Reinsmoen NL, Scott JP, Studer SM, Tazelaar HD, Wallwork JL, Westall G, Zamora MR, Zeevi A, Yousem SA. Revision of the 1996 working formulation for the standardization of nomenclature in the diagnosis of lung rejection. J Heart Lung Transplant. 2007 Dec;26(12):1229-42.

Hyperacute rejection presents with severe allograft dysfunction very early after reperfusion. It may be difficult to distinguish this from severe primary graft dysfunction (PGD) clinically. Preformed DSAs, which lead to hyperacute rejection, result in a positive direct donor-recipient crossmatch. Thus, the presence of preformed DSAs and a positive crossmatch are the distinguishing features between hyperacute rejection and PGD. The pathogenesis of hyperacute rejection is based on the binding of preformed DSA to HLA molecules on endothelial cells. This is followed by the activation of the complement cascade and infiltration of the allograft with myeloid cells, which result in endothelial cell necrosis, exposure of the basement membrane, and subsequent activation of the coagulation cascade.[41] The characteristic pathology demonstrates hyaline membrane formation, alveolar edema, intra-alveolar fibrin, and vascular injury with arteriolar fibrinoid necrosis and intravascular platelet and fibrin thrombi, with often noticeable neutrophilic capillary injury.[42] Advances in HLA antibody detection methods and improved specificity have allowed the precise identification of even low levels of HLA antibodies to avoid the reactive HLA in a prospective donor.[43,44] This practice, termed a "virtual crossmatch," makes it possible to predict a positive direct crossmatch and hyperacute rejection before donor organ acceptance, thereby improving donor selection and posttransplant outcomes. Consequently, hyperacute rejection has become rare. Nevertheless, it illustrates that antibodies can cause lung allograft failure and that the capillary endothelium is the focal point of initial injury.

Antibody-Mediated Rejection

Over the past 10 years, there has been increasing recognition of pulmonary AMR. To date, AMR has been recognized primarily in the context of allograft dysfunction, although a subclinical form, as is often seen in cellular rejection, may also exist. The pathogenesis of AMR is similar to hyperacute rejection, but the DSAs develop de novo instead of being preformed. The diagnosis of AMR is difficult and requires a high index of clinical suspicion. Unlike ACR, there is no specific histology, and the diagnosis requires a multidisciplinary approach. In 2016, the ISHLT developed a definition for AMR to standardize the nomenclature and promote multicenter research.[45] In this framework, the diagnosis requires multiple criteria, and the degree of clinical certainty is based on the number of criteria present. A diagnosis of definite AMR is made if all of the following criteria are present:

- Allograft dysfunction
- Circulating DSAs
- Abnormal lung histology
- C4d deposition in the capillary endothelium
- Exclusion of other potential causes of allograft dysfunction

A diagnosis of *probable* AMR is made if 1 of the criteria is absent, and a diagnosis of *possible* AMR is made if 2 of the criteria are absent.[45] However, the working group noted that a "confident" diagnosis of AMR could be made in the absence of C4d deposition. C4d deposition provides direct evidence of activation of the complement cascade and the effect of antibodies on the allograft. Indeed, C4d deposition was a breakthrough development in the identification of AMR after kidney transplantation.[46,47] However, C4d deposition has been problematic in lung transplantation. In fact, many cases of AMR were reported from multiple centers that were C4d-negative.[48,49] Similarly, 1 retrospective study that examined the role of C4d deposition in the diagnosis of AMR noted that most cases were C4d-negative.[50]

Furthermore, C4d-negative cases had similar clinical presentation, histologic findings, and clinical outcomes as C4d-positive cases.[50] Of note, all C4d-positive cases were associated with complement-binding DSAs (C1q-positive) whereas some C4d-negative cases were also C1q-negative, suggesting that AMR may occur without the activation of the complement cascade and that there may be different phenotypes of AMR.[50] Indeed, C4d-negative AMR is now widely recognized in kidney transplantation,[51,52] and the pathogenesis is believed to be mediated by natural killer cell interactions with DSAs bound to endothelial cells.[53,54] The role of complement activation in the pathogenesis of AMR has treatment implications if complement inhibitors are being considered.

Recent advances in donor-derived cell-free DNA (cfDNA) indicate that this is a sensitive marker of allograft injury, and the level of circulating cfDNA correlates well with the severity of injury and the likelihood of AMR.[55,56] Furthermore, elevated levels of cfDNA are detectable in peripheral blood approximately 3 months before the diagnosis of AMR,[55] making this assay a particularly appealing noninvasive screening tool for AMR. Although elevated levels of cfDNA are nonspecific markers of allograft injury, high levels are suggestive of AMR in the setting of DSAs and allograft dysfunction without an apparent alternative clinical cause.

General Management of Antibody-Mediated Rejection

Data to guide the management of AMR in lung transplantation are limited. Studies have focused on describing the characteristics of AMR, such as the characteristic histology and the associated DSA, and although management and outcomes are detailed, it is difficult to draw conclusions about the efficacy of a treatment or regimen without a control group. There have been no randomized controlled trials (RCTs) and no head-to-head comparisons of different regimens. Furthermore, regimens are often tailored to the severity of allograft dysfunction and clinical response to first-line treatments. In addition, no treatment has been developed specifically for AMR, and all treatments have been borrowed from the fields of oncology and rheumatology.

The goals of treatment for AMR are to deplete DSAs, suppress additional DSA production, and ameliorate allograft injury. Plasma exchange removes antibodies from the circulation, but does not suppress antibody production, and additional treatments that suppress B-cell or plasma cell proliferation and activity are needed. Although there are no RCTs in pulmonary AMR, there are 4 small RCTs of plasma exchange in kidney transplantation with conflicting results.[57–60] However, it is unclear if all patients in these older studies had AMR as defined today. In addition, intravenous immunoglobulin (IVIG), which is commonly used in combination with plasma exchange today, and other B-cell or plasma-cell–suppressing treatments were not used in any of these studies.

The use of rituximab in renal AMR has been studied in an RCT.[61] Rituximab is a monoclonal antibody to CD20, which is a cell surface molecule on mature B cells, but not plasma cells. Treatment with rituximab results in prolonged peripheral B-cell depletion. In this study, renal transplant recipients with AMR were randomized to standard of care with plasma exchange, IVIG, and high-dose corticosteroids or rituximab and standard of care.[61] There was no significant difference in the composite primary endpoint of allograft loss or lack of improvement in renal function between the 2 groups; however, more than 40% of patients randomized to the control group were treated with rituximab rescue therapy.[61] In addition to this high rate of crossover, only 38 patients were enrolled at 21 centers in France over 3 years. This illustrates the challenges of conducting clinical trials in AMR. In another RCT of patients with late AMR after kidney transplantation, there was no significant difference in renal function, DSA, or allograft survival between patients randomized to control or bortezomib (a proteasome inhibitor that promotes plasma cell apoptosis).[62] The findings of these RCTs are different from previous retrospective, single-arm studies.[63–65] Although these RCTs are small and probably not sufficiently powered, studies without a control group are biased and cannot define a treatment effect. Clearly, additional carefully designed and adequately powered controlled trials in AMR are needed, and this is especially true in lung transplantation.

Management of Pulmonary AMR and Outcomes

Multiple retrospective studies have reported single-center experiences with various treatment regimens for AMR after lung transplantation. In one study, 10 patients with AMR were treated with various combinations of plasma exchange, IVIG, high-dose corticosteroids, rituximab, and bortezomib; 5 patients died of refractory AMR, and 2 died of sepsis after treatment.[48] In another study, 9 patients were treated with plasma exchange, IVIG, high-dose corticosteroids, and rituximab; 6 died of progressive CLAD.[49] Similar outcomes were reported in another study of 21 patients with AMR.[66] Treatment consisted of various combinations of IVIG, plasma exchange, rituximab, bortezomib, antithymocyte globulin, and eculizumab.[66] Fifteen patients had an initial clinical response, but 15 died of refractory AMR or CLAD during the study period.[66] Those who had persistent DSA had significantly worse survival in this study.[66] In another study, 22 patients with AMR were treated with plasma exchange, IVIG, and rituximab, and 12 died during the study period.[67] In this study, DSA clearance after treatment was associated with better survival.[67] Carfilzomib is a second-generation proteasome inhibitor that binds irreversibly, resulting in permanent inhibition and plasma cell apoptosis. In one study, 14 patients with AMR were treated with carfilzomib, plasma exchange, and IVIG.[68] A carfilzomib response was defined as loss of C1q binding, and 10 patients were deemed responders. Responders were less likely to develop bronchiolitis obliterans than nonresponders, but there was no significant difference in freedom from restrictive allograft syndrome or survival between the 2 groups.[68] These experiences demonstrate that outcomes after AMR are exceedingly poor despite aggressive treatment, and although some patients may have a clinical response initially, there is a high incidence of subsequent CLAD development and death. Clearly, better treatment regimens are needed, and there is insufficient evidence to guide management, as the optimal treatment is unknown.

SUMMARY

Despite advances in immunosuppression, rejection remains a common problem after lung transplantation. Acute rejection and AMR are strong risk factors for the development of CLAD, which is the leading cause of death beyond the first year after transplantation and the main obstacle to better long-term outcomes. Mechanistic studies to better understand why lung allografts are more susceptible to rejection than other solid organs may provide insights to improve clinical management. Novel immunosuppressive protocols are needed to mitigate the risk of rejection with an acceptable toxicity profile. Ideally, these would be investigated using RCTs.

CLINICS CARE POINTS

- The best screening tool for acute rejection is spirometry. A drop of 10% or more in FEV1 should initiate a full evaluation to decipher

whether the decline in function is secondary to rejection, infection, airway issues, or other clinical diagnoses.

- If/when setting up a surveillance bronchoscopy program, schedule bronchoscopy primarily during the first year posttransplant, as the incidence of acute rejection is highest during this time. At least 5 pieces of alveolated lung parenchyma are recommended for the assessment of acute rejection.

- There is general consensus that patients with acute rejection grade A2 or higher should be treated with augmented immunosuppression. The management of asymptomatic acute rejection grade A1 remains controversial, despite its association with CLAD. Careful consideration of the risk/benefit ratio of therapy versus close follow-up (including a possible follow-up bronchoscopy) for the individual patient is imperative.

- In the setting of acute allograft dysfunction, consider the possibility of AMR. Initial evaluation should include testing for DSAs with further consideration for bronchoscopy and transbronchial lung biopsies depending on the results of the evaluation.

DISCLOSURE

R.R. Hachem has the following financial relationships to disclose: grant funding from Bristol Myers Squibb, grant funding from Mallinckrodt Pharmaceuticals, consulting for Transmedics, consulting for Natera, consulting for CareDx. D.J. Levine has the following financial relationships to disclose: grant funding from CareDx and consulting for Natera, consulting for CareDx.

REFERENCES

1. Chambers DC, Cherikh WS, Harhay MO, et al. International Society for Heart and Lung Transplantation. J Heart Lung Transplant 2019;38(10):1042–55.
2. Benjamin R, Koutsokera A, Cabanero M, et al. Acute rejection in the modern lung transplant era. Semin Respir Crit Care Med 2021;42:411–27.
3. Girgis RE, Tu I, Berry GJ, et al. Risk factors for the development of obliterative bronchiolitis after lung transplantation. J Heart Lung Transplant 1996;15(12):1200–8.
4. Hachem RR, Khalifah AP, Chakinala MM, et al. The significance of a single episode of minimal acute rejection after lung transplantation. Transplantation 2005;80(10):1406.
5. Burton CM, Iversen M, Carlsen J, et al. Acute cellular rejection is a risk factor for bronchiolitis obliterans

syndrome independent of post-transplant baseline FEV1. J Heart Lung Transplant 2009;28(09):888–93.

6. Hsiao HM, Scozzi D, Gauthier JM, et al. Mechanisms of graft rejection after lung transplantation. Curr Opin Organ Transplant 2017;22(01):29–35.

7. Snyder LD, Palmer SM. Immune mechanisms of lung allograft rejection. Semin Respir Crit Care Med 2006;27(5):534–43.

8. Gordon I, Bhorade VW, Vigneswaran WT, et al. SaLUTaRy: a survey of lung transplant rejection. J Heart Lung Transplant 2012;31(09):972–9.

9. De Vito Dabbs A, Hoffman LA, Iacono AT, et al. Are symptom reports useful for differentiating between acute rejection and pulmonary infection after lung transplantation? Heart Lung 2004;33:372–80.

10. Van Muylem A, Melot C, Antoine M, et al. Role of pulmonary function in the detection of allograft dysfunction after heart–lung transplantation. Thorax 1997; 52(7):643–7.

11. Martinu T, Pavlisko EN, Chen DF, et al. Acute allograft rejection: cellular and humoral processes. Clnics Chest Med 2011;32(2):295.

12. Park CH, Paik H, Haam S, et al. HRCT features of acute rejection in patients with bilateral lung transplantation: the usefulness of lesion distribution. Transplant Proc 2014;46(05):1511–6.

13. Kundu S, Herman S, Larhs A, et al. Correlation of chest radiographic findings with biopsy proven acute lung rejection. J Thorac Imaging 1999; 14(03):178–84.

14. Martinu T, Koutsokera A, Benden C, et al. Bronchoalveolar lavage standardization workgroup. ISHLT consensus statement for the standardization of bronchoalveolar lavage in lung transplant. J Heart Lung Transplant 2020;39(11):1171–90.

15. Stewart S, Fishbein MC, Snell GI, et al. Revision of the 1996 working formulation for the standardization of nomenclature in the diagnosis of lung rejection. J Heart Lung Transplant 2007;26(12): 1229–42.

16. Glanville AR, Aboyoun C, Klepetko W, et al. Three-year results of an investigator-driven multicenter, international, randomized open-label de novo trial to prevent BOS after lung transplantation. J Heart Lung Transplant 2015;34:16–25.

17. Hachem RR, Yusen RD, Chakinala MM, et al. A randomized controlled trial of tacrolimus versus cyclosporine after lung transplantation. J Heart Lung Transplant 2007;26:1012–8.

18. Hachem RR, Kamoun M, Budev MM, et al. Human leukocyte antigens antibodies. Primary results of the HALT study. Am J Transplant 2018;18(9): 2285–94.

19. Todd J, Neely M, Kopetskie H, et al. Risk factors for acute rejection in the first year after lung transplant. A multicenter study. Am J Respir Crit Care Med 2020;202(4):576–85.

20. Martinu T, Chen DF, Palmer SM. Acute rejection and humoral sensitization in lung transplant recipients. Proc Am Thorac Soc 2009;6(1):54–65.

21. Bando K, Paradis IL, Komatsu K, et al. Analysis of time-dependent risks for infection, rejection, and death after pulmonary transplantation. J Thorac Cardiovasc Surg 1995;109(01):49–57 [discussion 57–9].

22. Mangi AA, Mason DP, Nowicki ER, et al. Predictors of acute rejection after lung transplantation. Ann Thorac Surg 2011;91(06):1754–62.

23. Smith JD, Ibrahim MW, Newell H, et al. Pre-transplant donor HLA-specific antibodies: characteristics causing detrimental effects on survival after lung transplantation. J Heart Lung Transplant 2014; 33(10):1074–108.

24. Snell GI, Levy BJ, Paraskeva M, et al. The influence of clinical donor factors on acute rejection among lung and kidney recipients from the same multiorgan donor. Ann Transplant 2013;18:358–67.

25. Gammie JS, Pham SM, Colson YL, et al. Influence of panel-reactive antibody on survival and rejection after lung transplantation. J Heart Lung Transplant 1997;16(04):408–15.

26. Peltz M, Edwards LB, Jessen ME, et al. HLA mismatches influence lung transplant recipient survival, bronchiolitis obliterans and rejection: implications for donor lung allocation. J Heart Lung Transplant 2011; 30(04):426–34.

27. Glanville AR, Aboyoun CL, Morton JM, et al. Cyclosporine C2 target levels and acute cellular rejection after lung transplantation. J Heart Lung Transplant 2006;25(08):928–34.

28. Johansson I, Martensson G, Nyström U, et al. Lower incidence of CMV infection and acute rejections with valganciclovir prophylaxis in lung transplant recipients. BMC Infect Dis 2013;13:582.

29. Roux A, Mourin G, Fastenackels S, et al. CMV driven CD8(þ) T-cell activation is associated with acute rejection in lung transplantation. Clin Immunol 2013;148(01):16–26.

30. Hathorn KE, Chan WW, Lo W-K. Role of gastroesophageal reflux disease in lung transplantation. World J Transplant 2017;7(02):103–16.

31. Shah N, Force SD, Mitchell PO, et al. Gastroesophageal reflux disease is associated with an increased rate of acute rejection in lung transplant allografts. Transplant Proc 2010;42(07):2702–6.

32. Girnita AL, McCurry KR, Iacono AT, et al. HLA-specific antibodies are associated with high-grade and persistent-recurrent lung allograft acute rejection. J Heart Lung Transplant 2004;23(10):1135–41.

33. Sarahrudi K, Carretta A, Wisser W, et al. The value of switching from cyclosporine to tacrolimus in the treatment of refractory acute rejection and obliterative bronchiolitis after lung transplantation. Transpl Int 2002;15(01):24–8.

34. Ensor CR, Rihtarchik LC, Morrell MR, et al. Rescue alemtuzumab for refractory acute cellular rejection and bronchiolitis obliterans syndrome after lung transplantation. Clin Transplant 2017;31(04).

35. Valentine VG, Robbins RC, Wehner JH, et al. Total lymphoid irradiation for refractory acute rejection in heart-lung and lung allografts. Chest 1996;109(05):1184–9.

36. Isenring B, Robinson C, Buergi U, et al. Lung transplant recipients on long-term extracorporeal photopheresis. Clin Transplant 2017;31(10).

37. Keenan RJ, Iacono A, Dauber JH, et al. Treatment of refractory acute allograft rejection with aerosolized cyclosporine in lung transplant recipients. J Thorac Cardiovasc Surg 1997;113(02):335–40 [discussion 340–1].

38. Frost AE, Jammal CT, Cagle PT. Hyperacute rejection following lung transplantation. Chest 1996;110:559–62.

39. Bittner HB, Dunitz J, Hertz M, et al. Hyperacute rejection in single lung transplantation – case report of successful management by means of plasmapheresis and antithymocyte globulin treatment. Transplantation 2001;71:649–51.

40. Masson E, Stern M, Chabod J, et al. Hyperacute rejection after lung transplantation caused by undetected low-titer anti-HLA antibodies. J Heart Lung Transplant 2007;26:642–5.

41. Valenzuela NM, Reed EF. Antibody-mediated rejection across solid organ transplants: manifestations, mechanisms, and therapies. J Clin Invest 2017;127:2492–504.

42. Berry G, Burke M, Andersen C, et al. Pathology of pulmonary antibody-mediated rejection: 2012 update from the Pathology Council of the ISHLT. J Heart Lung Transplant 2013;32:14–21.

43. Tait BD, Süsal C, Gebel HM, et al. Consensus guidelines on the testing and clinical management issues associated with HLA and non-HLA antibodies in transplantation. Transplantation 2013;95:19–47.

44. Tambour AR, Campbell P, Claas FH, et al. Sensitization in transplantation: assessment of risk (STAR) 2017 working group meeting report. Am J Transplant 2018;18:1604–14.

45. Levine DJ, Glanville AR, Aboyoun C, et al. Antibody-mediated rejection of the lung: a consensus report of the International Society for Heart and Lung Transplantation. J Heart Lung Transplant 2016;35:397–406.

46. Feucht HE, Felber E, Gokel MJ, et al. Vascular deposition of complement-splint products in kidney allografts with cell-mediated rejection. Clin Exp Immunol 1991;86:464–70.

47. Feucht HE, Schneeberger H, Hillebrand H, et al. Capillary deposition of C4d complement fragment and early renal graft loss. Kidney Int 1993;43:1333–8.

48. Lobo LJ, Aris RM, Schmitz J, et al. Donor-specific antibodies are associated with antibody-mediated rejection, acute cellular rejection, bronchiolitis obliterans syndrome, and cystic fibrosis after lung transplantation. J Heart Lung Transplant 2013;32:70–7.

49. Otani S, Davis AK, Cantwell L, et al. Evolving experience of treating antibody-mediated rejection following lung transplantation. Transpl Immunol 2014;31:75–80.

50. Aguilar PR, Carpenter D, Ritter J, et al. The role of C4d deposition in the diagnosis of antibody-mediated rejection after lung transplantation. Am J Transplant 2018;18:936–44.

51. Haas M, Sis B, Racusen LC, et al. Banff 2013 meeting report: Inclusion of C4d-negative antibody-mediated rejection and antibody-associated arterial lesions. Am J Transplant 2014;14:272–83.

52. Orandi BJ, Alachkar N, Kraus ES, et al. Presentation and outcomes of C4d-negative antibody-mediated rejection after kidney transplantation. Am J Transplant 2016;16:213–20.

53. Hidalgo LG, Sis B, Sellarés J, et al. NK cell transcripts and NK cells in kidney biopsies from patients with donor-specific antibodies: evidence for NK cell involvement in antibody mediated rejection. Am J Transplant 2010;10:1812–22.

54. Sellarés J, Reeve J, Loupy A, et al. Molecular diagnosis of antibody-mediated rejection in human kidney transplants. Am J Transplant 2013;13:971–83.

55. Agbor-Enoh S, Jackson AM, Tunc I, et al. Late manifestation of alloantibody-associated injury and clinical pulmonary antibody-mediated rejection: evidence from cell-free DNA analysis. J Heart Lung Transplant 2018;37:925–32.

56. Agbor-Enoh S, Wang Y, Tunc I, et al. Donor-derived cell-free DNA predicts allograft failure and mortality after lung transplantation. EBioMedicine 2019;40:541–53.

57. Bonomini V, Vangelista A, Frasca GM, et al. Effects of plasmapheresis in renal transplant rejection: a controlled study. Trans Am Soc Artif Intern Organs 1985;31:698–703.

58. Blake P, Sutton D, Cardella CJ. Plasma exchange in acute renal transplant rejection. Prog Clin Biol Res 1990;337:249–52.

59. Allen NH, Dyer P, Geoghegan T, et al. Plasma exchange in acute renal allograft rejection: a controlled trial. Transplantation 1983;35:425–8.

60. Kirubakaran MG, Disney AP, Norman J, et al. A controlled trial of plasmapheresis in the treatment of renal allograft rejection. Transplantation 1981;32:164–5.

61. Sautenet B, Blancho G, Büchler M, et al. One-year results of the effects of rituximab on acute antibody-mediated rejection in renal transplantation: RITUX ERAH, a multicenter double-blind

randomized placebo-controlled trial. Transplantation 2016;100:391–9.

62. Eskandary F, Regele H, Baumann L, et al. A randomized trial of bortezomib in late antibody-mediated kidney transplant rejection. J Am Soc Nephrol 2018;29:591–605.

63. Faguer S, Kamar N, Guilbeaud-Frugier C, et al. Rituximab therapy for acute humoral rejection after kidney transplantation. Transplantation 2007;83: 1277–80.

64. Everly MJ, Everly JJ, Susskind B, et al. Bortezomib provides effective therapy for antibody and cell0me-diated acute rejection. Transplantation 2008;86: 1754–61.

65. Mulley WR, Hudson FJ, Tait BD, et al. A single low-fixed dose of rituximab to salvage renal transplants from refractory antibody-mediated rejection. Transplantation 2009;87:286–9.

66. Witt CA, Gaut JP, Yusen RD, et al. Acute antibody-mediated rejection after lung transplantation. J Heart Lung Transplant 2013;32:1034–40.

67. Roux A, Bendib Le Lan I, Holifanjaniaina S, et al. Antibody-mediated rejection in lung transplantation: clinical outcomes and donor-specific antibody characteristics. Am J Transplant 2016;16:1216–28.

68. Ensor CR, Yousem SA, Marrai M, et al. Proteasome inhibitor carfilzomib-based therapy for antibody-mediated rejection of the pulmonary allograft: use and short-term findings. Am J Transplant 2017;17: 1380–8.

Chronic Lung Allograft Dysfunction

Aida Venado, MD, MAS[a],*, Jasleen Kukreja, MD, MPH[b], John R. Greenland, MD, PhD[c]

KEYWORDS

- CLAD • BOS • RAS • PPFE

KEY POINTS

- Chronic lung allograft dysfunction (CLAD) is a syndrome of progressive lung function decline after lung transplant.
- CLAD develops as an obstructive—bronchiolitis obliterans syndrome (BOS), a restrictive—restrictive allograft syndrome (RAS), or a mixed phenotype with features of both. RAS typically progresses faster and has lower survival than BOS.
- Therapeutic approaches to CLAD include augmenting immunosuppression, immunomodulation, and antifibrotic medications. Because of their overall ineffectiveness, retransplantation is currently the only treatment that can extend survival for progressive CLAD.

CLAD DEFINITIONS

Chronic lung allograft dysfunction (CLAD) is a syndrome of progressive lung function decline after lung transplant largely attributed to chronic rejection that can manifest with obstructive and/or restrictive physiology. Our understanding of CLAD and its definitions has evolved over time. In 1993, the International Society of Heart and Lung Transplantation (ISHTL) sponsored a working formulation for the standardization of nomenclature of chronic dysfunction in lung allografts, which found forced expiratory volume in 1 second (FEV_1) to be the most reliable and consistent indicator of graft function.

Bronchiolitis obliterans syndrome (BOS) was defined as an unexplained deterioration of graft function secondary to progressive airways disease, a presumed manifestation of chronic rejection. BOS was staged in 4 categories based on FEV_1 decline and specifying the absence or presence of pathologic obliterative bronchiolitis as "a" and "b," respectively.[1] Subtypes "a" and "b"

are rarely used because of the low sensitivity of transbronchial biopsies to detect bronchiolitis obliterans.[2] In 2001, a potential BOS stage, BOS 0-p, was added, which included decline in mid expiratory flow rate (FEF_{25-75}) less than 75% of baseline,[3] later removed because of insufficient predictive utility.[4]

Around 2010, the term CLAD was introduced[5] and **restrictive allograft syndrome (RAS)** was proposed as a distinct subtype from BOS.[6] In 2014, the ISHLT defined CLAD as a decline in either FEV_1 or forced vital capacity (FVC) to 80% or lower than baseline, and recognized the obstructive and restrictive forms.[7] The term **acute lung allograft dysfunction** was introduced to indicate a 10% decline in FEV_1 that should prompt investigation for infection, rejection, or other reversible causes.

In 2019, the ISHLT defined CLAD as follows:

- "Possible CLAD" as an $FEV_1 \leq 80\%$ from baseline, which is the average of the 2 best

[a] Division of Pulmonary, Critical Care, Allergy, and Sleep Medicine, University of California, San Francisco, 505 Parnassus Ave, M1093A, San Francisco, CA 94143-2204, USA; [b] Division of Cardiothoracic Surgery, Univeristy of California, San Francisco, 500 Parnassus Ave, MU 405W Suite 305, San Francisco, CA 94143, USA; [c] Division of Pulmonary, Critical Care, Allergy, and Sleep Medicine, University of California, San Francisco, SF VAHCS Building 2, Room 453 (Mail stop 111D), 4150 Clement St, San Francisco CA 94121, USA

* Corresponding author.

E-mail address: aida.venado@ucsf.edu

Thoracic Surg Clin 32 (2022) 231–242
https://doi.org/10.1016/j.thorsurg.2021.11.004

- post-transplant FEV_1 measurements taken at least 3 weeks apart
- "Probable CLAD" if the FEV1 decline persists after 3 weeks
- "Definite CLAD" if it persists after 3 months.[8]

CLAD has 4 stages based on FEV_1 decline (**Table 1**). Mechanical and other factors that cause a persistent decline in FEV_1 are not considered part of the CLAD syndrome, including pleural effusions, airway stenosis, diaphragmatic dysfunction, and weight gain. When FEV_1 decline is attributed pathologies unlikely to be related to chronic rejection, a new baseline can be established once the FEV_1 remains stable for 6 months.

CLAD can be subdivided into BOS, RAS, mixed, or undefined patterns (**Table 2**).[8] Although there is some controversy over definitions:

- BOS can be diagnosed if there is airflow obstruction with FEV_1/FVC less than 70% and no persistent radiographic opacities.
- RAS is diagnosed if there is restriction with total lung capacity (TLC) $\leq$90% from baseline— the average of 2 best TLC measures at the same time or very close to the best FEV_1 values—with persistent parenchymal opacities on chest imaging.[9] As not all centers routinely perform serial TLC measurements, when restriction is suspected by FVC $\leq$ 80% from baseline—using the average of the 2 FVC measures at the time of the best FEV1 values post-transplant—the term "probable RAS" can be applied. Typical imaging findings of RAS include opacifications, fibrosis, and honeycombing, especially in the upper lobes and/or near the pleura, corresponding to pathologic features of **pleuroparenchymal fibroelastosis (PPFE).**

RAS accounts for 25% to 35% of CLAD cases and has a worse prognosis, with a median survival

of 8 to 10 months following diagnosis as compared with 35 months after diagnosis of BOS.[10,11] Although BOS is the predominant CLAD phenotype, 10% of cases that start as BOS evolve to RAS; this mixed phenotype has better survival than RAS, but worse than BOS.[12]

CLAD PATHOPHYSIOLOGY

Investigation of CLAD pathology dates back to the 1980s when autopsy findings from the first successful lung transplants became available.[13] Progressive obstructive pathology was observed, with some recipients having a superimposed restrictive defect. Autopsy findings consistently showed constrictive bronchiolitis, with a minority of patients also developing significant pleural fibrosis, consistent with contemporary BOS and RAS.[14]

CLAD pathogenesis likely reflects sequelae of alloimmune injury that have exceeded lung cell regenerative capacity, yet a comprehensive mechanistic understanding remains elusive. The physiologic and pathologic findings of the CLAD syndrome may have multiple causes. Indeed, constrictive bronchiolitis and PPFE are also observed even in the absence of alloimmunity. Our understanding of CLAD pathogenesis focuses on the mechanisms leading to these pathologic features:

Obliterative Bronchiolitis

Bronchioles are 1 to 10 mm, noncartilaginous airways connecting bronchi with alveoli. Given the large cross-sectional area of the peripheral airways, significant damage must occur to induce obstructive physiology. Constrictive or obliterative bronchiolitis, as seen in CLAD, is characterized by circumferential compression of airway lumen from submucosal and peribronchiolar fibrosis. There is heterogeneous small airway involvement, such that some airways will appear normal, even when neighboring airways have collapsed completely.[15] Obliterative bronchiolitis is irreversible and distinct from inflammatory bronchiolitis, which often occurs after viral infections, and proliferative bronchiolitis, also known as organizing pneumonia, in which bronchiolar injury of identifiable or cryptogenic etiology can lead to deposition of transluminal fibroblastic tissue (Masson bodies).

PPFE is a combination of fibrosis in the visceral pleura and fibroelastotic changes in the subpleural parenchyma. Outside of lung transplant, PPFE is an interstitial lung disease typically associated with idiopathic pulmonary fibrosis (IPF) and linked to telomere dysfunction.[16] Although PPFE is the most common pathology associated with RAS, nonspecific interstitial pneumonia, exudative

---

Table 1	
Chronic lung allograft dysfunction stages	
Stage	**Percent FEV1 from Baseline**
CLAD 0	>80%
CLAD 1	>65-80%
CLAD 2	>50-65%
CLAD 3	>35-50%
CLAD 4	FEV1 $\leq$ 35%

Adapted from Verleden GM, Glanville AR, Lease ED, et al. Chronic lung allograft dysfunction: Definition, diagnostic criteria, and approaches to treatment-A consensus report from the Pulmonary Council of the ISHLT. *J Heart Lung Transplant.* May 2019;38(5):493-503.

Table 2
Key characteristics of chronic lung allograft dysfunction phenotypes

CLAD Phenotype	Lung Function Defect	Chest CT Findings
BOS	Obstruction	Air trapping without persistent opacities.
RAS	Restriction	Persistent opacities consistent with pulmonary and/or pleural fibrosis.
Mixed	Obstruction and restriction	Persistent opacities consistent with pulmonary and/or pleural fibrosis. Air trapping may be present.
Undefined	Obstruction	Persistent opacities consistent with pulmonary and/or pleural fibrosis. Air trapping may be present.
Undefined	Obstruction and restriction	Air trapping without persistent opacities.

All CLAD phenotypes have persistent FEV1 decline to ≤80% from baseline, which is the average of the 2 best post-transplant FEV1 values, separated 3 or more weeks apart.
  Obstruction refers to FEV1/FVC less than 0.7.
  Restriction refers to TLC ≤90% from baseline, which is the average of the 2 best post-transplant TLC values at the time or close to the 2 best FEV1 values. The term "probable RAS" is used when TLC is not available and restriction is implied by FVC ≤80% from baseline and FEV1/FVC greater than 0.7, with the caveat that air trapping from BOS can lead to FVC decline. The baseline FVC is the average of the FVC values paired with the 2 best post-transplant FEV1 values.
  Persistent opacities are those present for 3 or more months.
  Adapted from[7–9].

fibrosis, and acute fibrinoid organizing pneumonia have also been observed.[17]

Alloimmune Activation

CLAD-like pathology and physiology are observed following allogeneic stem cell transplant and with major histocompatibility complex (MHC) antigen mismatch in lung transplant.[15] Although increasing number of donor-recipient HLA mismatches is a risk factor for CLAD in humans,[18] even a single antigen mismatch is sufficient to induce obliterative airway disease pathology in a CLAD mouse model.[19]

Acute cellular rejection (ACR) is thought to reflect alloimmune activation. Both perivascular lymphocytic inflammation and lymphocytic bronchitis, ISHLT A- and B- grade acute rejection, and acute inflammation in large airways are risk factors for CLAD.[20–22] However, minimal ACR does not appear to increase CLAD risk, and CLAD can occur without prior ACR.[22–24] These findings may reflect an insensitivity of transbronchial biopsies, as alloimmune response can be observed even when not detected by histopathologic examination of transbronchial biopsy tissue.[2,25]

Although type 1 immune responses are thought to predominate in CLAD, type 2 and type 17 alloimmunity have also been implicated.[26] Type 17 immune responses can drive neutrophilic inflammation. A syndrome of greater than 15% neutrophils in BAL and ≥10% decline in FEV$_1$ is termed neutrophilic reversible allograft dysfunction (NRAD) and can lead to CLAD unless reversed by azithromycin treatment.[27] Mechanistically, NRAD may be explained by the observation that calcineurin inhibition can increase IL-17–dependent neutrophil chemotaxis in airway epithelial cells, a process blocked by azithromycin.[28]

Humoral Immune Responses

Alloimmune CD4+ T cells can drive B and plasma cells to generate antibodies to donor MHC antigens, known as donor-specific antibodies (DSA). The syndrome of antibody-mediated rejection, including allograft dysfunction, DSA, complement (C4d) deposition, compatible lung histology, and the exclusion of other causes, conveys a significant increased risk of progression to CLAD, particularly RAS.[29–31] DSA can activate the complement cascade, resulting in C5a-mediated chemotaxis of neutrophils, monocytes, T cells, and activation of the membrane attack complex that causes direct cell lysis.[32] DSA can also stimulate natural killer (NK) cells leading to antibody-dependent cell-mediated cytotoxicity (ADCC).[33] Accordingly, recipients with genotypes that confer greater Fc-receptor binding to DSA have more rapid progression to CLAD, potentially because of greater ADCC.[34] DSA also directly stimulate airway epithelial cells, resulting in proliferative signals that could drive CLAD independent from other immune cells.[35] Overall, DSA confer an increased risk of CLAD and their resolution is a good prognostic sign.[36] As interventions to clear DSA do not necessarily result in improved outcomes, DSA may be both directly pathogenic and a biomarker of alloimmunity more broadly.[37,38]

Other Immune Responses

Autoimmune antibodies, such as type V collagen and K-α1 tubulin, can develop following lung transplant and are risk factors for progression to CLAD.[39] Innate immune gene polymorphisms are associated with differential CLAD risk either through direct immune activation or through increased susceptibility to infection.[40–42]

NK cells can have a variety of effects depending on the specific cell receptors that are activated. NK cells can target recipient antigen-presenting cells in the context of killer-cell immunoglobulin-like receptor (KIR) MHC mismatches, resulting in decreased risk of CLAD.[43] However, activation of NK cells to cytomegalovirus in the allograft via NKG2C, to stress molecules via NKG2D, or to antibodies via FcR would increase the risk of CLAD.[33,44]

Epithelial Cell Injury and Regeneration

CLAD pathology can be observed as a result of direct epithelial injury.[45] Primary graft dysfunction,[46] air pollution,[47] gastroesophageal reflux,[48] and infections[45,49,50] confer increased risk for CLAD. Although these insults may potentiate immune activation to some extent, they also drive epithelial cell damage and turnover.

Restoration of airway epithelium requires repopulation from epithelial cell precursors. Club cells serve both to protect the lung epithelium and repopulate bronchioles through differentiation into goblet and ciliated cells, and club cell loss is a hallmark of CLAD.[51] In a murine model of lung transplant with alloimmune mismatch, club cell depletion resulted in obliterative bronchiolitis pathology.[52] Increased turnover in the airway epithelium could be an important driver of CLAD if it exceeds the capacity of club cells to restore epithelial integrity. Telomere dysfunction in the allograft may explain why club cells could fail to keep up with the turnover from chronic alloimmune injury. A mouse model where telomeres were uncapped in club cells resulted in obliterative bronchiolitis pathology absent alloimmune responses.[53] Furthermore, allografts from donors with short telomeres are at increased risk for CLAD.[54] Mechanistically, epithelial cells actively signal to prevent mesenchymal proliferation, explaining how their loss could drive obliterative bronchiolitis.[55]

TREATMENT OF CLAD

Several therapies have been used to treat CLAD with variable results. Triple immunosuppression with steroid (prednisone), purine inhibitor (mofetil mycophenolate or azathioprine), and calcineurin inhibitor (CNI) (tacrolimus or cyclosporine) is standard after lung transplant. In the absence of strong evidence to guide management, a common approach to CLAD is to add therapies that fall into the categories of immunomodulation (azithromycin, montelukast, extracorporeal photopheresis (ECP), immunosuppression augmentation (mTOR inhibitors, alemtuzumab, antithymocyte globulin [ATG], inhaled cyclosporine), and more recently, antifibrotic medications (pirfenidone, nintedanib). Owing to the overall ineffectiveness of medical therapies to reverse or halt CLAD progression, currently retransplantation is the only treatment understood to extend survival (**Table 3**).

Azithromycin is a macrolide antibiotic that reduces airway neutrophilia and interleukin-8 mRNA expression in BOS patients, leading to improved FEV1 in the NRAD phenotype.[56] In 2014, the ISHLT issued the recommendation of a trial of azithromycin for at least 3 months in patients diagnosed with BOS.[57] Randomized controlled trials (RCTs) of azithromycin have shown variable results for treatment of established BOS versus prevention of BOS. For established BOS, FEV1 was on average 0.3 L higher among recipients taking azithromycin and a ≥10% increase in FEV1 from baseline, compared with placebo.[58] Recipients who started azithromycin early after transplant and took it for the first 2 years had better FEV1, lower prevalence of BOS (12.5% vs 44.2%), and improved BOS-free survival at 2 years compared with those taking placebo.[59] Azithromycin administered before transplant and on alternate days for 1 month following transplant had no effect in FEV1 at 3 months or CLAD-free survival compared with placebo.[60] A single-center study comparing outcomes before and after azithromycin for CLAD prevention reported improved survival but not reduction in the risk of CLAD or time to CLAD onset.[61] Azithromycin for CLAD prevention has been adopted in lung transplant centers worldwide, including ours.

Montelukast is a leukotriene receptor antagonist that decreases airway eosinophilic inflammation, used in the treatment of asthma. Reports of potential benefit in bronchiolitis obliterans associated with graft-versus-host disease after hematopoietic stem cell transplant led to the investigation of montelukast use for fibroproliferative BOS.[62] An open-label, pilot study showed attenuation of FEV1 decline in the 6 months following addition

Table 3
Current medical therapies for chronic lung allograft dysfunction

Therapy	Potential Mechanism of Action	Potential Adverse Events	References
Azithromycin	Macrolide antibiotic that reduces airway neutrophilia and interleukin-8 mRNA expression.	Diarrhea, nausea, vomiting, QT prolongation, arrhythmia, hearing loss.	56–61
Montelukast	Leukotriene receptor antagonist that decreases airway eosinophilic inflammation.	Nausea	62,63
Extracorporeal photopheresis	May promote effector lymphocyte apoptosis and/or stabilization of regulatory T cells.	Indwelling catheter infections, transient hypotension.	64–73
Sirolimus and everolimus	mTOR inhibitors decrease proliferation of B and T lymphocytes, NK cells, and fibroblasts. Associated with an increase in regulatory T cells.	Edema, hypertension, hypertriglyceridemia, anemia, leukopenia, wound dehiscence, pneumonitis.	75–79
Inhaled cyclosporine	Calcineurin inhibitor that reduces T cell activity by preventing cytokine transcription.	Conjunctivitis, pharyngitis, productive cough.	80–82
Alemtuzumab	Anti-CD52 antibody that induces B and T lymphocyte depletion by complement-mediated cell lysis, antibody-mediated cytotoxicity, and apoptosis.	Lymphopenia, infections.	83–87
Antithymocyte globulin	Antibodies derived from inoculation of rabbits and horses with human thymocytes with several targets against B and T cells that lead to lymphocyte depletion by complement-mediated-lysis, opsonization and phagocytosis, and apoptosis.	Lymphopenia, infections.	88,89
Total lymphoid irradiation	Targeted irradiation of supradiaphragmatic and infradiaphragmatic perivascular lymph nodes, spleen, and thymus that leads to depletion, impaired function, and abnormal maturation of T lymphocytes.	Bone marrow suppression, thrombocytopenia, leukopenia, infections.	90–92
Pirfenidone	Small molecule that inhibits the proliferation of lung fibroblasts and their differentiation into myofibroblasts by blocking TGF-β signaling.	Nausea, vomiting, diarrhea, weight loss, photosensitivity, hepatotoxicity.	93–97

(continued on next page)

Table 3 (continued)			
Therapy	Potential Mechanism of Action	Potential Adverse Events	References
Nintedanib	Tyrosine kinase inhibitor that inhibits TGF-β signaling in lung fibroblasts, myofibroblast differentiation, fibronectin, and collagen 1 expression.	Diarrhea, nausea vomiting, weight loss, hepatotoxicity.	98–101

of montelukast 10 mg daily.[62] A subsequent RCT of montelukast for 1 year in 30 patients with BOS already taking azithromycin found no difference in lung function or survival.[63] Although overall a negative trial, a post hoc analysis suggested stabilization of FEV1 in the year after the addition of montelukast in patients with early, stage 1 BOS.[63]

ECP is the induction of psoralen-mediated DNA crosslinks in white blood cells by exposure to ultraviolet A light, which causes apoptosis of lymphoid, NK, and T cells.[64] ECP was initially used in the 1980s to treat cutaneous T-cell lymphoma followed by other T cell-mediated conditions including Chron's disease, GVDH, and solid organ transplant rejection. ECP is considered an immunomodulatory rather than an immunosuppressive therapy, with less risk of infectious complications.[65] Although its immunomodulatory mechanisms remain unidentified, augmentation of regulatory T (Treg) cell responses has been proposed.[66–68] In BOS, ECP-induced increase or stabilization of peripheral Treg cells correlates with stabilization in FEV1, whereas absence of Treg response correlates with progressive FEV1 decline.[67] ECP has also been associated with increase in the inhibitory cytokines IL-4 and IL-10; decrease in the proinflammatory cytokines IL-1β, IL-2, IFN-γ, IL-17, IP-1, and MCP-1; and clearance of DSA in patients with BOS.[69]

Although ECP has been associated with decreased rate of FEV1 decline[65,67,69–72] and increased survival[65] in CLAD in nonrandomized studies, clinical responses are variable.[65] It is unclear if this variability may reflect the course of CLAD progression independent of ECP. Late development of BOS greater than 3 years after transplant, rapid FEV1 decline, start of ECP in more advanced BOS stages, and RAS phenotype have been associated with worse response.[65,73] Currently, ECP is recommended mainly for BOS, with duration of treatment guided by FEV1 response.[74] A randomized multicenter trial to assess the efficacy and tolerability of ECP to treat refractory and newly diagnosed BOS is ongoing (Clinical Trials.gov NCT02181257).

The **mTOR (mammalian target of rapamycin) inhibitors,** sirolimus and everolimus, prevent B and T lymphocyte proliferation,[75] decrease proliferation of NK cells, mesenchymal cells, and fibroblasts, and are associated with increase in Treg cells. These effects have led to the hypothesis of mTOR inhibition as a potential therapy for BOS.[76] Although mTOR inhibitors are commonly used to mitigate adverse events of other immunosuppressants—nephrotoxicity, leukopenia, gastrointestinal side effects—there is limited evidence on their effect on CLAD progression. The 4EVERLUNG randomized trial, which showed higher renal function 1-year post-transplant with everolimus-based quadruple low CNI immunosuppression compared with triple immunosuppression, found no difference in CLAD development.[77] A multicenter RCT of everolimus versus azathioprine in stable lung recipients taking prednisone and cyclosporine showed lower incidence of BOS at 12 months with everolimus, with no difference at 24 months.[78] Everolimus was discontinued more for adverse events, mainly infections and renal impairment. A retrospective study of everolimus added specifically for CLAD found FEV1 improvement at 6 months in BOS patients, but rapid decline in those with RAS.[79] The long-term effect of mTOR inhibitors on CLAD progression needs to be further assessed in RCTs, especially since their widespread effects, including enhanced activation of the native immune system (eg, macrophages and dendritic cells) can lead to inflammatory adverse events[75] such as pneumonitis.

Inhaled cyclosporine is a calcineurin inhibitor that reduces T lymphocyte effector function by preventing transcription of IL-2 and other cytokines upon activation of the T cell receptor. The side effects of systemic cyclosporine administration limited the concentration needed in the allograft, which led to the concept of regional immunosuppression—local drug delivery with higher graft and lower systemic effects. Animal studies found higher lung cyclosporine concentration by aerosolized than systemic route.[80] Small single-center studies in lung recipients with refractory rejection showed improvement in histologic ACR and FEV1 with inhaled cyclosporine deposition in the lungs in a dose-dependent manner.[81] In a randomized trial in 21 patients with BOS, twice daily inhaled liposomal cyclosporine led to stabilization of FEV1 and FVC, with ongoing decline in the standard of care group.[82] Median retransplant-free survival was better in patients taking cyclosporine at 4.1 years compared with 2.7 years in the standard of care group.[82] A large RCT to assess the efficacy of inhaled liposomal cyclosporine for BOS treatment was recently completed (ClinicalTrials.gov NCT03657342).

Alemtuzumab is a monoclonal antibody that binds to CD52 in the membrane of B and T lymphocytes, NK cells, dendritic cells, and macrophages.[83] Alemtuzumab induction is associated with improved survival after lung transplant and freedom from BOS versus no induction.[84] Although alemtuzumab improves refractory ACR, its use as rescue for established BOS has been associated with a transient increase in FEV1, particularly in stage 1 BOS, but no improvement in long-term outcomes.[85–87] Furthermore, the resulting profound and prolonged lymphopenia carries a significant risk of infection.

ATG is an anti–T-lymphocyte immunoglobulin, derived from horses and rabbits, that depletes circulating lymphocytes.[88] It is used for the induction and treatment of ACR. In a single-center study of 71 patients with CLAD treated with ATG, 23% had improved or stable FEV1, 40% had attenuated FEV1 decline, and 37% had worsening FEV1 decline.[89] CLAD phenotype was not associated with response. Infectious complications were common; a third of patients cultured positive and 4% were hospitalized for infections. Response was associated with better retransplant-free survival, though the contribution of other factors is unclear.

Total lymphoid irradiation involves targeted irradiation of all major supradiaphragmatic and infradiaphragmatic perivascular lymph nodes, spleen, and thymus that leads to depletion, impaired function, and abnormal maturation of T lymphocytes resulting in potent immunosuppression.[90] In several retrospective case series including over 150 patients with BOS, response, defined as stabilization of FEV1 or attenuation of its decline primarily in those with rapidly progressive BOS, was reported in 36% to 100% of patients.[91] The reasons for this variability are unclear.[91,92] Retransplant-free survival after total

lymphoid irradiation has been variable.[91] A protocol of 8 Gy administered over 10 fractions has been commonly used. Bone marrow suppression despite stopping antiproliferative agents and severe infections caused early discontinuation in up to a third of patients.

Pirfenidone is a small molecule that inhibits the proliferation of human lung fibroblasts and their differentiation into myofibroblasts.[93] Pirfenidone slows FVC decline and improves progression-free survival in patients with IPF.[94] Its antifibrotic effect has raised the question of whether pirfenidone could also slow the progression of CLAD.[95] Attenuation in FVC and FEV1 decline after initiation of pirfenidone in patients with RAS has been observed in the case series.[95–97] Though, half of the patients experienced side effects, mainly anorexia and nausea, requiring dose reduction and a 20% increase in CNI dose requirement was also reported.[97] A prospective open-label study to assess the safety and tolerability of 52 weeks of pirfenidone in patients with restrictive CLAD is ongoing (ClinicalTrials.gov identifier NCT03359863). Although the evidence of pirfenidone for CLAD is anecdotal at this time, 2 randomized, placebo-controlled studies are expected to provide robust data: the recently completed European Trial of Pirfenidone in BOS (EPOS; Clinical.Trials.gov identifier NCT02262299) and an ongoing trial assessing the effect of pirfenidone in CLAD by parametric response mapping (PRM), an emerging imaging diagnostic modality (ClinicalTrials.gov identifier NCT03473340).

Nintedanib is a multiple tyrosine kinase inhibitor that inhibits myofibroblast differentiation in human lung fibroblasts.[98] Nintedanib slows FVC decline in patients with IPF,[99] scleroderma-associated interstitial lung disease,[100] and progressive fibrosing interstitial lung disease.[101] Similar to pirfenidone, its antifibrotic effects could slow the progression of CLAD. A multicenter randomized trial to assess the effect of 6 months of nintedanib in FEV1 change in patients with BOS is ongoing (Clinical.Trials.gov identifier NCT03283007). Continuation of nintedanib after single lung transplant for IPF to preserve native lung function is also under investigation (Clinical.Trials.gov identifier NCT03562416).

Retransplantation for CLAD is currently the only treatment that can extend survival. However, survival after retransplant is inferior than after primary lung transplant at all time points.[102] A multicenter study reported a significantly worse survival after retransplant particularly for RAS compared with BOS.[103] Although the reasons for this difference are unclear, higher postoperative mortality and earlier redevelopment of CLAD were observed in patients retransplanted for RAS compared with BOS.

CONTROVERSIES

One fundamental area of uncertainty is the definition of CLAD itself[6,10]; thus, its incidence and estimates of CLAD-free survival remain uncertain. The natural history of CLAD remains poorly understood. Early biomarker abnormalities may shed light on the mechanisms and refine risk stratification.

Though lung function decline has been the main prognostic factor and the cornerstone of CLAD diagnosis, radiographic abnormalities, in particular RAS-like opacities, can precede functional changes and predict survival.[104,105] Using CT findings as an alternative to spirometry to diagnose RAS has been proposed.[106] Furthermore, the prognostic utility of routinely performed CT scans is expanding as new methods of image analysis emerge such as PRM.[107]

Beyond its utility to evaluate infection and ACR, bronchoscopy is emerging as a source of biomarker predictors of CLAD. Airway brushing analysis shows promise for detecting allograft rejection gene pathways, alterations in the microbiome, and other cellular and epigenetic changes in the course of CLAD.[25,49,108]

SUMMARY

CLAD is a syndrome of progressive lung function decline after lung transplant, which currently has no cure. Better definition of CLAD endotypes and prognostic biomarkers are needed to understand its pathobiology and develop effective therapies. Although single-center studies have been hypothesis-generating, large multicenter, RCTs are needed to assess the efficacy of current and future CLAD therapies.

DISCLOSURE

A. Venado: Pirfenidone for Restrictive Chronic Lung Allograft Dysfunction (PIRCLAD) study sponsored by Genentech (Principal Investigator). J. Kukreja: Lung Bioengineering (Data Safety Monitoring committee); Transmedics (research). John Greenland: Scientific Advisory Board for Atara Biotherapeutics, Theravance Biopharma, Boehringer Ingelheim; Research funding: Theravance Biopharma.

REFERENCES

1. Cooper JD, Billingham M, Egan T, et al. A working formulation for the standardization of nomenclature and for clinical staging of chronic dysfunction in lung allografts. International Society for Heart and Lung Transplantation. J Heart Lung Transpl 1993; 12(5):713–6.

2. Dugger DT, Fung M, Hays SR, et al. Chronic lung allograft dysfunction small airways reveal a lymphocytic inflammation gene signature. Am J Transpl 2021;21(1):362–71.

3. Estenne M, Maurer JR, Boehler A, et al. Bronchiolitis obliterans syndrome 2001: an update of the diagnostic criteria. J Heart Lung Transpl 2002; 21(3):297–310.

4. Hachem RR, Chakinala MM, Yusen RD, et al. The predictive value of bronchiolitis obliterans syndrome stage 0-p. Am J Respir Crit Care Med 2004;169(4):468–72.

5. Glanville AR. Bronchoscopic monitoring after lung transplantation. Semin Respir Crit Care Med 2010;31(2):208–21.

6. Sato M, Waddell TK, Wagnetz U, et al. Restrictive allograft syndrome (RAS): a novel form of chronic lung allograft dysfunction. J Heart Lung Transpl 2011;30(7):735–42.

7. Verleden GM, Raghu G, Meyer KC, et al. A new classification system for chronic lung allograft dysfunction. J Heart Lung Transplant 2014;33(2):127–33.

8. Verleden GM, Glanville AR, Lease ED, et al. Chronic lung allograft dysfunction: definition, diagnostic criteria, and approaches to treatment-A consensus report from the Pulmonary Council of the ISHLT. J Heart Lung Transpl 2019;38(5):493–503.

9. Glanville AR, Verleden GM, Todd JL, et al. Chronic lung allograft dysfunction: definition and update of restrictive allograft syndrome-A consensus report from the Pulmonary Council of the ISHLT. J Heart Lung Transpl 2019;38(5):483–92.

10. Verleden GM, Vos R, Verleden SE, et al. Survival determinants in lung transplant patients with chronic allograft dysfunction. Transplantation 2011;92(6):703–8.

11. Todd JL, Jain R, Pavlisko EN, et al. Impact of forced vital capacity loss on survival after the onset of chronic lung allograft dysfunction. Am J Respir Crit Care Med 2014;189(2):159–66.

12. Van Herck A, Verleden SE, Sacreas A, et al. Validation of a post-transplant chronic lung allograft dysfunction classification system. J Heart Lung Transpl 2019;38(2):166–73.

13. Tazelaar HD, Yousem SA. The pathology of combined heart-lung transplantation: an autopsy study. Hum Pathol 1988;19(12):1403–16.

14. Burke CM, Theodore J, Dawkins KD, et al. Post-transplant obliterative bronchiolitis and other late lung sequelae in human heart-lung transplantation. Chest 1984;86(6):824–9.

15. Greenland JR, Jones K, Singer JP. Bronchiolitis. In: Broaddus VC, Ernst JD, King TE, et al, editors.

Murray & Nadel's textbook of respiratory medicine, vol. 1, 7th edition. Philadelphia, PA: Elsevier; 2021. p. 994–1004.

16. Chua F, Desai SR, Nicholson AG, et al. Pleuroparenchymal fibroelastosis. A review of clinical, radiological, and pathological characteristics. Ann Am Thorac Soc 2019;16(11):1351–9.

17. Verleden SE, Von der Thusen J, Roux A, et al. When tissue is the issue: a histological review of chronic lung allograft dysfunction. Am J Transpl 2020;20(10):2644–51.

18. Belperio JA, Weigt SS, Fishbein MC, et al. Chronic lung allograft rejection: mechanisms and therapy. Proc Am Thorac Soc 2009;6(1):108–21.

19. Higuchi T, Maruyama T, Jaramillo A, et al. Induction of obliterative airway disease in murine tracheal allografts by CD8+ CTLs recognizing a single minor histocompatibility antigen. J Immunol 2005;174(4):1871–8.

20. Glanville AR, Aboyoun CL, Havryk A, et al. Severity of lymphocytic bronchiolitis predicts long-term outcome after lung transplantation. Am J Respir Crit Care Med 2008;177(9):1033–40.

21. Verleden SE, Scheers H, Nawrot TS, et al. Lymphocytic bronchiolitis after lung transplantation is associated with daily changes in air pollution. Am J Transpl 2012;12(7):1831–8.

22. Greenland JR, Jones KD, Hays SR, et al. Association of large-airway lymphocytic bronchitis with bronchiolitis obliterans syndrome. Am J Respir Crit Care Med 2013;187(4):417–23.

23. Levy L, Huszti E, Tikkanen J, et al. The impact of first untreated subclinical minimal acute rejection on risk for chronic lung allograft dysfunction or death after lung transplantation. Am J Transpl 2019;20(1):241–9.

24. Khalifah AP, Hachem RR, Chakinala MM, et al. Minimal acute rejection after lung transplantation: a risk for bronchiolitis obliterans syndrome. Am J Transpl 2005;5(8):2022–30.

25. Iasella CJ, Hoji A, Popescu I, et al. Type-1 immunity and endogenous immune regulators predominate in the airway transcriptome during chronic lung allograft dysfunction. Am J Transpl 2021;21(6):2145–60.

26. Lemaitre PH, Vokaer B, Charbonnier LM, et al. Cyclosporine A drives a Th17- and Th2-mediated posttransplant obliterative airway disease. Am J Transpl 2013;13(3):611–20.

27. Vos R, Verleden SE, Ruttens D, et al. Azithromycin and the treatment of lymphocytic airway inflammation after lung transplantation. Am J Transpl 2014;14(12):2736–48.

28. Vanaudenaerde BM, Wuyts WA, Geudens N, et al. Macrolides inhibit IL17-induced IL8 and 8-isoprostane release from human airway smooth muscle cells. Am J Transpl 2007;7(1):76–82.

29. Tikkanen JM, Singer LG, Kim SJ, et al. De Novo DQ donor-specific antibodies are associated with chronic lung allograft dysfunction after lung transplantation. Am J Respir Crit Care Med 2016;194(5):596–606.

30. Levine DJ, Glanville AR, Aboyoun C, et al. Antibody-mediated rejection of the lung: a consensus report of the International Society for Heart and Lung Transplantation. J Heart Lung Transpl 2016;35(4):397–406.

31. Roux A, Le Lan I, Holifanjaniaina S, et al. Antibody-mediated rejection in lung transplantation: clinical outcomes and donor-specific antibody characteristics. Am J Transpl 2016;16(4):1216–28.

32. Valenzuela NM, Reed EF. Antibodies in transplantation: the effects of HLA and non-HLA antibody binding and mechanisms of injury. Methods Mol Biol 2013;1034:41–70.

33. Calabrese DR, Lanier LL, Greenland JR. Natural killer cells in lung transplantation. Thorax 2019;74(4):397–404.

34. Paul P, Pedini P, Lyonnet L, et al. FCGR3A and FCGR2A genotypes differentially impact allograft rejection and patients' survival after lung transplant. Front Immunol 2019;10:1208.

35. Reznik SI, Jaramillo A, Zhang L, et al. Anti-HLA antibody binding to hla class I molecules induces proliferation of airway epithelial cells: a potential mechanism for bronchiolitis obliterans syndrome. J Thorac Cardiovasc Surg 2000;119(1):39–45.

36. Hachem RR, Yusen RD, Meyers BF, et al. Anti-human leukocyte antigen antibodies and preemptive antibody-directed therapy after lung transplantation. J Heart Lung Transpl 2010;29(9):973–80.

37. Islam AK, Sinha N, DeVos JM, et al. Early clearance vs persistence of de novo donor-specific antibodies following lung transplantation. Clin Transpl 2017;31(8):10.

38. Ius F, Sommer W, Tudorache I, et al. Preemptive treatment with therapeutic plasma exchange and rituximab for early donor-specific antibodies after lung transplantation. J Heart Lung Transpl 2015;34(1):50–8.

39. Hachem RR, Tiriveedhi V, Patterson GA, et al. Antibodies to K-alpha 1 tubulin and collagen V are associated with chronic rejection after lung transplantation. Am J Transpl 2012;12(8):2164–71.

40. Kastelijn EA, van Moorsel CH, Ruven HJ, et al. Genetic polymorphisms and bronchiolitis obliterans syndrome after lung transplantation: promising results and recommendations for the future. Transplantation 2012;93(2):127–35.

41. Calabrese DR, Wang P, Chong T, et al. Dectin-1 genetic deficiency predicts chronic lung allograft dysfunction and death. JCI Insight 2019;4(22):e133083.

42. Calabrese DR, Aminian E, Mallavia B, et al. Natural killer cells activated through NKG2D mediate lung

ischemia-reperfusion injury. J Clin Invest 2021; 131(3):e137047.

43. Greenland JR, Sun H, Calabrese D, et al. HLA mismatching favoring host-versus-graft NK cell activity via KIR3DL1 is associated with improved outcomes following lung transplantation. Am J Transpl 2017; 17(8):2192–9.

44. Calabrese DR, Chong T, Wang A, et al. NKG2C natural killer cells in bronchoalveolar lavage are associated with cytomegalovirus viremia and poor outcomes in lung allograft recipients. Transplantation 2019;103(3):493–501.

45. Weigt SS, Copeland CAF, Derhovanessian A, et al. Colonization with small conidia Aspergillus species is associated with bronchiolitis obliterans syndrome: a two-center validation study. Am J Transpl 2013;13(4):919–27.

46. Suzuki Y, Cantu E, Christie JD. Primary graft dysfunction. Semin Respir Crit Care Med 2013; 34(3):305–19.

47. Nawrot TS, Vos R, Jacobs L, et al. The impact of traffic air pollution on bronchiolitis obliterans syndrome and mortality after lung transplantation. Thorax 2011;66(9):748–54.

48. Biswas Roy S, Elnahas S, Serrone R, et al. Early fundoplication is associated with slower decline in lung function after lung transplantation in patients with gastroesophageal reflux disease. J Thorac Cardiovasc Surg 2018;155(6):2762–71.e1.

49. Dugger DT, Fung M, Zlock L, et al. Cystic fibrosis lung transplant recipients have suppressed airway interferon responses during pseudomonas infection. Cell Rep Med 2020;1(4):100055.

50. Khalifah AP, Hachem RR, Chakinala MM, et al. Respiratory viral infections are a distinct risk for bronchiolitis obliterans syndrome and death. Am J Respir Crit Care Med 2004;170(2):181–7.

51. Kelly FL, Kennedy VE, Jain R, et al. Epithelial clara cell injury occurs in bronchiolitis obliterans syndrome after human lung transplantation. Am J Transpl 2012;12(11):3076–84.

52. Liu Z, Liao F, Scozzi D, et al. An obligatory role for club cells in preventing obliterative bronchiolitis in lung transplants. JCI Insight 2019;5(9):e124732.

53. Naikawadi RP, Disayabutr S, Mallavia B, et al. Telomere dysfunction in alveolar epithelial cells causes lung remodeling and fibrosis. JCI Insight 2016; 1(14):e86704.

54. Faust HE, Golden JA, Rajalingam R, et al. Short lung transplant donor telomere length is associated with decreased CLAD-free survival. Thorax 2017; 72(11):1052–4.

55. Peng T, Frank DB, Kadzik RS, et al. Hedgehog actively maintains adult lung quiescence and regulates repair and regeneration. Nature 2015; 526(7574):578–82.

56. Verleden GM, Vanaudenaerde BM, Dupont LJ, et al. Azithromycin reduces airway neutrophilia and interleukin-8 in patients with bronchiolitis obliterans syndrome. Am J Respir Crit Care Med 2006; 174(5):566–70.

57. Meyer KC, Raghu G, Verleden GM, et al. An international ISHLT/ATS/ERS clinical practice guideline: diagnosis and management of bronchiolitis obliterans syndrome. Eur Respir J 2014;44(6): 1479–503.

58. Corris PA, Ryan VA, Small T, et al. A randomised controlled trial of azithromycin therapy in bronchiolitis obliterans syndrome (BOS) post lung transplantation. Thorax 2015;70(5):442–50.

59. Vos R, Vanaudenaerde BM, Verleden SE, et al. A randomised controlled trial of azithromycin to prevent chronic rejection after lung transplantation. Eur Respir J 2011;37(1):164–72.

60. Van Herck A, Frick AE, Schaevers V, et al. Azithromycin and early allograft function after lung transplantation: a randomized, controlled trial. J Heart Lung Transpl 2019;38(3):252–9.

61. Li D, Duan Q, Weinkauf J, et al. Azithromycin prophylaxis after lung transplantation is associated with improved overall survival. J Heart Lung Transpl 2020;39(12):1426–34.

62. Verleden GM, Verleden SE, Vos R, et al. Montelukast for bronchiolitis obliterans syndrome after lung transplantation: a pilot study. Transpl Int 2011;24(7):651–6.

63. Ruttens D, Verleden SE, Demeyer H, et al. Montelukast for bronchiolitis obliterans syndrome after lung transplantation: a randomized controlled trial. PLoS One 2018;13(4):e0193564.

64. Knobler R, Arenberger P, Arun A, et al. European dermatology forum - updated guidelines on the use of extracorporeal photopheresis 2020 - part 1. J Eur Acad Dermatol Venereol 2020;34(12): 2693–716.

65. Jaksch P, Scheed A, Keplinger M, et al. A prospective interventional study on the use of extracorporeal photopheresis in patients with bronchiolitis obliterans syndrome after lung transplantation. J Heart Lung Transpl 2012;31(9):950–7.

66. Lamioni A, Parisi F, Isacchi G, et al. The immunological effects of extracorporeal photopheresis unraveled: induction of tolerogenic dendritic cells in vitro and regulatory T cells in vivo. Transplantation 2005;79(7):846–50.

67. Meloni F, Cascina A, Miserere S, et al. Peripheral CD4(+)CD25(+) TREG cell counts and the response to extracorporeal photopheresis in lung transplant recipients. Transpl Proc 2007;39(1): 213–7.

68. Maeda A, Schwarz A, Kernebeck K, et al. Intravenous infusion of syngeneic apoptotic cells by

photopheresis induces antigen-specific regulatory T cells. J Immunol 2005;174(10):5968–76.

69. Baskaran G, Tiriveedhi V, Ramachandran S, et al. Efficacy of extracorporeal photopheresis in clearance of antibodies to donor-specific and lung-specific antigens in lung transplant recipients. J Heart Lung Transpl 2014;33(9):950–6.

70. Morrell MR, Despotis GJ, Lublin DM, et al. The efficacy of photopheresis for bronchiolitis obliterans syndrome after lung transplantation. J Heart Lung Transpl 2010;29(4):424–31.

71. Vazirani J, Routledge D, Snell GI, et al. Outcomes following extracorporeal photopheresis for chronic lung allograft dysfunction following lung transplantation: a single-center experience. Transpl Proc 2021;53(1):296–302.

72. Hage CA, Klesney-Tait J, Wille K, et al. Extracorporeal photopheresis to attenuate decline in lung function due to refractory obstructive allograft dysfunction. Transfus Med 2021.

73. Greer M, Dierich M, De Wall C, et al. Phenotyping established chronic lung allograft dysfunction predicts extracorporeal photopheresis response in lung transplant patients. Am J Transpl 2013;13(4): 911–8.

74. Knobler R, Arenberger P, Arun A, et al. European dermatology forum: updated guidelines on the use of extracorporeal photopheresis 2020 - Part 2. J Eur Acad Dermatol Venereol 2021;35(1):27–49.

75. Säemann MD, Haidinger M, Hecking M, et al. The multifunctional role of mTOR in innate immunity: implications for transplant immunity. Am J Transpl 2009;9(12):2655–61.

76. de Pablo A, Santos F, Solé A, et al. Recommendations on the use of everolimus in lung transplantation. Transpl Rev (Orlando) 2013;27(1):9–16.

77. Gottlieb J, Neurohr C, Muller-Quernheim J, et al. A randomized trial of everolimus-based quadruple therapy vs standard triple therapy early after lung transplantation. Am J Transpl 2019;19(6):1759–69.

78. Snell GI, Valentine VG, Vitulo P, et al. Everolimus versus azathioprine in maintenance lung transplant recipients: an international, randomized, double-blind clinical trial. Am J Transpl 2006;6(1):169–77.

79. Patrucco F, Allara E, Boffini M, et al. Twelve-month effects of everolimus on renal and lung function in lung transplantation: differences in chronic lung allograft dysfunction phenotypes. Ther Adv Chronic Dis 2021;12. 2040622321993441.

80. Mitruka SN, Won A, McCurry KR, et al. In the lung aerosol cyclosporine provides a regional concentration advantage over intramuscular cyclosporine. J Heart Lung Transpl 2000;19(10):969–75.

81. Iacono AT, Smaldone GC, Keenan RJ, et al. Dose-related reversal of acute lung rejection by aerosolized cyclosporine. Am J Respir Crit Care Med 1997;155(5):1690–8.

82. Iacono A, Wijesinha M, Rajagopal K, et al. A randomised single-centre trial of inhaled liposomal cyclosporine for bronchiolitis obliterans syndrome post-lung transplantation. ERJ Open Res 2019; 5(4):00167-2019–02019.

83. Zhao Y, Su H, Shen X, et al. The immunological function of CD52 and its targeting in organ transplantation. Inflamm Res 2017;66(7):571–8.

84. Furuya Y, Jayarajan SN, Taghavi S, et al. The impact of alemtuzumab and basiliximab induction on patient survival and time to bronchiolitis obliterans syndrome in double lung transplantation recipients. Am J Transpl 2016;16(8):2334–41.

85. Ensor CR, Rihtarchik LC, Morrell MR, et al. Rescue alemtuzumab for refractory acute cellular rejection and bronchiolitis obliterans syndrome after lung transplantation. Clin Transpl 2017;31(4):10.

86. Reams BD, Musselwhite LW, Zaas DW, et al. Alemtuzumab in the treatment of refractory acute rejection and bronchiolitis obliterans syndrome after human lung transplantation. Am J Transpl 2007; 7(12):2802–8.

87. Moniodis A, Townsend K, Rabin A, et al. Comparison of extracorporeal photopheresis and alemtuzumab for the treatment of chronic lung allograft dysfunction. J Heart Lung Transpl 2018;37(3):340–8.

88. Ippoliti G, Lucioni M, Leonardi G, et al. Immunomodulation with rabbit anti-thymocyte globulin in solid organ transplantation. World J Transpl 2015;5(4): 261–6.

89. Kotecha S, Paul E, Ivulich S, et al. Outcomes following ATG therapy for chronic lung allograft dysfunction. Transpl Direct 2021;7(4):e681.

90. Tochner Z, Slavin S. Immune modulation by ionized irradiation. Curr Opin Immunol 1988;1(2):261–8.

91. Lebeer M, Kaes J, Lambrecht M, et al. Total lymphoid irradiation in progressive bronchiolitis obliterans syndrome after lung transplantation: a single-center experience and review of literature. Transpl Int 2020;33(2):216–28.

92. Fisher AJ, Rutherford RM, Bozzino J, et al. The safety and efficacy of total lymphoid irradiation in progressive bronchiolitis obliterans syndrome after lung transplantation. Am J Transpl 2005;5(3): 537–43.

93. Conte E, Gili E, Fagone E, et al. Effect of pirfenidone on proliferation, TGF-beta-induced myofibroblast differentiation and fibrogenic activity of primary human lung fibroblasts. Eur J Pharm Sci 2014;58:13–9.

94. King TE Jr, Bradford WZ, Castro-Bernardini S, et al. A phase 3 trial of pirfenidone in patients with idiopathic pulmonary fibrosis. N Engl J Med 2014; 370(22):2083–92.

95. Vos R, Verleden SE, Ruttens D, et al. Pirfenidone: a potential new therapy for restrictive allograft syndrome? Am J Transpl 2013;13(11):3035–40.

96. Bennett D, Lanzarone N, Fossi A, et al. Pirfenidone in chronic lung allograft dysfunction: a single cohort study. Panminerva Med 2020;62(3):143–9.

97. Vos R, Wuyts WA, Gheysens O, et al. Pirfenidone in restrictive allograft syndrome after lung transplantation: a case series. Am J Transpl 2018;18(12):3045–59.

98. Rangarajan S, Kurundkar A, Kurundkar D, et al. Novel mechanisms for the antifibrotic action of nintedanib. Am J Respir Cell Mol Biol 2016;54(1):51–9.

99. Richeldi L, du Bois RM, Raghu G, et al. Efficacy and safety of nintedanib in idiopathic pulmonary fibrosis. N Engl J Med 2014;370(22):2071–82.

100. Distler O, Highland KB, Gahlemann M, et al. Nintedanib for systemic sclerosis-associated interstitial lung disease. N Engl J Med 2019;380(26):2518–28.

101. Flaherty KR, Wells AU, Cottin V, et al. Nintedanib in progressive fibrosing interstitial lung diseases. N Engl J Med 2019;381(18):1718–27.

102. Yusen RD, Edwards LB, Kucheryavaya AY, et al. The registry of the International Society for Heart and Lung Transplantation: thirty-first adult lung and heart-lung transplant report–2014; focus theme: retransplantation. J Heart Lung Transpl 2014;33(10):1009–24.

103. Verleden SE, Todd JL, Sato M, et al. Impact of CLAD phenotype on survival after lung retransplantation: a multicenter study. Am J Transpl 2015;15(8):2223–30.

104. Levy L, Huszti E, Renaud-Picard B, et al. Risk assessment of chronic lung allograft dysfunction phenotypes: validation and proposed refinement of the 2019 International Society for Heart and Lung Transplantation classification system. J Heart Lung Transpl 2020;39(8):761–70.

105. Dettmer S, Shin HO, Vogel-Claussen J, et al. CT at onset of chronic lung allograft dysfunction in lung transplant patients predicts development of the restrictive phenotype and survival. Eur J Radiol 2017;94:78–84.

106. Suhling H, Dettmer S, Greer M, et al. Phenotyping chronic lung allograft dysfunction using body plethysmography and computed tomography. Am J Transpl 2016.

107. Belloli EA, Degtiar I, Wang X, et al. Parametric response mapping as an imaging biomarker in lung transplant recipients. Am J Respir Crit Care Med 2017;195(7):942–52.

108. Dugger DT, Calabrese DR, Gao Y, et al. Lung allograft epithelium DNA methylation age is associated with graft chronologic age and primary graft dysfunction. Front Immunol 2021;12:704172.

Nonallograft Complications of Lung Transplantation

Tany Thaniyavarn, MD[a],*, Harpreet Singh Grewal, MD[b],
Hilary J. Goldberg, MD, MPH[a], Selim M. Arcasoy, MD, MPH[b]

KEYWORDS

- Lung transplantation • Nonallograft • Complications • Immunosuppression

KEY POINTS

- Nonallograft complications after lung transplantation have a major impact on short- and long-term outcomes.
- Chronic immunosuppression can lead to the exacerbation of existing medical comorbidities or may lead to the development of new medical comorbidities.
- Management of nonallograft complications requires close monitoring and a multidisciplinary team approach.

INTRODUCTION

Calcineurin inhibitors (CNI) are the backbone of modern immunosuppression that enable long-term survival in lung transplant recipients. According to the International Society for Heart and Lung Transplantation (ISHLT) Registry, in 2019 lung transplant recipients had a median survival of 10.2 and 6.5 years following bilateral and single lung transplantation (SLT), respectively, conditional on 1-year survival.[1] Long-term exposure to CNIs and other immunosuppressive agents, especially corticosteroids, may exacerbate preexisting medical conditions or result in new chronic diseases such as diabetes mellitus, hypertension, hyperlipidemia, cardiovascular disease, among others (**Table 1**). Moreover, the risk of malignancy is increased in the setting of long-term immunosuppression. Because polypharmacy is universal in transplant recipients, attention should be focused on drug–drug interactions, medication absorption, and adverse effects in this population. This article will focus on the most common medical disorders with highest impact following lung transplantation including diabetes mellitus, hypertension, hyperlipidemia, acute kidney injury (AKI) and chronic kidney disease (CKD), and malignancy.

Diabetes Mellitus

Epidemiology and risk factors

In lung transplant recipients, the prevalence of posttransplant diabetes mellitus (PTDM) is 20% to 43% in the first year, and approximately 33% to 60% of recipients will develop PTDM by 5 years.[1,2] One caveat to PTDM diagnosis is to distinguish transient hyperglycemia from PTDM. Transient hyperglycemia is common in the initial posttransplant phase as well as after corticosteroid treatment of rejection but is also a risk factor for PTDM. For this reason, the International Consensus Meeting on Posttransplantation Diabetes Mellitus 2013[3] and American Diabetes Association (ADA) Standards of Care 2021[4] have recommended that the diagnosis of PTDM be made in the outpatient setting when the patient is in a stable condition with immunosuppressive

T. Thaniyavarn and H.S. Grewal are Co-first authors.
[a] Brigham and Women's Hospital, Harvard Medical School, 75 Francis Street, PBB Clinic 3, Boston, MA 02115, USA; [b] Lung Transplant Program, Columbia University Irving Medical Center, 622 W 168th Street, PH 14E, Suite 104, New York, NY 10032, USA
* Corresponding author.
E-mail address: tthaniyavarn@bwh.harvard.edu

Thorac Surg Clin 32 (2022) 243–258
https://doi.org/10.1016/j.thorsurg.2022.01.004
1547-4127/22/© 2022 Elsevier Inc. All rights reserved.

Table 1
Nonallograft complications after lung transplantation

Organ System	Complications
Cardiovascular*	Atrial arrhythmia Coronary artery disease Acute pericarditis Hypertension*
Renal*	Acute kidney injury* Chronic kidney disease*
Neurologic	Tremors Seizure Cognitive dysfunction Posterior reversible encephalopathy syndrome (PRES) Stroke Progressive multifocal leukoencephalopathy (PML)
Musculoskeletal	Critical illness myopathy Rhabdomyolysis Avascular necrosis Osteoporosis Frailty
Hematological	Venous thromboembolism Cytopenia Immune hemolysis Thrombotic microangiopathy
Malignancy*	Skin cancer Posttransplant lymphoproliferative disorder Bronchogenic carcinoma Other solid and hematologic malignancies
Gastroesophageal, Intestinal, and Liver	Gastroesophageal reflux disease Gastroparesis Ileus Pneumatosis intestinalis Bowel ischemia and perforation Distal intestinal obstruction syndrome in cystic fibrosis Cholecystitis Diverticulitis Pancreatitis Nodular regenerative hyperplasia of the liver
Metabolic*	Diabetes mellitus* Dyslipidemia* Hypomagnesemia Hyperkalemia Obesity
Miscellaneous	Hyperammonemia Graft-versus-host disease Hypogammaglobulinemia Drug interactions

* indicate the complications that will be reviewed in this article.

therapy tapered to its maintenance level. Diagnostic criteria should be the same as those applied in nontransplant settings. Hemoglobin A1C should be used with caution in the first posttransplant year, especially in the initial posttransplant phase, as anemia can reduce the sensitivity of the test. The gold standard for PTDM diagnosis remains an oral glucose tolerance test. The risk factors for PTDM include both traditional and transplant-related factors as described in **Table 2**.

Prevention

Lifestyle modification (healthy diet, routine moderate-intensity physical activity at least

Table 2
Risk factors for posttransplant diabetes mellitus

Traditional Risk Factors	Transplant-Related Risk Factors
<ul><li>Age 45 or older</li><li>African American, Hispanic, American Indian, Asian American, or Pacific Islander</li><li>Family history of diabetes mellitus and genetic risk factors</li><li>History of gestational diabetes mellitus</li><li>Prediabetes mellitus</li><li>Polycystic ovary syndrome</li><li>Low HDL and/or high triglyceride</li><li>Obesity</li><li>Sedentary lifestyle</li><li>Cigarette smoking</li><li>Western diet</li></ul>	<ul><li>CNIs (Tacrolimus > cyclosporine)</li><li>Posttransplant transient hyperglycemia</li><li>Frequent rejection episodes</li><li>Hypomagnesemia</li><li>Hepatitis C (possible risk factor)</li><li>CMV infection (possible risk factor)</li></ul>

Abbreviations: CMV, cytomegalovirus; CNI, calcineurin inhibitor; HDL, High-density lipoprotein cholesterol.
Data from Refs.[3,4,73–75]

150 min/wk, and use of certified technology-assisted diabetes prevention programs) should be emphasized both before and after transplantation. Early detection of PTDM is key to management, and attention should be focused on patients with known risk factors, especially those with posttransplant hyperglycemia. Fasting glucose testing in combination with hemoglobin A1C level are recommended by the ADA for PTDM screening, though hemoglobin A1C may have lower sensitivity compared with that in the general population.[4]

Management

Irrespective of PTDM risk, the immunosuppressive regimen that leads to the best patient and allograft outcome should be adopted.[3,4] Tacrolimus is associated with higher incidence of PTDM as compared with cyclosporine;[5] however, tacrolimus-based regimens confer less rejection risk.[1] Therefore, one should not substitute tacrolimus with cyclosporine solely because of the increased potential for metabolic complications.

In the setting of acute illness and high corticosteroid dose such as in the early posttransplant phase and during therapy for rejection, insulin is the most reliable treatment of hyperglycemia. Initiation of basal insulin within 3 weeks for posttransplant hyperglycemia may prevent the development of PTDM.[6] ADA 2021 recommends starting insulin therapy for persistent hyperglycemia at a threshold of $\geq$ 180 mg/dL with a target glucose range of 140 to 180 mg/dL for hospitalized patients.[4] When patients are stable on maintenance immunosuppression, lifestyle modifications should be emphasized, and an oral hypoglycemic agent (OHA) can also be used. However, the evidence regarding the efficacy of OHAs in post lung transplant recipients is lacking. Metformin, thiazolidinedione, and dipeptidyl peptidase 4 (DPP-4) inhibitors have been used successfully in small studies.[7,8] Except for thiazolidinediones, which may result in decreased CNI and mTOR inhibitor levels, there is no significant drug–drug interaction between other OHAs and CNI or mTOR inhibitors. The decision to select an appropriate OHA, therefore, should be based on the side effect profile. For instance, metformin use may be limited by renal dysfunction and gastrointestinal side effects in the posttransplant patient. Thiazolidinedione is known to cause fluid retention, which may limit its use. DDP-4 inhibitors are appealing options as they generally have minimal side effects. For patients with atherosclerotic cardiovascular disease (ASCVD) or high ASCVD risk (age $\geq$ 55 years with coronary, carotid, or lower-extremity artery stenosis > 50% or left ventricular hypertrophy), established kidney disease, or heart failure, ADA recommends a sodium–glucose cotransporter 2 inhibitor or glucagon-like peptide 1 receptor agonist with demonstrated cardiovascular benefit as part of the treatment regimen.[4] However, these 2 medication classes may potentiate renal toxicity of CNI and mTOR inhibitors, and caution should be exercised in the transplant recipient population. Given the high prevalence of hypomagnesemia in transplant recipients and its implication on PTDM,[9] magnesium supplementation may be beneficial. Higher doses of magnesium, which can cause diarrhea, may be required to maintain normal or near-normal serum levels. Certain magnesium formulations that have fewer gastrointestinal side effects, such as magnesium glycinate or magnesium lactate, may be most appropriate.

Hypertension

Epidemiology and risk factors

Approximately 50% and 80% of lung transplant recipients are diagnosed with hypertension by year 1 and 5 posttransplant, respectively.[10] Risk factors for hypertension include but are not limited to advanced age, obesity, family history of hypertension, African–American race, high-sodium diet, and physical inactivity. CNIs and corticosteroids are known to cause hypertension.

Prevention

ACC/AHA recommends weight loss in those who are overweight or obese, institution of a heart-healthy diet, increased physical activity, sodium restriction, potassium supplementation in the form of dietary modification, and reduced alcohol consumption for the general population.[11] However, there are several important and unique differences in transplant recipients. Given the significant role of sodium and fluid retention in CNI and corticosteroid-induced hypertension, sodium restriction should be prioritized. Alcohol cessation before transplant is mandated by many programs; however, recipients who may have resumed alcohol consumption should be counseled, and clinicians should inquire about alcohol consumption posttransplant. Hyperkalemia induced by CNI inhibitors, trimethoprim-sulfamethoxazole use, and renal dysfunction often obviates the need for potassium supplementation in transplant recipients.

Management

The approach to the diagnosis of hypertension in transplant patients is similar to that in the general population. However, there is no evidence regarding blood pressure (BP) treatment goals or specific medication use in lung transplant recipients. Goal BP of less than 130/80 mm Hg has been used in kidney transplant recipients as it correlates with prolonged graft survival.[11,12] The pharmacologic management of hypertension in lung transplant recipients depends on the timing of hypertension development, medication side effects, and drug–drug interaction profile.

In the initial postlung transplant phase, fluid overload, development of atrial arrhythmia, and AKI contribute to the choice of pharmacologic agent for management. Fluid overload may result in BP elevation and fluid optimization with loop or thiazide diuretics should be emphasized. Atrial arrhythmia occurs in 30% to 50% of recipients in the immediate postlung transplant phase[13] and beta-blockers are frequently used for management, which often benefit BP control as well. Finally, AKI occurs in 52.5% of patients during this phase[14]; therefore, angiotensin-converting enzyme inhibitors (ACEI) and angiotensin receptor blockers (ARB) should be avoided. Moreover, ACEI may cause anemia through the inhibition of erythropoietin production. Although ACEI and ARB are known to have cardiovascular benefits, especially in the diabetic population, the evidence regarding patient survival is inconclusive in kidney transplant recipients.[15,16]

Dihydropyridine CCBs such as amlodipine exert more potent vasodilatory effects than nondihydropyridine CCBs and are frequently used to treat posttransplant hypertension. These agents counteract the vasoconstrictive effect of the CNI.[17] However, the drug–drug interaction modulated by CYP3A4 of the CCB with commonly prescribed medications for transplant, such as CNIs, statins, and azoles could result in increased toxicity of each medication. Rhabdomyolysis has been reported with such combinations[18] and dose adjustment of CCBs should be considered. Dihydropyridine CCBs and, to a greater degree, nondihydropyridine CCBs, result in increased CNI levels and warrant close monitoring of CNI trough level when deployed. In contrast, this combination could be useful in the rapid metabolizer to reduce the CNI dose required to achieve target levels. Other antihypertensive medications, such as alpha-1 blockers, have been safely used in posttransplant recipients but they should not be used as first-line agents.

Hyperlipidemia

Epidemiology and risk factors

Hyperlipidemia is another common comorbidity after lung transplantation with a prevalence of 26.7% and 58.2% at 1 and 5 years, respectively.[10] Risk factors for hyperlipidemia are similar to those of diabetes and hypertension. Dyslipidemia, which can happen in the absence of elevated total cholesterol levels, should be distinguished from hyperlipidemia. It includes other lipid abnormalities such as low high-density lipoprotein (HDL) cholesterol, elevated very low-density lipoprotein (VLDL), high apolipoprotein B, elevated small dense low-density lipoprotein (LDL) among others. In the study by Reed and colleagues, a decline in HDL was found in 89% of patients with COPD after lung transplantation.[19] However, the incidence of other dyslipidemias in lung transplant recipients is unknown.

Prevention

Hyperlipidemia usually accompanies other transplant-associated comorbidities, especially diabetes and hypertension. Lifestyle modification to prevent or improve those comorbidities could positively affect lipid levels.

Management

Treatment of hyperlipidemia for patients 40 to 75 years of age depends on 10-year ASCVD risk, which is calculated using the ASCVD Risk Estimator.[20] However, lung transplant survival remains the shortest among solid organ transplant cohorts, with conditional median survival of 10.2 years in bilateral lung transplant recipients.[1] Mortality due to cardiovascular disease accounts for 6.8% of deaths in those who are more than 10 years post-lung transplant.[1] Therefore, the benefit of treating hyperlipidemia to prevent ASCVD in lung transplant recipients remains debatable. On the other hand, there is evidence that hyperlipidemia is associated with a faster decline in kidney function after lung transplant.[21] In kidney transplant recipients, a low HDL is linked to increased cardiovascular events and all-cause mortality.[22] For patients 20 to 39 years of age, the initiation of statin therapy is recommended for those with a family history of premature ASCVD and LDL $\geq$ 160 mg/dL. The benefit of statin initiation in those who are older than 75 years is unclear and should be based on competing comorbidities.[23] However, if a patient is already on and tolerating a statin, it is reasonable to continue the therapy. The target lipid levels in patients posttransplant are not established, and American Heart Association/American College of Cardiology (AHA/ACC) guidelines for the general population are usually used.[23]

Regarding hypertriglyceridemia, AHA/ACC recommends initiating statin therapy in those with ASCVD risk $\geq$ 7.5% and modifying the risk factors for and addressing secondary causes of hypertriglyceridemia. Patients with fasting triglycerides $\geq$ 500 mg/dL and especially $\geq$ 1000 mg/dL despite the statin and modification of secondary causes should be started on a very low-fat diet, avoidance of refined carbohydrates and alcohol, omega-3 fatty acid, and if necessary, fibrate to prevent pancreatitis.

Medications used in the treatment of hyperlipidemia usually have drug–drug interactions or interfere with the absorption of the other commonly prescribed medications in the posttransplant setting. Statins are the most frequently used antihyperlipidemic agents and seem to be safe in combination with tacrolimus, but require dose reduction when combined with cyclosporine.[24]

Apart from immunosuppressive medications, dose adjustment needs to be taken into account when combining statins with other medications, especially azoles and CCBs. Patients with high ASCVD risk or diabetes require high-intensity statin therapy with high dose atorvastatin or rosuvastatin. However, this combination can result in major interactions if the patient is taking cyclosporine and, in this situation, other medications may be required to achieve the LDL target. Proprotein convertase subtilisin/kexin type 9 inhibitor, the newest agent for hyperlipidemia is considered very safe and needs no dose adjustment in the transplant patient.[25]

Acute Kidney Injury

Epidemiology and risk factors

Posttransplant AKI is a frequently reported the complication of lung transplantation and has been defined variably as doubling serum creatinine or using classification systems for AKI. Most commonly used classification systems in the lung transplant literature are AKIN (acute kidney injury network); RIFLE (risk, injury, failure, loss of kidney function, and end-stage kidney disease); and KDIGO (kidney disease: Improving global outcomes) criteria.[14,26,27] The incidence of AKI can be as high as 80% and varies widely among studies.[14,28,29] Despite the heterogeneity in the definition of AKI, the outcomes and risk factors reported in lung transplant recipients with AKI have remained consistent.[28–35] Risk factors associated with developing AKI include severity of illness at transplant, hemodynamic decompensation, utilization of cardiopulmonary support, type (single vs double), and duration of surgery (**Box 1**).[28,30–32,36,37] AKI in the immediate posttransplant period is associated with increased hospital length of stay, risk of CKD, duration of mechanical ventilation, and mortality.[31,34,35] Approximately 5% to 8% of recipients with AKI require renal replacement therapy, and this cohort has a nearly 10-fold increased risk of 30-day, and greater than 5-fold increased risk of 1-year mortality when compared with those not requiring renal replacement therapy.[37] Importantly, the meta-analysis by Lertjitabanjong and colleagues showed that the year of the study period did not affect the incidence of posttransplant AKI.[14]

Prevention and management

The above data highlight the importance of identifying patients at risk for developing AKI during the pretransplant phase of care. This can allow for the development of strategies tailored to reduce the risk for posttransplant AKI while ensuring secondary insult prevention. Longitudinally, it is important

Box 1
Risk factors for posttransplant acute kidney injury (AKI)

- High lung allocation score
- Pretransplant pulmonary artery mean pressure greater than 35 mm Hg
- Pretransplant systemic hypertension
- Extracorporeal membrane oxygenation support
- Mechanical ventilation bridge to transplant
- Prolonged mechanical ventilation after transplant
- Intraoperative cardiopulmonary bypass support
- Intra- and postoperative hypotension
- Posttransplant systemic infections
- Exposure to calcineurin inhibitors
- Indications other than COPD for lung transplantation
- Bilateral lung transplantation and redo lung transplantation

Data from Refs.[28,30–32,36,37]

to assess transplant candidacy in patients with baseline renal dysfunction and then reassess renal function regularly in this at-risk population.[28,31,37,38] Glomerular filtration rate (GFR) equations can be inaccurate to assess renal reserve in these patients and may even overestimate renal function in those with poor nutritional status or muscle wasting.[39] Early involvement of nephrology consultants for accurate diagnosis and classification of renal dysfunction, and consideration of renal transplantation in select candidates should be entertained.[40] A modified surgical approach to avoid or minimize the use of intraoperative cardio-pulmonary bypass in those

Box 2
Acute Kidney Injury

- AKI is associated with increased length of stay, risk of CKD, duration of mechanical ventilation, and risk of mortality
- The most common etiology of posttransplant AKI is the prerenal state leading to renal hypoperfusion and acute tubular necrosis
- Identifying modifiable risk factors and adopting strategies to mitigate risk can help reduce the frequency of posttransplant AKI and its adverse consequences

at risk of developing renal failure should be considered. Multidisciplinary engagement with anesthesia and perfusion teams during the surgery to minimize large swings in perfusion pressure can be beneficial. Appropriate fluid and hemodynamic resuscitation strategies to alleviate hemodynamic derangements in all phases of care are essential. The use of alternative immunosuppressive regimens relying on induction therapy may allow delay in the initiation of CNI therapy in patients at particularly high risk for early renal dysfunction. Pharmacy stewardship to ensure the appropriate selection and dosing of medications should be used.[29] Working with a multidisciplinary team to balance fluid status and kidney protective management strategies is also beneficial. Close monitoring of urine output is critical, as it can be the earliest sign of renal dysfunction, and interventions can improve mortality.[41] (**Box 2**)

Chronic Kidney Disease

Epidemiology and risk factors

Like AKI, CKD is a well-established complication after lung transplantation. CKD is defined as structural abnormalities on imaging or decreased function for more than 3 months according to KDIGO guidelines and consists of five stages. According to the most recent Scientific Registry for Transplant Recipients (SRTR) report, CKD with creatinine greater than 2.5 mg/dL, requiring chronic dialysis or renal transplant occurred in 6.2% at 1 year, and that number increased to 17.3% by 5 years.[35] AKI remains the most important risk factor for CKD development.[14,42] Early decline in GFR in the first month after lung transplantation can predict CKD.[42] Further, a biphasic loss of renal function has been reported with rapid loss in the first 6 months after transplantation and a slower decline afterward.[43] The incidence of doubling of serum creatinine as a marker for CKD in the SRTR report was noted to be 34% and 53% at 1 year and 5 years after transplantation, respectively.[26,27] Preoperative hypertension, development of posttransplant hypertension, especially elevated diastolic BP greater than 90 mm Hg, and the use of cyclosporine are risk factors for CKD and end-stage renal disease.[27,44,45]

Prevention and management

The cornerstone of CKD prevention rests on the prevention of AKI and assessing modifiable risk factors. Hypertension is an important contributor to CKD and appropriate management as described in the prior section should be used. Consideration should be given to the avoidance of nephrotoxic medications (ie, nonsteroidal anti-inflammatory agents), adjustment of therapeutic

CNI target levels when feasible, along with a possible transition to alternative immunosuppression strategies such as sirolimus, while balancing the adverse effects and risk of rejection with this strategy.[46,47] Canales and colleagues reported that recipients who survived greater than 6 years after transplant had similar GFR at less than 1 year and greater than 6 years. This association suggests that early renal insults after lung transplantation may have a long-term impact on renal function.[27,47,48] Involving a nephrologist in the management of these patients may be helpful and in select cases with advanced CKD, renal transplantation may be considered (**Box 3**).

Malignancy

Epidemiology and risk factors

Malignancy is the second most common cause of death after bronchiolitis obliterans syndrome in lung transplant recipients who survive more than 5 years, accounting for approximately 17% of deaths.[1] The incidence of malignancy is higher in transplant recipients as compared with that in the general population.[49] Among solid organ transplants, lung transplant recipients have the highest risk for cancer, likely related to the intensity of immunosuppressive therapy.[50] Risk factors for developing posttransplant malignancy include both general and transplant-specific risk factors as summarized in **Table 3**. Various types of malignancy have been reported in lung transplant recipients. We will focus on the most common malignancies in this population, including cutaneous squamous cell carcinoma (SCC), posttransplant lymphoproliferative disorder (PTLD), and lung cancer.[49,50]

There are several mechanisms for postlung transplant cancer development, including new infections and reactivation of oncogenic viruses, mutation burden from ultraviolet light exposure, direct effects of immunosuppression, and rarely donor-derived malignancies. The most important

Table 3
Risk factors for posttransplant malignancy

General Risk Factors	Transplant-Specific Risk Factors

- Advanced age
- Genetic predisposition
- Family history of malignancy
- Personal history of malignancy
- Pretransplant tobacco exposure
- Alcohol use
- Environmental factors such as sun exposure
	- Use of T-cell depleting agent (Muromonab (no longer in use), Alemtuzumab, and ATG) as opposed to non–T-cell depleting agents such as Basiliximab and Daclizumab
	- Immunosuppressive agent (except mTOR inhibitor which may have a protective effect), duration and magnitude
	- Skin cancer
	  ∘ Azathioprine as opposed to Mycophenolate mofetil
	  ∘ Voriconazole use
	- PTLD
	  ∘ EBV D+/R-
	  ∘ White race
	  ∘ Age < 40 y
	  ∘ CMV D+/R-
	  ∘ Any pretransplant malignancy
	  ∘ Recipient with HLA Bw22, B18, or B21
	  ∘ Fewer HLA matches
	- Lung cancer
	  ∘ Single lung transplant (native lung malignancy in IPF and COPD)
	- Transfer of donor malignancy

ATG, Antithymocyte globulin; EBV D+/R-, Epstein–Barr virus donor seropositive/recipient seronegative; CMV D+/R-, Cytomegalovirus donor seropositive/recipient seronegative; COPD, chronic obstructive pulmonary disease; HLA, human leukocyte antigen; IPF, idiopathic pulmonary fibrosis; mTOR, mammalian target of rapamycin; PTLD, posttransplant lymphoproliferative disorder
Data from Refs[49,50,52,58–60]

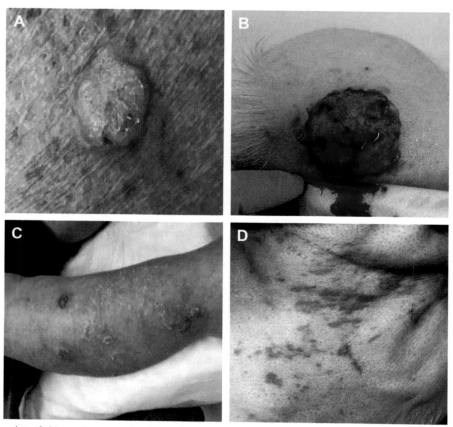

Fig. 1. Examples of skin malignancy. (*A*) Cutaneous SCC on the arm; (*B*) Large bleeding scalp SCC following rapid growth; (*C*) Multifocal pleomorphic dermal sarcoma following panniculitis with multiple ulcerated and bleeding nodules; (*D*) Kaposi's sarcoma involving the chest wall and lung transplant incision site.

risk for posttransplant malignancy is the impairment of antitumor and antiviral T-cell immune surveillance from induction and chronic immunosuppressive therapy.[51]

Skin Cancer

Though usually not fatal, skin cancer is the most common malignancy following solid organ transplantation, including after lung transplantation. The cumulative incidence of skin cancer is 31% at 5 years and 47% at 10 years post-lung transplantation.[52] (**Fig. 1**) SCC and basal cell carcinoma (BCC) account for 95% of all skin cancers.[53,54] Cutaneous SCC and BCC primarily affect the sun-exposed areas. BCC favors face and upper torso and SCC tends to involve arms along with upper torso and face.[54] Melanomas are usually pigmented lesions which can be assessed with the ABCDE (asymmetry, border, color, diameter, and evolution) technique.[55] Among these skin cancers, SCC has the highest incidence and is the most aggressive. Cutaneous SCC in lung

transplant recipients tends to be poorly differentiated and invasive compared with that in the general population.[56] In a study of in-transit metastatic SCC at 2-year follow-up, one-third of transplant recipients had died and one-third had metastatic disease; in comparison, 80% of nonimmunocompromised patients were free of disease at 2 years, and no deaths were observed.[57] The risk of recurrence and metastatic disease in lung transplant recipients after the treatment of cutaneous SCC at 1.5 years can be as high as 14% and 8%, respectively.[56]

Posttransplant Lymphoproliferative Disorder

PTLD affects 1.8% to 9.4% of lung transplant recipients but the incidence may be as high as 20% to 30% in Epstein–Barr virus (EBV)-seronegative recipients who receive lungs from EBV-seropositive donors (EBV D+/R-).[50,58,59] Most PTLD occurs in the first posttransplant year and is most often seen in patients with EBV D+/R- serostatus; 6.2% of those with EBV D+/R-

Table 4
Cancer screening recommendations[a]

Cancer	Condition	Screening Recommendation
Breast	Women 50–74 y	Biennial screening mammography
Cervical	< 21 y	No screening
	21–29 y	Cervical cytology alone every 3 y
	30–65 y	Cervical cytology alone every 3 y or hrHPV testing every 5 y or hrHPV with cervical cytology every 5 y
	> 65 y	No screening
Colorectal	First-degree relative with CRC or advanced polyp at age < 60 y or More than 2 first-degree relatives with CRC or advanced polyp at any age	Colonoscopy at age 40 or 10 y before the youngest affected relative, whichever is earlier
	45–49 y	Colonoscopy may be recommended
	50–75 y	Colonoscopy every 10 y[b]sea
	CF pretransplant	Colonoscopy beginning at age 40 y Rescreen every 5 y Any adenomatous polyp to be rescreened every 3 y
	CF posttransplant	Age ≥ 30 y, colonoscopy within 2 y after transplant unless negative colonoscopy within the past 5 y. Rescreen every 5 y Any adenomatous polyp to be rescreened every 3 y

Abbreviations: CF, cystic fibrosis; CRC, colorectal cancer; hrHPV, High-risk human papillomavirus.
[a] This table does not include special circumstances, such as those with a genetic disorder prone to having malignancy. Certain malignancies such as prostate, liver, ovarian, or pancreatic cancer screening are not recommended in the general population.
[b] Colonoscopy has the highest sensitivity in detecting colorectal cancer and polyps, as well as allowing lesion removal. Therefore, it is preferred over other screening modalities in the preand posttransplant setting.
Data from Refs.[76–79]

serostatus develop PTLD and 60.8% of those who develop PTLD do so within the first posttransplant year.[58] Most of these early PTLDs originate from B-lymphocytes of the recipients, are EBV-related, involve the lung allograft, and respond to reduction in immunosuppression.[50,60] Late PTLD that occurs after 1 year post-lung transplantation can originate from other cells such as T-cell and NK-cell, is more likely to be EBV-negative and may be extrapulmonary as well as disseminated at the time of diagnosis.[50]

Lung Cancer

Postlung transplant lung cancers may develop in the allograft (as donor transmitted or *de novo* malignancy), in the native lung, or may represent recurrence of the recipient's primary lung cancer if lung transplant is performed for this indication. Lung cancer may also be an incidental finding in the explanted lung. Compared with the general population, the incidence of lung cancer is increased by 4.8-fold in lung transplant recipients. Those with SLT experience a 13-fold increase in lung cancer incidence, with most occurring in the native right lung possibly due to the larger size of the right lung.[50,61] The median time to diagnosis is 3.9-years posttransplant.[61]

Prevention and Screening

Pretransplant cancer screening, especially in those with risk factors, is mandatory. ISHLT consensus guidelines for candidate selection recommend at least 5 years of disease-free interval for those with most types of pre-existing malignancy before proceeding with transplantation.[62] However, despite meeting this requirement, the risk of malignancy recurrence should be taken into account, and candidacy should be based on a multidisciplinary decision. On the other hand, a 2-year disease-free interval combined with low predicted risk of cancer recurrence may be reasonable for certain malignancies such as localized prostate cancer or nonmelanoma skin cancer. There is no lung transplant-specific guideline for post transplant cancer screening except for colorectal cancer screening in the cystic fibrosis (CF)

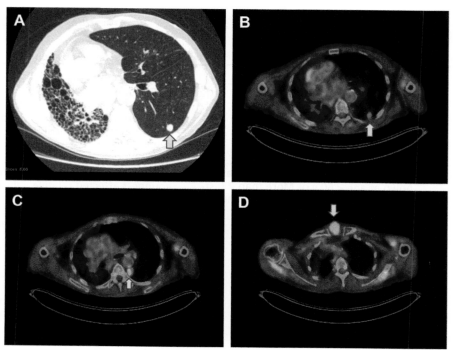

Fig. 2. Metastatic cutaneous SCC. (*A*) CT scan of the chest with a rounded pulmonary nodule in the left lower lobe of the allograft; (*B*) The nodule showing FDG avidity on PET scan; (*C*) An additional FDG avid pulmonary nodule juxtaposed to the descending aorta; (*D*) A large, intensely FDG-avid subcutaneous SCC mass in the suprasternal region.

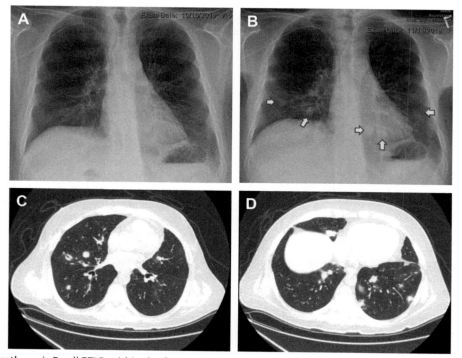

Fig. 3. Intrathoracic B-cell PTLD within the first year of lung transplantation. (*A*) Baseline chest X-ray with no pulmonary nodules; (*B*) Subtle, bilateral pulmonary nodular opacities (yellow *arrows*) observed 4 weeks after the baseline chest X-ray; (*C, D*) Chest CT scan reveals bilateral pulmonary nodules of different shapes and sizes.

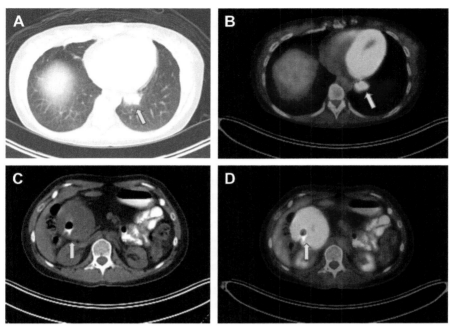

Fig. 4. T-cell PTLD with pulmonary and gastrointestinal involvement leading to the duodenal obstruction 8 years after lung transplant. (*A*) Chest CT scan reveals a left lower lobe paracardiac lung mass; (*B*) PET scan shows FDG avidity of this mass; (*C*) Abdominal CT scan shows a circumferential soft tissue mass around the second portion of the duodenum; (*D*) Duodenal mass reveals intense FDG avidity on PET scan.

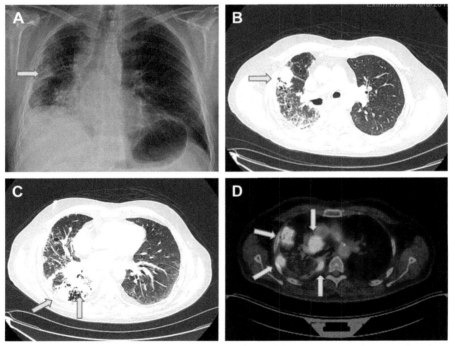

Fig. 5. Nonsmall cell bronchogenic carcinoma in the native lung. (*A*) A new triangular, peripheral opacity in the fibrotic native lung on chest X-ray; (*B*) CT scan of the chest confirms a peripheral mass lesion; (*C*) Additional mass lesions are seen in the right lower lobe centrally and peripherally on the same chest CT; (*D*) PET scan reveals multiple hypermetabolic lung lesions and mediastinal adenopathy.

population (**Table 4**). General guidelines for malignancy screening are usually used. **Table 4** summarizes malignancy screening recommendations that are usually implemented in the pre- and post-lung transplant periods. Many transplant centers perform a yearly chest CT scan for routine allograft evaluation, which also serves as lung cancer screening, especially in those following SLT.

Pretransplant education and screening should be routinely used. For skin cancer risk assessment, a recent Delphi panel recommended risk-stratifying candidates using an evidence-based risk stratification tool and having dermatologists perform full-body examinations in transplant patients.[63] An example of an evidence-based skin cancer screening tool is the Skin and Ultraviolet Neoplasia Transplant Risk Assessment Calculator (SUNTRAC). It has been developed to risk-stratify patients based on race, age, sex, prior history of skin cancer, and type of organ transplant. The SUNTRAC tool classifies patients into 4 tiers ranging from low to very high risk. This type of risk stratification may help clinicians institute skin cancer screening based on the risk of skin cancer development tailored to each patient.[64]

Patients should be advised to use sunscreen with sun protective factor 30 or higher, clothing that covers the body adequately, wearing hats and sunglasses, having a routine self-examination regimen, and seeing a dermatologist at least once a year.[53,54] Regarding PTLD, patients with EBV D+/R-serostatus should have close EBV viral load monitoring. Lower intensity immunosuppression should be considered, when possible, especially in those with EBV viremia. Ganciclovir prophylaxis has been shown to reduce PTLD risk by up to 83%.[65]

Evaluation and Treatment

Skin cancer

In those with a diagnosis of skin cancer, reduction in the intensity of immunosuppression is commonly undertaken but should always be weighed against the risk of graft rejection.[54] When able in precancerous or early noninvasive skin cancers, resection or destructive techniques, such as Mohs procedure, are available for treatment.[54] Other therapies include topical treatments and systemic therapies. A multi-disciplinary approach with early involvement of dermatology, oncology, and surgery specialists when indicated and close monitoring should be used to ensure optimal outcomes. Patients should be monitored for recurrent or metastatic disease (**Fig. 2**).

Posttransplant lymphoproliferative disorder

PTLD has a variable presentation. Nonspecific constitutional symptoms include fever, fatigue, and weight loss. Single or multiple pulmonary nodules, masses, or lobar consolidation and pleural effusions may be observed with intrathoracic PTLD.[54] (**Fig. 3**) Other signs and symptoms depend on the particular organ involved; examples include new cough with pulmonary involvement, constipation with abdominal pain in gastrointestinal PTLD, altered mentation or focal neurologic findings with central nervous system disease, or urosepsis with bladder PTLD.[54,66] (**Fig. 4**) General approach to the management of PTLD includes a careful reduction in immunosuppression, typically by stopping cell cycle inhibitors, anti-B cell therapy with Rituximab, chemotherapy, and radiation.[67,68] Effective treatment of PTLD requires the close collaboration of transplant and oncology teams.[54]

Lung cancer

Broadly, lung cancer is separated into small cell and nonsmall cell carcinoma. Both types can present with constitutional symptoms such as anorexia, fatigue and weight loss, or with pulmonary symptoms including new-onset cough, dyspnea, chest pain, or rarely hemoptysis. The presentation may also be asymptomatic with incidental finding of lung nodule(s) or lymphadenopathy on routine chest imaging.[54] (**Fig. 5**) Lung cancer commonly progresses rapidly under the influence of immunosuppression, and this rapid progression may at times mimic infection.[69,70] Diagnostic and staging strategies remain the same as in the nontransplant population but may be limited due to nodal resection at the time of transplantation.[54] Curative resection should be attempted when possible.[54] Chemotherapeutic options are limited by recipient comorbidities and in the case of immune checkpoint inhibitors, increased risk of rejection.[50,54] Reduction in immunosuppression as with PTLD and skin cancers is commonly undertaken, although benefits remain unclear.[50,54]

SUMMARY

In summary, although rejection and infection are the main concerns following lung transplantation, there is a multitude of medical complications that may develop and require careful multidisciplinary care. Long-term exposure to immunosuppression may exacerbate existing diseases, lead to the development of new acute and chronic conditions and increase the risk of malignancy. These complications have a negative impact on short- and long-term outcomes independent of lung allograft health.

CLINICS CARE POINTS

- Diagnosis of postlung transplant diabetes mellitus should be made while the patient is in a stable condition and is on maintenance immunosuppressive therapy.[3,4]

- Hemoglobin A1C has reduced sensitivity in the diagnosis of post-lung transplant diabetes mellitus, especially in the first posttransplant year.[3,4]

- Insulin is the main treatment of post-lung transplant hyperglycemia and early initiation could prevent the development of true diabetes mellitus.[4,6]

- Oral antihyperglycemic agent should only be used when the patient is on stable maintenance immunosuppressive therapy.[4]

- Antihypertensive medications are generally safe for posttransplant patients. Choice of the medication mostly depends on other clinical perspectives such as using diuretics in the setting of fluid overload, beta-blocker in the setting of atrial arrhythmia, or dihydropyridine calcium channel blocker to mitigate the vasoconstrictive effect of the CNI.[13,17]

- Calcium channel blockers especially nondihydropyridine may increase the level of the CNIs and its use warrants close monitoring and CNI dose adjustment

- Management of hyperlipidemia in post-lung transplant patients is based on ASCVD risk similar to the general population using the same guidelines recommended by AHA/ACC, though one should pay close attention to avoid drug–drug interactions.[23]

- Initiation of CNI therapy may be delayed relying on induction therapy in lung transplant recipients with development of AKI after lung transplantation.[28,46]

- Pharmacy stewardship will ensure appropriate dosing of peri and posttransplant medication dosing.[29]

- Close monitoring of urine output is critical as it can be the earliest sign of renal dysfunction and can alert the medical team to modify management strategies early.[28,37,41,71]

- Early renal insults after lung transplantation can impact long-term renal function.[27,47,48]

- Malignancy is the second most common cause of death after bronchiolitis obliterans syndrome in lung transplant recipients who survive more than 5 years.[1]

- Skin cancer especially squamous cell carcinoma is the most common cancer in the post-lung transplant recipient.[52]

- Most posttransplant lymphoproliferative disorders occur in the first posttransplant year in EBV-seronegative patients who receive lungs from EBV-seropositive donor.[58]

- Colonoscopy is recommended to begin at age 40 for patients with cystic fibrosis pretransplant and at the age of 30 within 2 years of surgery posttransplant.[72]

- Education about malignancy risk, preventive strategies and screening of malignancies using evidence -based guidelines and tools such as the SUNTRAC calculator should be routinely utilized in all phases of transplant care.[53,54,62,63]

DISCLOSURE

None of the author have any commercial or financial conflicts of interest or funding associated with this project.

REFERENCES

1. Chambers DC, Cherikh WS, Harhay MO. The international thoracic organ transplant registry of the international society for heart and lung transplantation: thirty-sixth adult lung and heart-lung transplantation report – 2019; focus theme: donor and recipient size match. J Heart Lung Transplant 2019;38(10):1042–55.

2. Hackman KL, Snell GI, Back LA. Prevalence and predictors of diabetes after lung transplantation: a prospective, longitudinal study. Diabetes Care 2014;37(11):2919–25.

3. Sharif A, Hecking M, Vries APJ. Proceedings from an international consensus meeting on posttransplantation diabetes mellitus: recommendations and future directions. Am J Transplant 2014;14(9):1992–2000.

4. Classification and Diagnosis of Diabetes. Standards of Medical Care in Diabetes—2021. Diabetes Care 2021;44:S15–33.

5. Vincenti F, Friman S, Scheuermann E. Results of an international, randomized trial comparing glucose metabolism disorders and outcome with cyclosporine versus tacrolimus. Am J Transplant 2007;7(6). 1606-1514.

6. Hecking M, Haidinger M, Döller D. Early basal insulin therapy decreases new-onset diabetes after renal transplantation. J Am Soc Nephrol 2012;23(4):739–49.

7. Kurian B, Joshi R, Helmuth A. Effectiveness and long-term safety of thiazolidinediones and metformin

in renal transplant recipients. Endocr Pract 2008; 14(8):979–84.

8. Halden TAS, Åsberg A, Vik K. Short-term efficacy and safety of sitagliptin treatment in long-term stable renal recipients with new-onset diabetes after transplantation. Nephrol Dial Transplant 2014;29(4): 926–33.

9. Peled Y, Ram E, Lavee J. Hypomagnesemia is associated with new-onset diabetes mellitus following heart transplantation. Cardiovasc Diabetol 2019; 18(1):132.

10. Yusen RD, Edwards LB, Dipchand AI. The registry of the international society for heart and lung transplantation: thirty-third adult lung and heart-lung transplant report – 2016; focus theme: primary diagnostic indications for transplant. J Heart Lung Transplant 2016;35(10):1170–84.

11. Whelton PK, Carey RM, Aronow WS. ACC/AHA/ AAPA/ABC/ACPM/AGS/APhA/ASH/ASPC/NMA/ PCNA guideline for the prevention, detection, evaluation, and management of high blood pressure in adults: executive summary: a report of the american college of cardiology/american heart association task force on clinical practice guidelines. Hypertension 2017;71(6):1269–324.

12. Weir MR, Burgess ED, Cooper JE. Assessment and management of hypertension in transplant patients. J Am Soc Nephrol 2015;26. Published online June.

13. Fan J, K Z, S L. Incidence, risk factors and prognosis of postoperative atrial arrhythmias after lung transplantation: a systematic review and meta-analysis. Interact Cardiovasc Thorac Surg 2016;23(5): 790–9.

14. Lertjitbanjong P, Thongprayoon C, Cheungpasitporn W, et al. Acute kidney injury after lung transplantation: a systematic review and meta-analysis. J Clin Monit 2019;8(10):1713. https://doi.org/10.3390/jcm8101713.

15. Heinze G, Mitterbauer C, Regele H. Angiotensin-converting enzyme inhibitor or angiotensin II type 1 receptor antagonist therapy is associated with prolonged patient and graft survival after renal transplantation. J Am Soc Nephrol 2006;17(3): 889–99.

16. Opelz G, Zeier M, Laux G. No improvement of patient or graft survival in transplant recipients treated with angiotensin-converting enzyme inhibitors or angiotensin II type 1 receptor blockers: a collaborative transplant study report. J Am Soc Nephrol 2006; 17(11):3257–62.

17. Grześk G, Wiciński M, Malinowski B. Calcium blockers inhibit cyclosporine A-induced hyperreactivity of vascular smooth muscle cells. Mol Med Rep 2012;5(6):1469–74.

18. Khan S, Khan I, Novak M. The concomitant use of atorvastatin and amlodipine leading to rhabdomyolysis. Cureus 2018;10(1):e2020.

19. Reed RM, Hashmi S, Eberlein M, et al. Impact of lung transplantation on serum lipids in COPD. Respir Med 2011;105(12):1961–8.

20. Estimator ASCVDR.; 2021. Available at: https://tools. acc.org/ldl/ascvd_risk_estimator/index.html#!/ calulate/estimator/.

21. Stephany BR, Alao B, Budev M. Hyperlipidemia is associated with accelerated chronic kidney disease progression after lung transplantation. Am J Transplant 2007;7(11):2553–60.

22. Barn K, Laftavi M, Pierce D. Low levels of high-density lipoprotein cholesterol: an independent risk factor for late adverse cardiovascular events in renal transplant recipients. Transpl Int 2010;23(6):574–9.

23. Grundy SM, Stone NJ, Bailey AL. AHA/ACC/ AACVPR/AAPA/ABC/ACPM/ADA/AGS/APhA/ASPC/ NLA/PCNA guideline on the management of blood cholesterol: executive summary. Circulation 2018; 139(25):1082–143.

24. Migliozzi DR, Asal NJ. Clinical controversy in transplantation: tacrolimus versus cyclosporine in statin drug interactions. Ann Pharmacother 2020;54(2): 171–7.

25. Uyanik-Uenal K, Stoegerer-Lanzenberger M, Auersperg K. Treatment of Therapy-resistant hyperlipidemia after heart transplant with PCSK9-inhibitors. J Heart Lung Transplant 2019;38(4):S213–4.

26. Hingorani S. Chronic kidney disease after liver, cardiac, lung, heart–lung, and hematopoietic stem cell transplant. Pediatr Nephrol 2008;23(6):879–88.

27. Ishani A, Erturk S, Hertz MI, et al. Predictors of renal function following lung or heart-lung transplantation. Kidney Int 2002;61(6):2228–34.

28. Puttarajappa CM, Bernardo JF, Kellum JA. Renal complications following lung transplantation and heart transplantation. Crit Care Clin 2019;35(1):61–73.

29. Du WW, Wang XX, Zhang D, et al. Retrospective analysis on incidence and risk factors of early onset acute kidney injury after lung transplantation and its association with mortality. Ren Fail 2021;43(1): 535–42.

30. Xue J, Wang L, Chen CM, et al. Acute kidney injury influences mortality in lung transplantation. Ren Fail 2014;36(4):541–5.

31. Rocha PN, Rocha AT, Palmer SM, et al. Acute renal failure after lung transplantation: incidence, predictors and impact on perioperative morbidity and mortality. Am J Transplant 2005;5(6):1469–76.

32. Jacques F, El-Hamamsy I, Fortier A, et al. Acute renal failure following lung transplantation: risk factors, mortality, and long-term consequences. Eur J Cardio-Thoracic Surg 2011. https://doi.org/10.1016/ j.ejcts.2011.04.034.

33. Logan AT, Casale JP, Doligalski CT. Early acute kidney injury in lung transplantation is associated with significant mortality. The J Heart Lung Transplant 2016;35(4):S235.

34. Fidalgo P, Ahmed M, Meyer SR, et al. Incidence and outcomes of acute kidney injury following orthotopic lung transplantation: a population-based cohort study. Nephrol Dial Transplant 2014;29(9):1702–9. https://doi.org/10.1093/ndt/gfu226.

35. Valapour M, Lehr CJ, Skeans MA, et al. OPTN/SRTR 2019 Annual data report: lung. Am J Transplant 2021;21(S2):441–520.

36. Atchade E, Barour S, Tran-Dinh A, et al. Acute kidney injury after lung transplantation: perioperative risk factors and outcome. Transplant Proc 2020; 52(3):967–76.

37. Banga A, Mohanka M, Mullins J, et al. Characteristics and outcomes among patients with need for early dialysis after lung transplantation surgery. Clin Transplant 2017;31(11):e13106. https://doi.org/10.1111/ctr.13106.

38. Osho AA, Castleberry AW, Snyder LD, et al. Assessment of different threshold preoperative glomerular filtration rates as markers of outcomes in lung transplantation. The Ann Thorac Surg 2014;98(1):283–90.

39. Barraclough K, Menahem S, Bailey M, et al. Predictors of decline in renal function after lung transplantation. J Heart Lung Transplant 2006;25(12):1431–5.

40. Yerokun BA, Mulvihill MS, Osho AA, et al. Simultaneous or sequential lung-kidney transplantation confer superior survival in renal-failure patients undergoing lung transplantation: a national analysis. J Heart Lung Transplant 2017;36(4):S95.

41. Jin K, Murugan R, Sileanu FE, et al. Intensive monitoring of urine output is associated with increased detection of acute kidney injury and improved outcomes. Chest 2017;152(5):972–9.

42. Wehbe E, Brock R, Budev M, et al. Short-term and long-term outcomes of acute kidney injury after lung transplantation. J Heart Lung Transplant 2012; 31(3):244–51.

43. Pattison JM, Petersen J, Kuo P, et al. The incidence of renal failure in one hundred consecutive heart-lung transplant recipients. Am J Kidney Dis 1995; 26(4):643–8.

44. Kunst H, Thompson D, Hodson M. Hypertension as a marker for later development of end-stage renal failure after lung and heart-lung transplantation: a cohort study. J Heart Lung Transplant 2004;23(10): 1182–8.

45. Esposito C, De Mauri A, Vitulo P, et al. Risk factors for chronic renal dysfunction in lung transplant recipients. Transplantation 2007;84(12):1701–3.

46. Naesens M, Kuypers DRJ, Sarwal M. Calcineurin inhibitor nephrotoxicity. Clin J Am Soc Nephrol 2009; 4(2):481–508.

47. Ivulich S, Westall G, Dooley M, et al. The evolution of lung transplant immunosuppression. Drugs 2018; 78(10):965–82.

48. Canales M, Youssef P, Spong R, et al. Predictors of chronic kidney disease in long-term survivors of lung and heart-lung transplantation. Am J Transplant 2006;6(9):2157–63.

49. Engels EA, Pfeiffer RM, Fraumeni JF. Spectrum of cancer risk among U.S. solid organ transplant recipients: The transplant cancer match study. J Am Med Assoc 2011;306(17):1891–901.

50. Shtraichman O, Ahya VN. Malignancy after lung transplantation. Ann Transl Med 2020;8(6):416. https://doi.org/10.21037/atm.2020.02.126.

51. Cangemi M, Montico B, Faè DA. Dissecting the multiplicity of immune effects of immunosuppressive drugs to better predict the risk of de novo malignancies in solid organ transplant patients. Front Oncol 2019;9. Published online March.

52. Rashtak S, Dierkhising RA, Kremers WK. Incidence and risk factors for skin cancer following lung transplantation. J Am Acad Dermatol 2015;72(1):92–8.

53. Tejwani V, Deshwal H, Ho B, et al. Cutaneous complications in recipients of lung transplants. Chest 2019;155(1):178–93.

54. Benvenuto L, Aversa M, Arcasoy SM. Malignancy following lung transplantation. In: Reference module in biomedical sciences. Elsevier; 2021. https://doi.org/10.1016/B978-0-08-102723-3.00120-7. B9780081027233001000.

55. Abbasi NR, Shaw HM, Rigel DS, et al. Early diagnosis of cutaneous melanoma: revisiting the ABCD criteria. J Am Med Assoc 2004;292(22):2771–6.

56. Mittal A, Colegio OR. Skin cancers in organ transplant recipients. Am J Transplant 2017;17(10): 2509–30.

57. Carucci JA, Martinez JC, Zeitouni NC, et al. In-Transit metastasis from primary cutaneous squamous cell carcinoma in organ transplant recipients and nonimmunosuppressed patients: clinical characteristics, management, and outcome in a series of 21 patients. Dermatol Surg 2004;30(4p2):651–5.

58. Courtwright AM, Burkett P, Divo M. Posttransplant lymphoproliferative disorders in epstein-barr virus donor positive/recipient negative lung transplant recipients. Ann Thorac Surg 2018;105(2):441–7.

59. Cheng J, Moore CA, Iasella CJ. Systematic review and meta-analysis of post-transplant lymphoproliferative disorder in lung transplant recipients. Clin Transplant 2018;32(5):e13235.

60. Neuringer IP. posttransplant lymphoproliferative disease after lung transplantation. Clin Dev Immunol 2013;2013:1–11.

61. Triplette M, Crothers K, Mahale P. Risk of lung cancer in lung transplant recipients in the United States. Am J Transplant 2019;19(5):1478–90.

62. Weill D, Benden C, Corris PA, et al. A consensus document for the selection of lung transplant candidates: 2014—an update from the pulmonary transplantation council of the international society for heart and lung Transplantation. J Heart Lung Transplant 2015;34(1):1–15.

63. Crow LD, Jambusaria-Pahlajani A, Chung CL, et al. Initial skin cancer screening for solid organ transplant recipients in the United States: Delphi method development of expert consensus guidelines. Transpl Int 2019;32(12):1268–76.

64. Jambusaria-Pahlajani A, Crow LD, Lowenstein S, et al. Predicting skin cancer in organ transplant recipients: development of the SUNTRAC screening tool using data from a multicenter cohort study. Transpl Int 2019;32(12):1259–67.

65. Funch DP, Walker AM, Schneider G. Ganciclovir and acyclovir reduce the risk of post-transplant lymphoproliferative disorder in renal transplant recipients. Am J Transplant 2005;5(12):2894–900.

66. Grewal HS, Lane C, Highland KB, et al. Post-transplant lymphoproliferative disorder of the bladder in a lung transplant recipient. Oxford Med Case Rep 2018;2018(3).

67. Trappe R, Oertel S, Leblond V, et al. Sequential treatment with rituximab followed by CHOP chemotherapy in adult B-cell post-transplant lymphoproliferative disorder (PTLD): the prospective international multicentre phase 2 PTLD-1 trial. Lancet Oncol 2012;13(2):196–206.

68. Choquet S. Efficacy and safety of rituximab in B-cell post-transplantation lymphoproliferative disorders: results of a prospective multicenter phase 2 study. Blood 2006;107(8):3053–7.

69. Arcasoy SM, Hersh C, Christie JD, et al. Bronchogenic carcinoma complicating lung transplantation. J Heart Lung Transplant 2001;20(10):1044–53.

70. Grewal AS, Padera RF, Boukedes S, et al. Prevalence and outcome of lung cancer in lung transplant recipients. Respir Med 2015;109(3):427–33.

71. Ollech JE, Kramer MR, Peled N. Post-transplant diabetes mellitus in lung transplant recipients: incidence and risk factors. Eur J Cardiothorac Surg 2008;33(5):844–8.

72. Maldonado F, Tapia G, Ardiles L. Early hyperglycemia: a risk factor for posttransplant diabetes mellitus among renal transplant recipients. Transplant Proc 2009;41(6):2664–7.

73. Hjelmesæth J, Sagedal S, Hartmann A. Asymptomatic cytomegalovirus infection is associated with increased risk of new-onset diabetes mellitus and impaired insulin release after renal transplantation. Diabetologia 2004;47(9):1550–6.

74. Shaukat A, Kahi CJ, Burke CA. ACG clinical guidelines: colorectal cancer screening 2021. Am J Gastroenterol 2021;116(3):458–79.

75. Siu AL, USPST Force. Screening for breast cancer: u.s. preventive service task force recommendation statement. Ann Intern Med 2016;164(4):279–96.

76. Curry SJ, Krist AH, Owens DK. Screening for cervical cancer: us preventive service task force recommendation statement. J Am Med Assoc 2018; 320(7):674–86.

77. Bibbins-Domingo K, Grossman DC, Curry SJ. Screening for colorectal cancer: us preventive services task force recommendation statement. J Am Med Assoc 2016;315(23):2564–75.

78. Bennett D, Fossi A, Marchetti L, et al. Postoperative acute kidney injury in lung transplant recipients. Interact Cardiovasc Thorac Surg 2019;28(6):929–35.

79. Hadjiliadis D, Khoruts A, Zauber AG, et al. Cystic fibrosis colorectal cancer screening consensus recommendations. Gastroenterology 2018;154(3):736–45. e14.

Lung Retransplantation

Eriberto Michel, MD[a], Matthew Galen Hartwig, MD, MHS[b],*,
Wiebke Sommer, MD[c]

KEYWORDS

- Lung transplantation • Retransplantation • Redo lung transplant • Chronic lung allograft dysfunction

KEY POINTS

- Acute graft failure, chronic lung allograft dysfunction, and airway complications are the indications for lung retransplantation.
- Careful recipient and donor selection is paramount to achieve satisfactory patient outcomes.
- Minimally invasive surgical techniques are promising but the ultimate goal of conducting a safe operation is of greatest importance.
- Outcomes for lung retransplantation have improved over time and in some recipients are similar to primary lung transplantation.

BACKGROUND

As the first human lung transplant was performed by Hardy and colleagues at the University of Mississippi in 1963 and the initial successful series in the 1980s, the clinical application of lung transplantation for patients suffering from end-stage lung disease continues to grow and expand. Unfortunately, acute graft failure and chronic lung allograft dysfunction (CLAD) remain common and graft failure is the most significant limitation to long-term survival. Lung retransplantation is the only treatment of irreversible lung allograft failure. Initial reports of retransplantation were discouraging as they showed lower survival for patients who underwent early retransplantation and decreased allograft function several years postoperatively.[1,2] Fortunately, more contemporary reports have shown improving outcomes, with increasing demand for lung retransplantation[3] (**Fig 1**).

CLAD is the most common cause of late mortality and indication for retransplantation, which develops in approximately 40% of primary lung allografts within 5 years.[4] Although CLAD is common and the median survival for lung transplantation remains around 6 years, lung retransplantation accounts for only 4% of all lung transplants performed in the current era, with no notable change over the years.[5] This gap in the number of recipients who suffer from CLAD and those that eventually undergo redo lung transplantation likely reflects a complex mixture of candidate, health care system, outcome, and ethical factors.

INDICATIONS FOR LUNG RETRANSPLANTATION

There are 3 main conditions leading to allograft failure in primary lung transplant recipients; acute graft failure secondary to primary graft dysfunction (PGD), CLAD, and postoperative airway complications.[6,7]

Acute Graft Failure

PGD following initial lung transplantation can occur due to extensive ischemia/reperfusion injury. Hyperacute allograft rejection can also occur, albeit infrequently, causing early acute allograft failure. Acute allograft dysfunction is typically self-limited and does not result in graft failure. For this reason, many centers avoid urgent retransplantation, reserving it for exceptional circumstances whereby it can be a life-saving measure.

[a] Division of Cardiac Surgery, Department of Surgery, Massachusetts General Hospital, 55 Fruit Street, Cox 630, Boston, MA 02114, USA; [b] Division of Cardiovascular and Thoracic Surgery, Department of Surgery, Duke University School of Medicine, DUMC 3863, Durham, NC 27710, USA; [c] Department of Cardiac Surgery, University of Heidelberg, Im Neuenheimer Feld 420, 69120 Heidelberg, Germany
* Corresponding author.
E-mail address: matthew.hartwig@duke.edu

Thorac Surg Clin 32 (2022) 259–268
https://doi.org/10.1016/j.thorsurg.2021.12.001

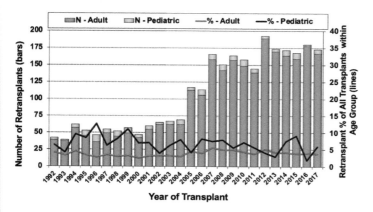

Fig. 1. Adult and pediatric lung retransplants by year and age group. (*From* The International Society for Heart and Lung Transplantation. International Thoracic Organ Transplant (TTX) Registry Data Slides. 2019 Slides: Overall Lung Transplantation Statistics. https://ishlt.org/research-data/registries/ttx-registry/ttx-registry-slides.)

However, early lung retransplantation, regardless of the etiology, has consistently shown poor outcomes with 1-year survival of less than 50%.[7–10] Treatment of severe acute graft failure often is supportive in nature with either prolonged mechanical ventilation, sedation, and/or with extracorporeal membrane oxygenation (ECMO) support. Early retransplantation recipients are at high risk for infectious complications due to prolonged mechanical ventilation, sedation, paralysis and ICU-related procedures, renal failure related to immunosuppression and hemodynamic instability, and other end-organ impairments (eg, ischemic cholangiopathy, bowel ischemia, and so forth). These multitude of factors further increase the risk of subsequent interventions and hence the risk of complications. Likewise, it can be clinically difficult to discern when early allograft failure is irreversible or not, thereby delaying the decision for retransplantation until multiorgan system failure develops. Therefore, many centers avoid urgent retransplantation for acute graft failure outside of exceptional circumstances.

Chronic Lung Allograft Dysfunction

The majority of recipients undergoing pulmonary retransplantation suffer from the chronic rejection of their primary allograft. CLAD can further be divided into obstructive allograft dysfunction (BOS; bronchiolitis obliterans syndrome) and a restrictive phenotype (rCLAD; restrictive allograft syndrome, RAS). The phenotype of CLAD has a significant impact on the course of the disease, as well as prognosis following lung retransplantation, and should be considered in the decision to pursue retransplantation.

CLAD is characterized as a persistent decline in FEV1 (≥20%) from a posttransplant baseline value, which is defined as the mean of the 2 best postoperative measurements. BOS, which affects about 70% of all patients with CLAD, presents with progressive airflow obstruction caused by the fibrous obliteration of the small airways. BOS typically shows no pulmonary opacities in radiologic imaging and the course of the disease varies widely[11,12] (**Fig. 2**). In experienced centers, outcome after lung retransplantation for BOS has been shown to be similar to primary lung transplantation.[7,12]

The RAS presents with persistent radiologic opacities and pleural thickening, a decline in FEV1 and FVC, and a decrease in total lung capacity (**Fig. 3**). During the course of the disease, interstitial reticular shadows, and traction bronchiectasis may develop.[13] Histology of RAS

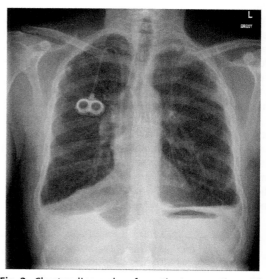

Fig. 2. Chest radiography of a patient presenting with Bronchiolitis Obliterans Syndrome following bilateral lung transplantation. The chest X-ray shows no significant lung field opacities and flattening of the diaphragms suggestive of hyperinflation.

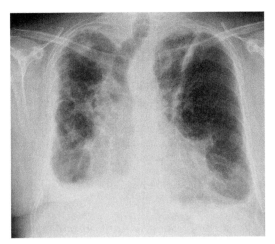

Fig. 3. Chest radiography of a patient presenting with restrictive allograft syndrome (rCLAD) following bilateral lung transplantation. The chest X-ray shows typical pleural thickening, interstitial reticular shadows and tracheal shift.

lungs typically shows pulmonary pleuro-parenchymal fibroelastosis with collagen deposition in the alveolar septal structure.[14] RAS typically shows a more rapid disease progression, with median survival after onset of disease being half of that for patients with BOS.[15] Similarly, survival after lung retransplantation for RAS has been reported to be inferior when compared with retransplantation for BOS.[12]

Multiple reports have shown that a minority of patients develop a mixed form of CLAD with a combined obstructive and restrictive pattern, with or without radiological findings such as parenchymal opacities and/or pleural thickening.[16] For both pure and mixed phenotypes, lung retransplantation remains the only treatment option in patients with advanced CLAD given the absence of reliable pharmacologic therapeutics.[12]

Airway Complications

Complications of bronchial anastomosis following lung transplantation are uncommon, but if severe may require retransplantation when broncho-scopic and conventional surgical therapies fail. The overall incidence of severe airway complications, which include stenosis and dehiscence, differ across centers between 1.5% and 13%.[7,17,18] Overall, the incidence of severe airway complication has decreased over time, most likely due to improved surgical technique and endobronchial therapeutic options. The number of retransplantation for bronchial complications has decreased substantially and shown good mid-

and long-term results in more recent publications.[7,17]

PATIENT EVALUATION AND SELECTION FOR LUNG RETRANSPLANTATION

Patient selection for lung retransplantation is critical to achieve acceptable outcomes and must take into account the perioperative mortality risk. In addition, the ethical dilemma of donor organ scarcity should be considered, requiring a broader perspective from a multidisciplinary team when evaluating patients for lung retransplantation.

In general, patient selection for retransplantation should apply the same criteria as for primary lung transplantation.[19] Therefore, malignancies, severe advanced nonpulmonary diseases, and uncontrolled infections are typically contraindications for lung retransplantation. Special attention should be paid to the patient's overall compliance and adherence to previous medical therapy. The overall clinical status prior to lung retransplantation is an important consideration as patients awaiting retransplantation at home have significantly better outcomes compared with those waiting in the hospital with or without mechanical support.[12] CLAD phenotype is relevant as the determinants for survival following lung retransplantation are different in patients with RAS and BOS. In patients with RAS, lower BMI had a negative impact on survival compared with BOS recipients.[12] In contrast, obese patients (BMI >29.9) requiring retransplantation had lower postoperative survival in a large SRTR registry analysis.[20] Early retransplantation—within the first year—after primary transplantation and the diagnoses of acute rejection and PGD has been associated with poor postoperative survival.[5,6,21–23] Similarly, those requiring preoperative mechanical ventilation and/or extracorporeal support bridge to retransplantation have even worse survival.[3,6,7,24]

While a UNOS registry study of recipients requiring ECMO bridge to lung retransplantation showed an overall increase in the use of extracorporeal support for bridging purposes over time, the 90-day and 1-year survival after ECMO bridge to retransplantation were significantly lower when compared with retransplantation without ECMO bridging. Preoperative high serum bilirubin, ICU stay, mechanical ventilation, and PGD were all associated with higher mortality in the ECMO cohort. Therefore, retransplantation with extracorporeal bridging strategies is associated with significant mortality and must be considered with extreme caution.[20] Further, age, specifically greater than 65 years old, and end-organ dysfunction such as chronic renal failure (GFR <50–60 mL/

min) have been identified as other important independent risk factors for postoperative mortality and reduced 1-year survival.[25,26] Renal function is nearly always impaired in the retransplantation setting due to the ubiquitous use of calcineurin inhibition as standard maintenance immunosuppression. The lung retransplantation procedure type (single vs double) has also been analyzed in multiple publications with mixed results.[6,10,21,22,27,28] Finally, multiple lung retransplantations show particularly poor outcomes.[22,23]

IMMUNOLOGIC ASPECTS OF LUNG RETRANSPLANTATION

Primary lung transplantation represents an immunizing event for the recipient which leads to the existence of alloreactive memory T cells, that may transform into effector T cells on antigen reexposure with the capability of provoking allograft rejection.[29]

Donor Selection

Donor selection in the presence of preformed human leukocyte antigen (HLA) antibodies requires HLA typing of the donor as well as specifications of circulating HLA antibodies to recognize potential donor-specificity.[30,31] A virtual crossmatch using donor HLA typing and recipient's HLA antibody specifications may predict donor–recipient compatibility. Therefore, donor selection for sensitized recipients must be made with full knowledge of the full HLA typing of the donor to avoid a crossmatch positive transplantation. Of note, in the absence of circulating HLA antibodies in the recipient, the selection of a donor that does not have an identical HLA typing as the first lung donor does not seem to impact postoperative outcome. Therefore, such donors need not be avoided during donor:recipient matching.[32]

The Sensitized Recipient

Preexisting circulating HLA antibodies are known to cause hyperacute rejection by binding to mismatched HLA, leading to sudden graft failure very early after or even on the operative table with hemorrhagic lung edema and severe parenchymal infiltrates.[33,34] Therefore, testing for existing HLA antibodies before transplantation is essential for primary transplantation as well as retransplantation. Current diagnostic standards are regular serum screenings using solid-phase assays, which use single antigen beads for the specification of the antibodies. Regular retesting, especially after immunizing events such as blood transfusions, is recommended before

retransplantation.[35] Donor HLA profiles should be selected to avoid preformed donor-specific antibodies in the recipient. Sensitized recipients have a higher risk of developing severe PGD, acute cellular rejection (ACR), and antibody-mediated rejection (AMR) after transplantation with a negative impact on survival.[36–39] Preoperative desensitization protocols including therapeutic plasma exchange, intravenous immunoglobulin (IVIg), and B-cell depleting agents such as rituximab or bortezomib have been used. Unfortunately, postoperative outcomes have not been significantly different between treated and untreated sensitized patients.[40]

De-Novo Donor-Specific Antibodies After Retransplantation

Development of de novo donor-specific HLA antibodies (DSA) after transplantation occurs in 12% to 40% of all recipients, with retransplantation being an independent risk factor for de novo DSA.[41–43] Therefore, regular monitoring of recipients after lung retransplantation for de novo DSA, especially within the first postoperative year is recommended to improve transplant outcomes.[42–44] Given the negative impact of persistent DSA after lung transplantation on CLAD-free survival, multiple centers have published their protocols for the perioperative treatment of sensitized patients, achieving CLAD-free survival similar to recipients without DSA.[41–43,45,46] Importantly, in the absence of DSA, lung retransplantation does not carry a higher risk of acute allograft rejection or developing CLAD.[3,5,7]

SURGICAL TECHNIQUES

Reoperative thoracic transplant surgery is a significant technical undertaking. Adhesive disease manifested as dense pleural thickening, vascular adhesions to the chest wall (**Fig. 4**), significant hemorrhage, and underlying renal dysfunction is only a few of the factors that contribute to this difficult and arduous operation. There are several key issues that must be considered when performing lung retransplantation.

Clamshell Versus Lateral Thoracotomy

Given the technical challenges associated with retransplantation, a generous bilateral trans-thoracosternotomy (clamshell) incision has historically been the incision of choice for many centers. It provides excellent access to bilateral pleural spaces, the pulmonary hila, and the anterior mediastinum. However, the clamshell incision can be associated with pain, prolonged recovery, and

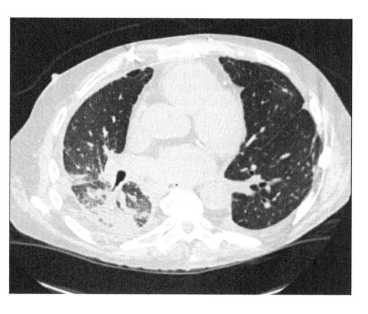

Fig. 4. Computed Tomography scan of lung retransplant candidate who underwent bilateral pleurodesis showing thickened pleura.

potential wound complications. These limitations have driven some centers to adopt alternative approaches.

Bhama and colleagues reported their early experience using a sternal-sparing approach to bilateral lung retransplantation. In this retrospective review of a small patient sample, they showed no significant difference in postoperative outcomes and a trend toward a reduced duration of postoperative mechanical ventilation and length of hospital stay.[47] In a larger series, the Hannover group reported their experience with a minimally invasive protocol for lung retransplantation which included favoring bilateral lung transplantation, avoidance of allograft size reduction, minimally invasive sternum-sparing anterior thoracotomies, avoidance of extracorporeal circulation, avoidance of heparin, and prophylactic coagulation factor transfusion. They showed reduced rates of postoperative dialysis, mechanical ventilation, need for tracheostomy, ICU length of stay and showed superior in-hospital, 30-day, and 1 year survival.[7] Although a less invasive approach to lung retransplantation is attractive for many reasons, ultimately, the safety and exposure of the operation remains paramount. The conduct of the first operation or intervening procedures before the retransplant procedure (eg, surgical pleurodesis for recurrent effusions or decortication for trapped lung) can play a considerable role in the approach and conduct of retransplantation. Anecdotally, any pleural operation following the first transplant makes the retransplant procedure technically more difficult and more likely to require

massive transfusions. Routinely, we often close the superior portion of the pericardium over the aortic cannulation site to void catastrophic reentry hemorrhage. The pericardium is not closed in its entirety to avoid pericardial effusions or pericardial constriction, an uncommon but morbid complication. With regards to the hilum, placing soft tissue, often thymic fat, between the pulmonary artery (PA) and the bronchial anastomoses can facilitate their dissection at the time of retransplantation. Closing the peribronchial soft tissue may also help the separation of the bronchus and PA during retransplantation dissection.

Single Versus Bilateral Orthotopic Lung Retransplant

Over the last 3 decades, there has been a trend toward bilateral primary lung transplantation for nearly all indications.[5] Suppurative lung disease and severe idiopathic pulmonary hypertension have been the classic absolute indications for bilateral transplantation in primary recipients. Though the same tenets apply to retransplantation, the use of bilateral or single lung retransplantation has been less clear. In a review of the United Network for Organ Sharing (UNOS) registry between 2005 and 2013, Shumer and colleagues identified 410 patients who underwent lung retransplantation. They observed no significant difference in survival between retransplant recipients regardless of their initial transplant or retransplant type and they concluded that single lung retransplants should be performed regardless of previous transplant type in an effort to maximize limited organ resources.[28] In another UNOS study, Kon and colleagues reviewed outcomes for 325 patients who had undergone lung retransplantation after single lung transplant. They found that ipsilateral single lung retransplantation carried an increased risk of early and midterm mortality when compared with contralateral and bilateral lung retransplantation. In fact, contralateral and bilateral lung retransplantation had comparable survival to initial lung transplantation at 30 days and 1 year.[48] These findings should not be surprising, in that the decision to perform an ipsilateral retransplant suggests a bias toward avoiding the contralateral side for reasons that cannot be gathered from national registries. The Duke group has previously published their experience with staged bilateral transplant in patients with interstitial lung disease who were deemed to have higher surgical risk.[49] This included patients over the age of 65, those with significant coronary artery disease, and patients demonstrating diminished functional status. The patients underwent single lung transplantation, reevaluated after a period of recovery, relisted for their native lung disease subsequently underwent contralateral single lung transplant. These patients were found to have comparable short-term survival and pulmonary function test at 1 year with decreased incidence of renal injury. A contralateral single transplant after a previous single lung transplant for native lung disease (ie, a "staged bilateral lung transplant") should not be misconstrued as a retransplantation that is performed for allograft failure.

Our practice has been to preferentially perform bilateral retransplantation in patients who previously received a bilateral transplant. For patients who previously received a single lung transplant the answer is more nuanced. For example, for patients who underwent a single primary lung transplant instead of bilateral because of a "hostile" contralateral hemithorax, our choice would be to perform an ipsilateral single lung retransplant. In patients who received a single lung transplant due to frailty, acute exacerbation of their chronic illness, and otherwise have an anatomically adequate contralateral hemithorax, we would proceed with contralateral single lung retransplantation. Rarely have we performed a bilateral lung retransplant in a patient with a previous single lung transplant; however, this may be necessary depending on the microbiologic environs of the recipient and other considerations. Each case requires careful review and scrutiny to maximize the opportunity for a successful outcome.

Extracorporeal Circulation

The use of extracorporeal circulation for lung transplantation has evolved over time. Cardiopulmonary bypass (CPB) was the early mainstay for support of intraoperative hemodynamics and respiratory function during lung transplantation. However, the use of CPB is associated with higher transfusion requirements and increased systemic inflammatory response associated with higher rates of PGD. While many programs opt to perform lung transplantation "off pump," an increasing number of centers are now routinely using intraoperative ECMO which has been shown to be safe and effective with a reduction in PGD, transfusion requirements and postoperative end-organ dysfunction.[50,51] Furthermore, if the patient requires postoperative support, ECMO can be easily reconfigured and continued in the ICU.[51]

There is a paucity of data on the use of intraoperative extracorporeal support for lung retransplantation. Wallinder and colleagues reported similar rates of extracorporeal circulation use during primary procedures and retransplants. However, most of their cases were performed without circulatory support.[21] As extracorporeal circulation generally requires systemic anticoagulation, the increased risk of bleeding must be weighed against the need for cardiopulmonary support. The risk for inadvertent injury to the PA or pulmonary veins during dissection is higher during retransplantation and may require mechanical support in the form of CPB. Otherwise, staying off mechanical support can often be advantageous during the pleural dissection to minimize blood loss from vascular adhesions.

Hematological Management

Perioperative hematological management is of utmost importance in the setting of lung retransplantation. Given the technical challenges of this tour-de-force operation, it is not surprising that lung retransplantation is associated with higher transfusion requirements.[52,53] As increased transfusion rate has been associated with higher incidence of PGD and lower survival, efforts to reduce transfusions in this patient population are imperative.[52-56] However, high-quality data regarding the impact of transfusion on lung transplant outcomes are lacking. In a systematic review of blood transfusion and outcomes in lung transplantation, Klapper and colleagues highlighted the need for transplant programs to develop algorithmic approaches to perioperative hematological management in lung transplant recipients.[57]

Smith and colleagues showed that implementing a point of care rotational thromboelastometry

(ROTEM) and protocolized bleeding management led to significantly decreased transfusion of packed red blood cells, fresh frozen plasma, and platelets.[58] Another promising avenue to decrease the perioperative transfusion requirement is the use of recombinant and reconstituted factor concentrates.[59] These treatments also avoid the volume load that is associated with the use of traditional products.

POSTOPERATIVE MANAGEMENT AND OTHER IMPORTANT CONSIDERATIONS

The postoperative management of primary and retransplantation is effectively the same with some important differences.

The "Open" Chest

The partial closure of the surgical incision or "leaving the chest open" with a temporary sterile dressing is important adjuncts in challenging lung transplantation operations, which do not uncommonly include retransplantation. Though our goal is to definitively close the surgical incision, the higher likelihood of hemorrhage, donor–recipient size mismatch, and higher rates of PGD requiring the continuation of extracorporeal support, occasionally it may be safer to leave the chest open at the end of the initial operation. In cases of continuation of central cannulation for venoarterial ECMO or significant coagulopathic hemorrhage requiring ongoing resuscitation our practice is to not "over pack" the chest but achieve the primary goal of hemostasis. We then suture in place a temporary dressing made of tailored Esmarch bandage and Ioban drapes. The chest is reexplored and dressing is changed every 24 to 48 hours until the hemorrhage is controlled or extracorporeal circulation support can be weaned and definitive closure is appropriate.

Donor – Recipient Size Match

Another important consideration is the relatively fixed nature of the thoracic cavity in redo operations due to scar tissue. Careful attention should be paid to size matching with an emphasis on avoiding significant oversizing. The restrictive physiology of a fixed and rigid thoracic cavity in combination with donor lung oversizing and the overall decrease in compliance that is commonly seen during and immediately after lung transplantation can lead to significant respiratory difficulty. This is another situation in which leaving the chest temporarily open can be beneficial, with an addition of a temporary "strut" allowing for additional thoracic cavity dimension. The critical care and

nursing teams must be diligent in monitoring the integrity of the dressing and paying close attention to pressure sores, given the patients obligate supine bed rest.

LONG-TERM RESULTS
Survival

Historically, retransplantation has shown inferior results as compared with primary lung transplantation with the highest mortality occurring within the first year. Registry data from 1992 to 2017 show a 1-year survival for recipients of lung retransplantation of 69.8%, whereas primary transplants in the same time frame have a 1-year survival of 89.9%. Similarly, the 5-year survival for retransplantation is 41.9% compared with 56.4% for primary transplantation.[60]

However, when looking at the underlying diagnosis for retransplantation, recipients with CLAD at experienced centers show a similar survival to the primary transplantation, with 1-year survival greater than 85%.[7,10,61] In contrast, recipients receiving a second lung transplantation early after primary lung transplantation for severe PGD show a significantly worse outcome, with multiple publications reporting a 1-year survival between 38% and 44%.[7,25,27]

The phenotype of CLAD also impacts postoperative survival. One-year survival for patients with RAS after retransplantation has been significantly lower than for BOS patients, 59% versus 84%, respectively.[12] There is no significant difference in the main causes of death within the first year after lung retransplantation, with graft failure and infectious complications reported as the main reasons for patient death.[62] After the first postoperative year, chronic allograft rejection represents the major cause of death, similar to patients after primary transplantation.[62]

Chronic Lung Allograft Dysfunction After Lung Retransplantation

Chronic rejection occurs after the first year following lung retransplantation, with the majority being diagnosed with CLAD between postoperative years 3 and 5. Median CLAD-free survival for contemporary lung retransplant cohorts ranges between 59 and 63 months, which is similar to primary transplants.[7,62] However, the phenotype of CLAD also impacts the postoperative CLAD-free survival, patients with RAS developing earlier and more frequent chronic allograft dysfunction after retransplantation. A multi-center study reported a CLAD-free survival of 51% for patients with RAS at 3 years after retransplantation, whereas

CLAD-free survival in patients with BOS was 69% at the same time point.[12]

SUMMARY

Lung retransplantation remains the standard treatment of irreversible lung allograft failure. Though early experience showed near prohibitive outcomes, improvements in patient selection, surgical technique, intraoperative and perioperative management, as well as the use of safe adjuncts, such as ECMO and thromboelastogram informed transfusion management, have made it a viable and important therapy for patients and programs.

CLINICS CARE POINTS

- Acute graft failure, chronic lung allograft dysfunction, and air complications are the most important indications for lung retransplantation.
- Careful recipient and donor selection is paramount in achieving satisfactory patient outcomes.
- Minimally invasive surgical techniques are promising in improving patient outcomes
- Postoperative management of primary and lung retransplantation is similar.

DISCLOSURE

EM: No disclosures.
  WS: No disclosures.
  MGH: Intuitive Surgical (consulting and research), Paragonix (consulting and research), BiomedInnovations (consulting and research), Mallinckrodt (research).

REFERENCES

1. Miller JD, Patterson GA. Retransplantation following isolated lung transplantation. Semin Thorac Cardiovasc Surg 1992;4(2):122–5.
2. Novick RJ, Schafers HJ, Stitt L, et al. Seventy-two pulmonary retransplantations for obliterative bronchiolitis: predictors of survival. Ann Thorac Surg 1995;60(1):111–6.
3. Halloran K, Aversa M, Tinckam K, et al. Comprehensive outcomes after lung retransplantation: a single-center review. Clin Transplant 2018;32(6):e13281.
4. Yusen RD, Edwards LB, Kucheryavaya AY, et al. The registry of the international society for heart and lung transplantation: thirty-second official adult lung and heart-lung transplantation report–2015; focus theme: early graft failure. J Heart Lung Transplant 2015;34(10):1264–77.
5. Yusen RD, Edwards LB, Kucheryavaya AY, et al. The registry of the International Society for Heart and Lung Transplantation: thirty-first adult lung and heart-lung transplant report–2014; focus theme: retransplantation. J Heart Lung Transplant 2014; 33(10):1009–24.
6. Kawut SM, Lederer DJ, Keshavjee S, et al. Outcomes after lung retransplantation in the modern era. Am J Respir Crit Care Med 2008;177(1):114–20.
7. Sommer W, Ius F, Kuhn C, et al. Technique and outcomes of less invasive lung retransplantation. Transplantation 2018;102(3):530–7.
8. Harringer W, Wiebe K, Struber M, et al. Lung transplantation–10-year experience. Eur J Cardiothorac Surg 1999;16(5):546–54.
9. Wekerle T, Klepetko W, Wisser W, et al. Lung retransplantation: institutional report on a series of twenty patients. J Heart Lung Transplant 1996;15(2):182–9.
10. Osho AA, Castleberry AW, Snyder LD, et al. Differential outcomes with early and late repeat transplantation in the era of the lung allocation score. Ann Thorac Surg 2014;98(6):1914–20 [discussion 1911–20].
11. Godinas L, Van Raemdonck D, Ceulemans LJ, et al. Lung retransplantation: walking a thin line between hope and false expectations. J Thorac Dis 2019; 11(11):E200–3.
12. Verleden SE, Todd JL, Sato M, et al. Impact of CLAD phenotype on survival after lung retransplantation: a multicenter study. Am J Transplant 2015;15(8): 2223–30.
13. Sato M, Hwang DM, Waddell TK, et al. Progression pattern of restrictive allograft syndrome after lung transplantation. J Heart Lung Transplant 2013; 32(1):23–30.
14. Ofek E, Sato M, Saito T, et al. Restrictive allograft syndrome post lung transplantation is characterized by pleuroparenchymal fibroelastosis. Mod Pathol 2013;26(3):350–6.
15. Sato M, Hirayama S, Matsuda Y, et al. Stromal activation and formation of lymphoid-like stroma in chronic lung allograft dysfunction. Transplantation 2011;91(12):1398–405.
16. Yoshiyasu N, Sato M. Chronic lung allograft dysfunction post-lung transplantation: the era of bronchiolitis obliterans syndrome and restrictive allograft syndrome. World J Transpl 2020;10(5):104–16.
17. Schweiger T, Nenekidis I, Stadler JE, et al. Single running suture technique is associated with low rate of bronchial complications after lung transplantation. J Thorac Cardiovasc Surg 2020;160(4): 1099–108.e3.
18. Moreno P, Alvarez A, Algar FJ, et al. Incidence, management and clinical outcomes of patients with

airway complications following lung transplantation. Eur J Cardiothorac Surg 2008;34(6):1198–205.

19. Orens JB, Estenne M, Arcasoy S, et al. International guidelines for the selection of lung transplant candidates: 2006 update–a consensus report from the Pulmonary Scientific Council of the International Society for Heart and Lung Transplantation. J Heart Lung Transplant 2006;25(7):745–55.

20. Hayanga JW, Aboagye JK, Hayanga HK, et al. Extracorporeal membrane oxygenation as a bridge to lung re-transplantation: Is there a role? J Heart Lung Transplant 2016;35(7):901–5.

21. Wallinder A, Danielsson C, Magnusson J, et al. Outcomes and long-term survival after pulmonary retransplantation: a single-center experience. Ann Thorac Surg 2019;108(4):1037–44.

22. Thomas M, Belli EV, Rawal B, et al. Survival after lung retransplantation in the united states in the current era (2004 to 2013): better or worse? Ann Thorac Surg 2015;100(2):452–7.

23. Dubey GK, Hossain A, Dobrescu C, et al. Repeat lung retransplantation and death risk. J Heart Lung Transplant 2020;39(8):841–5.

24. Collaud S, Benden C, Ganter C, et al. Extracorporeal life support as bridge to lung retransplantation: a multicenter pooled data analysis. Ann Thorac Surg 2016;102(5):1680–6.

25. Ren D, Kaleekal TS, Graviss EA, et al. Retransplantation outcomes at a large lung transplantation program. Transpl Direct 2018;4(11):e404.

26. Osho AA, Castleberry AW, Snyder LD, et al. Determining eligibility for lung transplantation: a nationwide assessment of the cutoff glomerular filtration rate. J Heart Lung Transplant 2015;34(4):571–9.

27. Hall DJ, Belli EV, Gregg JA, et al. Two decades of lung retransplantation: a single-center experience. Ann Thorac Surg 2017;103(4):1076–83.

28. Schumer EM, Rice JD, Kistler AM, et al. Single versus double lung retransplantation does not affect survival based on previous transplant type. Ann Thorac Surg 2017;103(1):236–40.

29. Abou-Daya KI, Tieu R, Zhao D, et al. Resident memory T cells form during persistent antigen exposure leading to allograft rejection. Sci Immunol 2021; 6(57):eabc8122.

30. Bosanquet JP, Witt CA, Bemiss BC, et al. The impact of pre-transplant allosensitization on outcomes after lung transplantation. J Heart Lung Transplant 2015; 34(11):1415–22.

31. Hulbert AL, Pavlisko EN, Palmer SM. Current challenges and opportunities in the management of antibody-mediated rejection in lung transplantation. Curr Opin Organ Transpl 2018;23(3):308–15.

32. Sommer W, Hallensleben M, Ius F, et al. Repeated human leukocyte antigen mismatches in lung retransplantation. Transpl Immunol 2017;40:1–7.

33. Frost AE, Jammal CT, Cagle PT. Hyperacute rejection following lung transplantation. Chest 1996; 110(2):559–62.

34. Kulkarni HS, Bemiss BC, Hachem RR. Antibody-mediated rejection in lung transplantation. Curr Transpl Rep 2015;2(4):316–23.

35. Levine DJ, Glanville AR, Aboyoun C, et al. Antibody-mediated rejection of the lung: a consensus report of the International Society for Heart and Lung Transplantation. J Heart Lung Transplant 2016; 35(4):397–406.

36. Hadjiliadis D, Chaparro C, Reinsmoen NL, et al. Pre-transplant panel reactive antibody in lung transplant recipients is associated with significantly worse post-transplant survival in a multicenter study. J Heart Lung Transplant 2005;24(7 Suppl):S249–54.

37. Brugiere O, Suberbielle C, Thabut G, et al. Lung transplantation in patients with pretransplantation donor-specific antibodies detected by Luminex assay. Transplantation 2013;95(5):761–5.

38. Kim M, Townsend KR, Wood IG, et al. Impact of pretransplant anti-HLA antibodies on outcomes in lung transplant candidates. Am J Respir Crit Care Med 2014;189(10):1234–9.

39. Lau CL, Palmer SM, Posther KE, et al. Influence of panel-reactive antibodies on posttransplant outcomes in lung transplant recipients. Ann Thorac Surg 2000;69(5):1520–4.

40. Snyder LD, Gray AL, Reynolds JM, et al. Antibody desensitization therapy in highly sensitized lung transplant candidates. Am J Transplant 2014;14(4): 849–56.

41. Verleden SE, Vanaudenaerde BM, Emonds MP, et al. Donor-specific and -nonspecific HLA antibodies and outcome post lung transplantation. Eur Respir J 2017;50(5):1701248.

42. Ius F, Sommer W, Tudorache I, et al. Early donor-specific antibodies in lung transplantation: risk factors and impact on survival. J Heart Lung Transplant 2014;33(12):1255–63.

43. Ius F, Muller C, Sommer W, et al. Six-year experience with treatment of early donor-specific anti-HLA antibodies in pediatric lung transplantation using a human immunoglobulin-based protocol. Pediatr Pulmonol 2020;55(3):754–64.

44. Hachem RR. Donor-specific antibodies in lung transplantation. Curr Opin Organ Transpl 2020;25(6): 563–7.

45. Tinckam KJ, Keshavjee S, Chaparro C, et al. Survival in sensitized lung transplant recipients with perioperative desensitization. Am J Transplant 2015;15(2):417–26.

46. Courtwright AM, Cao S, Wood I, et al. Clinical outcomes of lung transplantation in the presence of donor-specific antibodies. Ann Am Thorac Soc 2019;16(9):1131–7.

47. Bhama JK, Bansal A, Shigemura N, et al. Sternal-sparing approach for reoperative bilateral lung transplantation. Interact Cardiovasc Thorac Surg 2013;17(5):835–7.

48. Kon ZN, Bittle GJ, Pasrija C, et al. The optimal procedure for retransplantation after single lung transplantation. Ann Thorac Surg 2017;104(1):170–5.

49. Hartwig MG, Ganapathi AM, Osho AA, et al. Staging of bilateral lung transplantation for high-risk patients with interstitial lung disease: one lung at a time. Am J Transplant 2016;16(11):3270–7.

50. Ius F, Kuehn C, Tudorache I, et al. Lung transplantation on cardiopulmonary support: venoarterial extracorporeal membrane oxygenation outperformed cardiopulmonary bypass. J Thorac Cardiovasc Surg 2012;144(6):1510–6.

51. Hoetzenecker K, Schwarz S, Muckenhuber M, et al. Intraoperative extracorporeal membrane oxygenation and the possibility of postoperative prolongation improve survival in bilateral lung transplantation. J Thorac Cardiovasc Surg 2018;155(5):2193–206. e3.

52. Grande B, Oechslin P, Schlaepfer M, et al. Predictors of blood loss in lung transplant surgery-a single center retrospective cohort analysis. J Thorac Dis 2019;11(11):4755–61.

53. Cernak V, Oude Lansink-Hartgring A, van den Heuvel ER, et al. Incidence of massive transfusion and overall transfusion requirements during lung transplantation over a 25-year period. J Cardiothorac Vasc Anesth 2019;33(9):2478–86.

54. Ong LP, Thompson E, Sachdeva A, et al. Allogeneic blood transfusion in bilateral lung transplantation: impact on early function and mortality. Eur J Cardiothorac Surg 2016;49(2):668–74 [discussion 674].

55. Hayes D Jr, Higgins RS, Kilic A, et al. Extracorporeal membrane oxygenation and retransplantation in lung transplantation: an analysis of the UNOS registry. Lung 2014;192(4):571–6.

56. Diamond JM, Lee JC, Kawut SM, et al. Clinical risk factors for primary graft dysfunction after lung transplantation. Am J Respir Crit Care Med 2013;187(5): 527–34.

57. Klapper JA, Hicks AC, Ledbetter L, et al. Blood product transfusion and lung transplant outcomes: a systematic review. Clin Transplant 2021;35(10): e14404.

58. Smith I, Pearse BL, Faulke DJ, et al. Targeted bleeding management reduces the requirements for blood component therapy in lung transplant recipients. J Cardiothorac Vasc Anesth 2017;31(2): 426–33.

59. Bhaskar B, Zeigenfuss M, Choudhary J, et al. Use of recombinant activated Factor VII for refractory after lung transplant bleeding as an effective strategy to restrict blood transfusion and associated complications. Transfusion 2013;53(4):798–804.

60. Chambers DC, Cherikh WS, Harhay MO, et al. The International Thoracic Organ Transplant Registry of the International Society for Heart and Lung Transplantation: thirty-sixth adult lung and heart-lung transplantation report-2019; Focus theme: donor and recipient size match. J Heart Lung Transplant 2019;38(10):1042–55.

61. Biswas Roy S, Panchanathan R, Walia R, et al. Lung retransplantation for chronic rejection: a single-center experience. Ann Thorac Surg 2018;105(1): 221–7.

62. Lund LH, Edwards LB, Kucheryavaya AY, et al. The registry of the International Society for Heart and Lung Transplantation: thirty-first official adult heart transplant report–2014; focus theme: retransplantation. J Heart Lung Transplant 2014;33(10): 996–1008.

Moving?

Make sure your subscription moves with you!

To notify us of your new address, find your **Clinics Account Number** (located on your mailing label above your name), and contact customer service at:

Email: journalscustomerservice-usa@elsevier.com

800-654-2452 (subscribers in the U.S. & Canada)
314-447-8871 (subscribers outside of the U.S. & Canada)

Fax number: 314-447-8029

Elsevier Health Sciences Division
Subscription Customer Service
3251 Riverport Lane
Maryland Heights, MO 63043

*To ensure uninterrupted delivery of your subscription,
please notify us at least 4 weeks in advance of move.

Printed and bound by CPI Group (UK) Ltd, Croydon, CR0 4YY

08/05/2025

01864715-0014